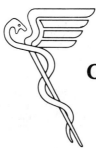

1981
YEAR BOOK OF
OBSTETRICS AND GYNECOLOGY

THE 1981 YEAR BOOKS

The YEAR BOOK series provides in condensed form the essence of the best of the recent international medical literature. The material is selected by distinguished editors who critically review more than 500,000 journal articles each year.

Anesthesia: *Drs. Eckenhoff, Bart, Brunner, Holley, and Linde.*

Cancer: *Drs. Clark, Cumley, and Hickey.*

Cardiology: *Drs. Harvey, Kirkendall, Kirklin, Nadas, Sonnenblick, and Resnekov.*

Clinical Pharmacy: *Dr. Woolley.*

Dentistry: *Drs. Hale, Hazen, Moyers, Redig, Robinson, and Silverman.*

Dermatology: *Drs. Dobson and Thiers.*

Diagnostic Radiology: *Drs. Whitehouse, Adams, Bookstein, Gabrielsen, Holt, Martel, Silver, and Thornbury.*

Drug Therapy: *Drs. Hollister and Lasagna.*

Emergency Medicine: *Dr. Wagner.*

Endocrinology: *Drs. Schwartz and Ryan.*

Family Practice: *Dr. Rakel.*

Medicine: *Drs. Rogers, Des Prez, Cline, Braunwald, Greenberger, Bondy, and Epstein.*

Neurology and Neurosurgery: *Drs. De Jong and Sugar.*

Nuclear Medicine: *Drs. Hoffer, Gottschalk, and Zaret.*

Obstetrics and Gynecology: *Drs. Pitkin and Zlatnik.*

Ophthalmology: *Dr. Hughes.*

Orthopedics: *Dr. Coventry.*

Otolaryngology: *Drs. Strong and Paparella.*

Pathology and Clinical Pathology: *Dr. Brinkhous.*

Pediatrics: *Drs. Oski and Stockman.*

Plastic and Reconstructive Surgery: *Drs. McCoy, Brauer, Haynes, Hoehn, Miller, and Whitaker.*

Psychiatry and Applied Mental Health: *Drs. Romano, Freedman, Friedhoff, Kolb, Lourie, and Nemiah.*

Sports Medicine: *Drs. Krakauer, Shephard and Torg, Col. Anderson, and Mr. George.*

Surgery: *Drs. Schwartz, Najarian, Peacock, Shires, Silen, and Spencer.*

Urology: *Drs. Gillenwater and Howards.*

The YEAR BOOK of

Obstetrics and Gynecology
1981

Editor

ROY M. PITKIN, M.D.
Professor and Head, Department of Obstetrics and Gynecology,
University of Iowa College of Medicine

Associate Editor

FRANK J. ZLATNIK, M.D.
Associate Professor and Vice-Chairman,
Department of Obstetrics and Gynecology,
University of Iowa College of Medicine

YEAR BOOK MEDICAL PUBLISHERS, INC.
CHICAGO • LONDON

Table of Contents

The material covered in this volume represents literature reviewed up to August 1980.

Introduction

It is surely not possible to identify with any confidence the "high points' of such a large body of current literature as that represented by a volume of the YEAR BOOK. Yet, from my perspective of having just put the finishing touches on the manuscript, it is tempting for me to try. In obstetrics, the first to come to mind are several papers describing methods of achieving the type of rigid metabolic control generally regarded as representing the hallmark of modern management of diabetic pregnancy. In particular, the use of home glucose analyses in patient self-regulation is an exciting new development now demonstrated to be practical and feasible.

In endocrinology, a number of new advances have been made, but perhaps the most intriguing is the technique of ultrasound visualization of follicular growth developed and reported virtually simultaneously by several groups. With this methodology, many possibilities for physiologic and clinical studies come to mind. In gynecologic oncology, refinements of recent studies documenting improved survival in advanced ovarian cancer with combination chemotherapy now appear to indicate that the improvement occurs in those tumors of certain histologic grades only, permitting more precise selection of proper therapy.

These represent but a few of the important papers abstracted in this edition of the YEAR BOOK. As the volume of medical literature continues its inexorable growth, this mechanism of "keeping abreast" increases proportionately in value.

The first of two special articles in the 1981 YEAR BOOK OF OBSTETRICS AND GYNECOLOGY is "Prenatal Diagnosis of Congenital Malformations," written by Dr. Maurice J. Mahoney of Yale University. It represents a concise "state of the art" summary of the current status of an area that in just a few short years has come to represent a major effect in obstetric practice. In the second special article, "Urinary Incontinence," Dr. Douglas J. Marchant of Tufts University has prepared an excellent review. Writing from the perspective of a vast personal experience and a thorough knowledge of the literature, the article by Douglas Marchant clearly outlines his approach to the diagnosis of this common and distressing symptom. His paper will be appreciated by many of us who are as distressed as our patients as we attempt to evaluate and treat this many-faceted symptom complex.

ROY M. PITKIN, M.D.

Current Literature Quiz

The questions below are an informal test of your knowledge before and/or after reading the YEAR BOOK. The questions are answered by locating the appropriate article in the text by its reference number, which appears in parentheses after each question. The reference numbers indicate the chapter in which the article appears and its numerical order within the chapter.

1. What is the amount of fat normally stored during pregnancy and when is it laid down? (1–1)
2. What is the relationship between circadian rhythms of free estriol and cortisol at 34 weeks' gestation and at term? (1–12)
3. What is the effect of dehydroepiandrosterone sulfate intravenously on maternal prolactin levels? (1–14)
4. What happens to the number of uterine adrenergic nerves during gestation? (1–20)
5. What is the pattern of endogenous creatinine clearance in late pregnancy? (1–22)
6. Describe the alterations in the fasting and residual gallbladder volumes in late pregnancy. (1–24)
7. Is fetal growth impaired in women with acyanotic cardiac disease? (2–2)
8. List the adverse effects of anticoagulation during pregnancy. (2–3)
9. What is the significance of C_3 and C_4 complement levels in patients with systemic lupus erythematosus? (2–6)
10. How often is pancreatitis in pregnancy associated with gallstones? (2–7)
11. What is class H diabetes mellitus? (2–19)
12. How does chronic persistent hepatitis affect pregnancy outcome? (2–25)
13. What percentage of pregnant women have antibody against all four types of group B streptococci implicated in early-onset disease? (2–33)
14. What is the obstetric significance of in utero diethylstilbestrol exposure? (3–7)
15. How might prostaglandins of the A series be related to toxemia? (3–19)
16. How do hydrostatic factors affect the roll-over test? (3–21)
17. Are β-adrenergic agents effective in lengthening gestation when used prophylactically in patients with twins? (3–29)
18. Does maternal aminophylline administration affect fetal lung maturation? (3–35)
19. What is the best ultrasonic means of identifying intrauterine growth retardation? (4–3)
20. What is the prognostic significance of the length of the latency period (the time from the start of a uterine contraction to the beginning of the late deceleration) in a patient with a positive oxytocin challenge test? (4–7)
21. What is saturated phosphatidylcholine? (4–21)
22. What adverse maternal effect of tocolytic therapy with betamimetic agents has recently been emphasized? (5–10)
23. What is relaxin? (5–15)

24. What periodic fetal heart rate change is associated with delivery as an occiput posterior? (5–17)
25. What happens to fetal breathing activity in labor? (5–23)
26. Macrosomic fetuses are predisposed to fetal distress in labor. True or false? (5–17)
27. What factors are involved in water intoxication associated with oxytocin infusion? (5–27)
28. What differences in the neonatal period would you predict in a comparison between infants delivered by the Leboyer method vs. a gentle conventional delivery? (6–1)
29. How should mepivacaine intoxication of the neonate be treated? (6–4)
30. In the laboratory animal, the aspiration of an antacid has what effects? (6–9)
31. How do the odds of having a fetus with open spina bifida in the face of an elevated amniotic fluid α-fetoprotein value vary according to the reason for the amniocentesis? (7–5)
32. Amniotic fluid 3,3′,5′-triiodothyronine determinations are not reliable in diagnosing intrauterine hypothyroidism. True or false? (7–12)
33. Maternal ingestion of what common drug has been associated with neonatal pulmonary hypertension? (7–18)
34. What is a chimera? (7–20)
35. What is the most important variable concerning the development of puerperal infection? (8–3)
36. Should patients routinely have anticoagulation after cesarean section? (8–10)
37. How does preeclampsia affect cord prolactin levels? (8–11)
38. Most children with cerebral palsy weighed less than 2,500 gm at birth. True or false? (8–14)
39. What is the postulated mechanism of neonatal hyperbilirubinemia allegedly related to oxytocin induction of labor? (8–18)
40. What is the prognostic significance of retinal hemorrhages in the newborn? (8–19)
41. How does diet influence plasma prolactin levels in lactating women? (8–25)
42. Is it safe for women taking propylthiouracil to nurse their babies? (8–30)
43. Does the use of washed packed red blood cells prevent posttransfusion hepatitis? (9–7)
44. List drugs that may be useful in the management of the "unstable bladder" with non-stress incontinence. (10–4)
45. What structure is used to close a vesicovaginal fistula by the Martius technique? (10–6)
46. What is the effect of pneumoperitoneum on cardiac output? (10–11)
47. What is the comparative efficacy of systemic dexamethasone and promethazine and intraperitoneal 10% dextran 40 and 32% dextran 70 in preventing tubal adhesions postoperatively? (10–21)
48. What factor is most important in determining recurrence-risk in vulvar carcinoma in situ? (11–2 and 11–3)
49. What advantages does laser offer over cryotherapy in treatment of cervical intraepithelial neoplasia? (11–10)
50. Compare the frequency of lung metastases in cervical and endometrial cancer. (11–16)
51. What type of endometrial hyperplasia is most likely to lead to carcinoma? (11–20)
52. How does the prognosis with endometrial cancer compare in patients who did and did not take exogenous estrogens? (11–23)

53. What characteristics indicate increased likelihood of endometrial adeno-carcinoma responding to progestational agents? (11–28)
54. What is the relationship between histologic grade and response to combination chemotherapy in ovarian cancer? (11–33)
55. Following treatment for ovarian cancer, what type of patient is a candidate for a "second-look" operation? (11–37 and 11–38)
56. What is citrovorum factor and how is it useful in trophoblastic disease? (11–43)
57. What is the correlation between periurethral bacterial colonization and recurrent urinary tract infections? (12–3)
58. What is Reiter's syndrome? (12–10)
59. How could tubo-ovarian abscess lead to falsely positive pregnancy tests? (12–14)
60. What could explain elevation in estrogen and progesterone levels immediately after intense exercise? (13–4)
61. When is polytomography indicated in amenorrheic patients? (13–8)
62. What is the responsible mechanism in menopausal hot flushes? (13–15)
63. How does estrogen absorption from vaginal creams differ in premenopausal and postmenopausal women? (13–18)
64. How are risk of osteoporosis and body weight correlated? (13–22)
65. What is the effect of spironolactone on plasma testosterone levels? (13–27)
66. How is luteal-phase deficiency diagnosed? (14–2)
67. What is the relationship between body weight and clomiphene dosage needed for ovulation induction? (14–10)
68. What is the effect on conception rates of insemination with mixed and infertile husband semen? (14–17)
69. What is the effect of oral contraceptives on serum and urinary levels of copper and zinc? (15–5)
70. What drugs apparently lower the efficacy of oral contraceptives? (15–7 and 15–8)
71. What is the relationship between estrogen level in oral contraceptives and carbohydrate metabolism? (15–12)
72. What factors of oral contraceptive usage correlate with hepatocellular adenoma? (15–16)
73. How does type of intrauterine contraceptive device (copper vs. inert) relate to volume of menstrual bleeding? (15–20)
74. When does ovulation resume after induced abortion? (16–3)
75. What amount of radiation does the breast receive with the new low-dose mammography? (17–2)
76. What is the relationship between estrogen receptor status and prognosis in breast cancer? (17–7 and 17–8)

PART ONE

OBSTETRICS

1. Maternal and Fetal Physiology

Changes in Fat, Fat-Free Mass, and Body Water in Human Normal Pregnancy. Studies in rats have shown a considerable increase in body fat during pregnancy, but studies on human pregnancy have produced varying results.

N. G. J. Pipe, T. Smith, D. Halliday, C. J. Edmonds, C. Williams, and T. M. Coltart[1-1] (Guy's Hosp., London) performed serial measurements of body weight, total body water, total body potassium, skinfold thickness, and fat cell diameter during pregnancy and post partum in 27 normal women aged 19 to 40 years. Body weights in early pregnancy were 48 to 66 kg and did not differ from expected by more than 20%. Nineteen subjects were primigravidas. The pregnancies were uncomplicated, and none ended before 38 weeks. Adipose tissue was sampled from over the upper outer part of the right buttock.

Total body fat increased during pregnancy, reaching a maximum toward the end of the second trimester before declining. Fat cell diameter measurements correlated poorly with estimated total body fat values, but skin-fold thickness values showed good correlation. Total body potassium showed a highly significant increase during pregnancy. Total body water post partum was very similar to that found in early pregnancy. Increases in free fat mass and excess water were delayed in relation to the increase in maternal body fat, with maximum values in late pregnancy. There was no significant net accumulation of fat in the last three months of pregnancy.

The general trend for fat deposition in pregnancy is that of accumulation of fat reserve in the second trimester. There is apparently no further net accumulation of fat in the last trimester of pregnancy. In the puerperium, total body fat decreases to early pregnancy levels. The findings support the view that fat is accumulated in pregnancy and may act as a nutrient reserve during times of food deprivation.

▶ [The indices of body composition utilized in this study were necessarily indirect and therefore subject to some degree of error. Nevertheless, this is an important piece of work that extends our knowledge of maternal physiology. The major finding is that pregnant women normally store substantial amounts of fat, averaging 2.4 kg, during the second trimester, mostly as a result of fat cell hypertrophy (ie, enlargement of size of individual cells) rather than as a consequence of hyperplasia. Teleologically, it would seem that the reason for this appreciable storage is the laying down of energy reserves against a future time when caloric needs may exceed available sources, such as during the third trimester, and particularly during lactation when energy requirements approximate 750 kcal/day.] ◀

Weight Gain and Outcome of Pregnancy. Studies in both the United States and England have shown that perinatal mortality is lowest when maternal pregnancy weight gain is between 24 and 27

(1-1) Br. J. Obstet. Gynaecol. 86:929–940, December 1979.

lb, but these studies have not fully considered the possible role of maternal nutritional reserves. Richard L. Naeye[1-2] (Pennsylvania State Univ.) examined the relationship of maternal weight gain to pregnancy outcome by analyzing data from the Collaborative Perinatal Project of the National Institute of Neurologic and Communicative Disorders and Stroke, which prospectively followed the course of 53,518 pregnancies in 12 American hospitals during 1959–1966. The offspring had follow-up to age 8 years. Only single-born infants were included in the analysis.

In mothers with optimal or less than optimal prepregnancy body weights, perinatal mortality was lowest when pregnancy weight gains were 80%–120% of optimal values, and a fivefold increase in fetal and neonatal losses occurred when weight gains were less than 25% of the optimal values. Thin mothers had the highest perinatal mortality with low weight gains and had the lowest mortality with optimal weight gains. At term, their lowest perinatal mortality correlated with a 30-lb weight gain (Fig 1–1). The most overweight mothers had the lowest perinatal mortality when they gained only 24%–54% of optimal amounts. In term pregnancies, their most favorable weight gain was 15 to 16 lb. Weight gain correlated most closely with the outcome of pregnancy when the offspring were male and had blood group B and the mothers had 1 + or greater acetonuria during pregnancy. Only modest increases in the rates of most common placental and fetal disorders were noted with low or high pregnancy weight gains; however, once a disorder was established, the risk of death usually increased severalfold with a low or high pregnancy

Fig 1–1.—Relation of weight gain and perinatal mortality in overweight, underweight, and normally proportioned mothers. (Courtesy of Naeye, R. L.: Am. J. Obstet. Gynecol. 135:3–9, Sept. 1, 1979.)

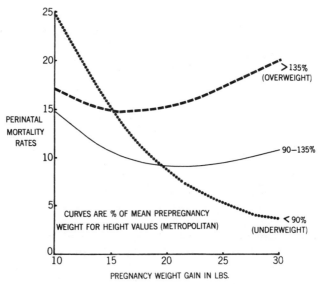

weight gain. Only 13% of the excess perinatal mortality seen in the less than 25% weight gain group were attributable to large placental infarcts, abruptio placentae, or marked placental growth retardation.

A mother's optimal weight gain in pregnancy depends on her body build. The optimal gain for an overweight mother is only about half that for a thin one. The fetus may be more vulnerable to maternal dietary deficiencies and excesses than has often been thought.

▶ [This report addresses the important question of what range of pregnancy weight gain is associated with optimal outcome. The results imply that the value varies with prepregnancy weight-for-height status. Naeye suggests, for pregnancies carried to term, 20 lb for normally proportioned patients, 30 lb for those underweight and 16 lb for overweight women. However, translating these figures into recommendations strikes us as deceptively simplistic. Inspection of Figure 1–1 indicates relatively flat curves for normal and overweight patients and we would question the statistical significance of any difference between points along either curve. Indeed, the data presented in the paper seem to confirm this suspicion in that perinatal mortality rates for weight gains greater than 50% of "optimal values" lack statistical significance. By contrast, there appears to be a clear inverse relationship between perinatal mortality and weight gain in underweight subjects. The implication seems clear that the aim in patients entering pregnancy more than 10% under ideal weight for height should be a gain of at least 30 lb. Beyond this, we do not feel that this article provides sufficient data on which to base recommendations.] ◀

Effects of Maternal Undernutrition and Heavy Physical Work During Pregnancy on Birth Weight. Both maternal body weight and dietary intake during pregnancy have been reported to strongly influence fetal growth rates. N. Tafari, R. L. Naeye, and A. Gobezie[1-3] attempted to determine whether the level of physical activity during pregnancy also affects fetal growth. Women with low caloric intakes in Addis Ababa, Ethiopia, were studied in 1976–1977. A total of 181 patients with pregnancies before 12 weeks' gestation were included and 130 completed the study. The mothers were given dietary advice and intakes were evaluated by home dietary surveys in 42 women at 20–24 and 36–38 weeks of pregnancy.

Maternal intakes of calories and protein were similar in the high- and low-physical activity groups and in both were below recommended levels. This was due in part to a fear that a large infant would lead to an obstructed labor. Full-term infants of mothers engaging in heavy labor weighed 3,068 gm at birth compared with 3,-270 gm for infants of less active mothers. Adjustment of data for early-pregnancy body weight and the nonfetal component of the pregnancy weight gain did not change the apparent effects of heavy work on weight gain. The influence of early-pregnancy body weight on birth weight was small. Mothers who did heavy work during pregnancy had much smaller pregnancy weight gains than less active mothers, independent of the weights of their fetuses. Placental abnormalities were comparably frequent in the two groups.

Women in this study who engaged in hard physical labor and had subnormal caloric intakes during pregnancy had lower early-pregnancy body weights and gestational weight gains and lighter infants than less active mothers on similarly low caloric intakes. Metabolic

(1–3) Br. J. Obstet. Gynaecol. 87:222–226, March 1980.

adjustments must partially protect the fetus from inadequate maternal food intake and heavy energy output during pregnancy. No evidence of uteroplacental underperfusion was found but further studies are needed to confirm this. Efforts to improve fetal growth through dietary supplementation need to be coupled with efforts to reduce muscular work during pregnancy.

▶ [Not surprisingly, in these Ethiopian women heavy work, when coupled with low caloric intake in pregnancy, resulted in lower birth weights of offspring than when low caloric intake was not associated with heavy work. Either decreased uterine blood flow or decreased substrate concentration in the maternal blood, or both, may have been involved.

Certain "super-jock" obstetric patients of our acquaintance, despite excellent general health and high socioeconomic status, have gained weight poorly in pregnancy and have delivered babies of less than average size. We need to know more about the effects of running and serious jogging during pregnancy.] ◀

Effects of Low-Protein Diet During Pregnancy of the Rhesus Monkey: III. Growth of Infants. Studies in subprimate species suggest that fetal growth retardation associated with protein-calorie deficiency during pregnancy may continue in postnatal life despite availability of an adequate diet. Mary Bess Kohrs, George R. Kerr, and Alfred E. Harper[1-4] studied the effects of gestational protein deficiency on subsequent growth of infant monkeys. An experimental diet with 25% as much protein as a control diet was fed, starting 30 days after conception. The diet was made isocaloric by substituting lactose for protein.

Average body weight of infants whose mothers received the low-protein diet was significantly less at birth and 180 days after birth than that of controls. Head circumferences were smaller in the prenatally malnourished infants at birth, but no significant difference was found on day 180. Average body length of the experimental group was consistently less than that of controls, but the differences were not significant. Eight of 16 malnourished infants died perinatally. Prenatally malnourished infant animals consumed significantly greater volumes of formula than controls starting on day 130.

The weight and head circumference of newborn animals may be affected more than body length by prenatal malnutrition. Decreased utilization of food by infant animals subjected to malnutrition prenatally may be due to impaired nutrient absorption. Reduced postnatal growth of these infants may also reflect hormonal aberrations related to prenatal malnutrition.

▶ [In this primate study, maternal protein restriction during pregnancy resulted in offspring of lower birth weight. The monkeys in the experimental group did not "catch up" to controls by six months of age. These findings are consistent with those of several studies in subprimates, but differ from those of another study in monkeys (Riopelle, A. J., et al.: Am. J. Clin. Nutr. 28:989, 1975).

The significance of various levels of dietary protein in human pregnancy is poorly understood as well. Read on.] ◀

A Randomized Controlled Trial of Prenatal Nutritional Supplementation in New York City was performed by David Rush, Zena Stein, and Mervyn Susser[1-5] (New York) because of literature

---

(1–4) Am. J. Clin. Nutr. 33:625–630, March 1980.
(1–5) Pediatrics 65:683–697, April 1980.

reviews relating maternal nutrition to low birth weight and mental competence. The study, performed in a poor black urban population, was aimed at increasing birth weights and improving postnatal development of offspring of mothers at high risk of having low birth weight infants. Women in New York City who weighed less than 140 lb at conception were recruited into the study. In addition, they either had to weigh less than 110 lb at conception, have low weight gain, have had at least one previous low birth weight infant, or have a history of protein intake below 50 gm in the preceding 24 hours. Study subjects received a beverage complement of 6 gm of animal protein and 322 calories daily, or a supplement of 40 gm of animal protein and 470 calories daily. Vitamins and minerals were supplied to both study groups and the nonintervention group.

The only favorable effect of supplementation noted at birth was the prevention of depressed birth weight in offspring of mothers who smoked heavily. With balanced protein-calorie supplementation, length of gestation was increased, percentage of low birth weight infants was reduced, and mean birth weight was raised by 41 gm (not significant). High-protein supplementation was associated with an excess of very early premature births and associated neonatal deaths, and there was significant growth retardation up to 37 weeks' gestation. High-protein supplementation was also associated with higher scores for visual habituation, visual dishabituation, and length of free-play episodes at age 1 year. These measures were unrelated to measures of growth at birth and at age 1 year. No adverse effects of high-protein supplementation were noted at age 1 year.

High-protein supplementation apparently accelerated weight gain in all women at the outset and later inhibited weight gain in those who were delivered prematurely. The psychologic effects of high-protein supplementation are assumed to be favorable. Continued observations and animals studies of high-protein supplementation are indicated at present, rather than further human intervention studies.

▶ [In this large-scale intervention study, protein supplementation was associated with *adverse* perinatal outcome. This finding is most surprising when one considers the socioeconomic gradients concerning both protein intake and birth weight. Although the patients were assigned "randomly" to the three experimental groups, we wonder whether inadvertent differences apart from the nutritional intervention existed among the groups. The reported protein intake in the control group of "poor" women (79.3 gm/day) is higher than we would have guessed.] ◀

Folic Acid Supplement and Intrauterine Growth. Folic acid metabolites are necessary for nucleic acid formation and growth, but red blood cell folic acid content falls throughout pregnancy. A prospective study in Denmark showed a significant reduction in numbers of placental cells in early summer and a corresponding reduction in fetal weight. A lack of uncooked green vegetables was implicated. J. Rolschau, J. Date, and K. Kristoffersen[1-6] (Odense Univ.) examined the effects of a folic acid supplement on birth and placental weights in women delivering in early summer. Thirty-six consecutive women were supplied with 5 mg of folic acid daily or control tablets from

(1–6) Acta Obstet. Gynecol. Scand. 58:343–346, 1979.

week 23 of gestation; 20 received folic acid. Gestational ages were similar in the two groups.

The average fetal weight was 12.7% higher in the folic acid group, a significant effect. Placental weight was increased by 11.9% on average and the DNA content by 11.1%; these effects were not significant. Red blood cell folic acid concentration at delivery correlated significantly with birth weight, and there was a trend toward positive correlations with placental weight and placental DNA and RNA. Plasma folic acid levels were 105% higher at delivery and the red blood cell folic acid concentration was 34% greater in the folic acid group than in the control group. Weight increase during pregnancy was 1.7 kg greater in the folic acid group; this was not significant. Hemoglobin levels were comparable in the two groups.

Birth and placental weights increased in folic acid-supplemented women in this study. The effects of folic acid on intrauterine growth must be related to folic acid deficiency. Even if the effect is confined to a few months, a reduction in the rate of infants small for dates would be expected.

▶ [Folic acid is important in reproduction, but how often folic acid deficiency accounts for adverse obstetric outcome is controversial. Several years ago, it was suggested by workers in England that placental abruption and other problems were due to folic acid deficiency. Several subsequent studies in the United States failed to confirm this view. The recommended daily allowance for folic acid in pregnancy is 800 μg. Most typical prenatal vitamin-mineral preparations meet or exceed this recommendation.

The authors of the present study note that fresh green vegetables are uncommon in Denmark in the winter. They therefore studied a 5-mg folic supplement vs. no supplement in patients due to deliver in June. The reported results are striking! Birth weight was 400 gm heavier in the supplemented group. Other differences between the two groups did not readily explain the heavier babies and placentas in those patients given folic acid supplements. Different populations have different dietary habits, of course. Green salads are common in the winter in the United States (even in Iowa). Nonetheless, this report may rekindle an interest in the topic of folic acid consumption and obstetric performance.] ◀

Fetal Malnutrition: Price of Upright Posture? Ander Briend[1-7] (Dakar, Senegal) points out that the pattern of preterm fetal growth faltering, the usual finding in man, differs from that observed in animals. Rather than representing an adaptation to facilitate birth, the phenomenon is much more likely to be due to rapid evolution and imperfect adaptation to the upright posture. Gruenwald postulated that transfer of nutrients across the placenta is limited at the end of pregnancy by a maternal factor as yet unknown. An infant increases growth rapidly soon after birth, and those of short gestation do not experience a dip in growth at the time they normally should have been delivered. The morphological changes associated with intrauterine malnutrition are the reverse of what would be expected had they appeared under selective pressure to improve the outcome of delivery.

Maternal cardiovascular changes occur in late pregnancy that tend to reduce uterine blood flow and, as a consequence, fetal nutrition. Assumption of the upright posture decreases the space available to the pregnant uterus, leading it to interfere with maternal hemody-

(1–7) Br. Med. J. 2:317–319, Aug. 4, 1979.

namics near term. Aortic compression causes a fall in arterial pressure distal to the lumbar lordosis. Compression of the inferior cava decreases blood volume, leading to a fall in cardiac output. The amount of bed rest at the end of pregnancy could be a limiting factor in fetal nutrition and growth. A heavy demand on the cardiovascular system at this time might well further impair the mother's capacity to sustain fetal growth up to birth. Heavier work and less bed rest in socially deprived groups would limit cardiovascular function more than the norm. This finding helps to explain the observed social distribution of intrauterine malnutrition. Good maternal nutrition during pregnancy is not the only prerequisite for normal fetal growth.

▶ [All those who find this speculation interesting, stand up and be counted!] ◀

Fetal Growth Retardation in Cigarette-Smoking Mothers Is Not Due to Decreased Maternal Food Intake. The cause of fetal growth retardation in cigarette-smoking mothers is unclear. Besides the effects of nicotine and carbon monoxide, it has been suggested that smoking may reduce the mother's appetite and result in undernutrition, which may lead to restricted fetal growth. J. C. Haworth, J. J. Ellestad-Sayed, Jean King, and Louise A. Dilling[1-8] (Univ. of Manitoba) compared diets toward the end of pregnancy in smoking and nonsmoking women of different socioeconomic groups. Of the 536 women interviewed at the last antepartum visit or just after delivery in 1975 and 1976, 302 were smokers, and 153 were public patients. Dietary intake was assessed from the average daily nutrient intake in the diet history and from recall of all foods and drinks taken in the past 24 hours or in a typical day.

Public patients were younger and shorter than private patients, had less pregnancy weight gain and greater parity, and consumed less of most of the assessed nutrients. Infants of smoking mothers had lower birth weights and, in the private group, smaller head circumferences. In the private group, smokers consumed significantly more energy, total fat, and niacin than nonsmokers, but significantly less vitamin C. More eating between meals rather than larger meals appeared to be responsible. Coffee and alcohol consumption was greater in the smokers. A similar pattern was seen in the public group. In the private group only, the amount of smoking correlated with the dietary intakes of energy and fat, and dietary intake correlated with pregnancy weight gain. Pregnancy weight gain correlated with birth weight in both groups.

Fetal growth retardation among women who smoke during pregnancy is not due to their lower intake of food compared with nonsmokers. It is unlikely that the harmful effect of smoking could be reversed by increasing the mother's dietary intake.

▶ [Studies abstracted in earlier editions of the YEAR BOOK have suggested that the fetal growth retardation accompanying maternal smoking reflects, at least partially, diminished food intake by the smoking gravida. This report reaches a contrary conclusion, based on a lack of difference between smokers and nonsmokers with respect to nutrient intake and weight gain. The issue of whether the effect of smoking on fetal growth is mediated through nutrition is an important one because of its implications for clinical management.] ◀

(1–8) Am. J. Obstet. Gynecol. 137:719–723, July 15, 1980.

Estriol in Pregnancy: VI. Experience With Unconjugated Plasma Estriol Assays and Antepartum Fetal Heart Rate Testing in Diabetic Pregnancies. Martin J. Whittle, Dennis Anderson, Richard I. Lowensohn, Jorge H. Mestman, Richard H. Paul, and Uwe Goebelsmann[1-9] (Univ. of Southern California) assessed the reliability of daily unconjugated plasma estriol (E_3) determinations as a first-line test for fetal surveillance in the management of 70 consecutive diabetic pregnancies over a 1-year period. All patients were insulin dependent. Only when the lecithin-sphingomyelin ratio exceeded 2.0 was the pregnancy ended at 38 weeks' gestation. Antepartum fetal heart rate testing was carried out weekly or whenever the plasma E_3 concentration fell by 40% or more.

Forty patients (57%) were delivered electively at 38 weeks' gestation. Seven were delivered early for presumed fetal distress and 3 on maternal indications. Cesarean section delivery was performed in 5 of 20 women with spontaneous labor and in 31 of 50 who were delivered electively. The 70 infants were delivered at a mean gestational age of 38 weeks and had an average birth weight of 3,602 gm. The rate of termination for presumed or documented fetal distress was 10% in this series. Delivery was indicated in 2 cases because both E_3 values and heart rate tests became abnormal. Four other patients had falling E_3 concentrations. Twenty-six of 317 nonstress tests were nonreactive in 18 women. Seven of 9 nonreactive tests were followed by a negative contraction stress test and 2 by a positive contraction stress test. The latter 2 patients were the only ones in whom the plasma E_3 concentration fell by more than 50%, and fetal distress was documented at delivery.

Daily unconjugated plasma E_3 assays are a highly effective first-line test for fetal surveillance in diabetic pregnancies, but a single test is inadequate. Increasing experience with the combination of E_3 determinations and fetal heart rate tests will allow the obstetrician to minimize the impact of a falsely abnormal biochemical or biophysical test.

▶ [The University of Southern California group has been the principal advocate of estriol measurements in management of diabetic pregnancy, pointing out the need for daily studies in order to detect the occasional case of rapid deterioration. Their earlier studies were based on 24-hour urine assays and in this report they note similar findings with free estriol measurements in plasma, overcoming a number of the disadvantages of 24-hour urine collection. Nevertheless, the need for daily samples and rapid "turnaround" time in the laboratory poses substantial problems for many units. An interesting and potentially important observation is the occurrence of significant free estriol drops in several patients with normal fetal heart rate studies during the past week, implying that weekly nonstress tests or contraction stress tests (the interval used by most) as a *sole* technique of fetal surveillance in diabetes is inadequate.] ◀

▶ ↓ Time of sampling for plasma estriol studies is of critical importance, as indicated by the following article. ◀

Estriol Determinations in Diabetic Pregnancies Complicated by Nephropathy. Although estriol measurements appear to be of value in assessing fetal well-being, erroneously low urinary estriol excretion may occur in patients without fetal distress. Suzanne B.

(1–9) Am. J. Obstet. Gynecol. 135:764–772, Nov. 15, 1979.

Rothchild, Dan Tulchinsky, Montserrat deM. Fencl, Wanda Metcalf, and Fredric D. Frigoletto, Jr.[1-10] (Harvard Med. School) examined the effects of decreased renal function on urinary and plasma estriol levels in patients at 28–38 weeks' gestation. Forty-four diabetic patients had normal endogenous creatinine clearance rates, whereas 25 others had rates below 100 ml/minute. The study included 7 patients with class A diabetes complicated by hypertension or mild preeclampsia, 15 with class B, 25 with class C, 13 with class D, 7 with class F/R and F, 1 with class R, and 1 with class T diabetes.

No correlation was found between creatinine clearance rates and estriol clearance rates in the overall group, and estriol clearance rates were comparable in the patients with normal and those with subnormal creatinine clearance rates. Good correlation was found between plasma unconjugated estriol and urinary estriol excretion. Plasma estriol also correlated well with the 24-hour urinary estriol excretion. Early morning spot urine estriol-creatinine ratios correlated well with the 24-hour urinary estriol excretion. All 7 patients with subnormal or falling creatinine clearances who were studied serially had rising or normal plasma and urinary estriol concentrations and a normal plasma-urinary estriol concentration ratio.

Decreased creatinine clearance had no apparent effect on urinary estriol excretion in these diabetic patients, possibly because renal tubular function remained intact. Either plasma or urinary estriol can be used to assess fetoplacental function in patients with diabetic nephropathy. Plasma and urinary estriol levels do not necessarily correlate with one another in a given patient.

▶ [The standard teaching is that in pregnant patients with renal disease the urinary estriol concentration may be artifactually low and plasma level artifactually high. This is not so in diabetic nephropathy, according to this report. Plasma and urinary levels were highly correlated in patients with low as well as with normal creatinine clearances. The authors suggest that this reflects the nature of the renal lesion (tubular function important in estriol excretion is generally preserved). Therefore, this finding in diabetic nephropathy should not be extrapolated to other renal diseases. The authors also caution that their general observations may not hold in an individual patient.] ◄

Screening for Fetal Risk with Urinary Estrogen-Creatinine Ratio at 34 Weeks. Measurement of the estrogen-creatinine (E-C) ratio in first morning urine samples avoids the delay and potential inaccuracy of prolonged collection, and the results correlate well with 24-hour estrogen values. C. O'Herlihy and R. H. Martin[1-11] (Leeds, England) determined the accuracy of a single E-C ratio determination at 34 weeks' gestation in detecting fetoplacental insufficiency and in predicting birth weight. First morning specimens were collected at 34 weeks from 261 women with reliable menstrual dates, excluding those with chronic renal disease and those receiving ampicillin or corticosteroids. Urinary total estrogen and creatinine concentrations were measured; an all-aqueous, automated, continuous-flow method was used for estrogens.

A urinary E-C ratio below 0.78 was found in 16.1% of subjects (ta-

(1–10) Am. J. Obstet. Gynecol. 134:772–775, Aug. 1, 1979.
(1–11) Br. J. Obstet. Gynaecol. 87:388–392, May 1980.

FETAL MORTALITY, MORBIDITY, AND BIRTH WEIGHT AMONG
PATIENTS WITH LOW AND NORMAL URINARY ESTROGEN-CREATININE
(O/C) RATIOS AT 34 WEEKS' GESTATION

	Low O/C ratio	Normal O/C ratio	Statistical significance
No. of patients	42	219	
Stillbirths	3	0	$p < 0.01$
Small-for-dates infants	19 (45.2%)	21 (9.6%)	$p < 0.001$
Fetal distress in labour	10 (27.0%) (n = 37)	14 (6.6%) (n = 211)	$p < 0.001$
Birth weight (kg) Mean ± SD	2.90 ± 0.69	3.32 ± 0.47	$p < 0.001$

ble). All 3 stillbirths due to fetal hypoxia occurred at 36 to 37 weeks in patients with low E-C ratios. One neonatal death occurred in the face of a normal ratio; a neural tube defect was present. Significantly more women with low E-C ratios delivered small for dates infants or infants with fetal distress in labor. The mean birth weight was reduced in this group. Birth weight correlated well with the urinary E-C ratio at 34 weeks' gestation. The measurement suggested fetal growth retardation significantly more often than did abdominal examination. Preeclampsia was equally frequent in the normal and low E-C groups. Neither preterm delivery nor cigarette smoking correlated with the E-C ratio.

An E-C ratio more than 1 SD below the normal mean at 34 weeks' gestation can identify patients likely to develop placental insufficiency in late pregnancy or in labor more accurately than can clinical methods. There is no significant diurnal variation, in contrast to the serum estriol concentration. By obtaining weekly estimates or cardiotocograms in patients with a low E-C ratio at 34 weeks, the physician should be able to distinguish "false positives" from true placental insufficiency.

▶ [The 1979 YEAR BOOK contained both positive and negative reports concerning the value of the estrogen-creatinine ratio determined on a single voiding at 32–34 weeks' gestation as a screening test for fetal risk. The results of the current study look good. The issue remains open.] ◀

Circadian Rhythms in Maternal Plasma Cortisol, Estrone, Estradiol, and Estriol at 34 to 35 Weeks' Gestation. John Patrick, John Challis, Renato Natale, and Bryan Richardson[1-12] (Univ. of Western Ontario) examined the relationship between circadian rhythms in different steroids by determining cortisol (F), estrone (E_1), estradiol (E_2), and estriol (E_3) concentrations by radioimmunoassay in maternal venous plasma at 30 to 60 minute intervals during 24 hour periods. Studies were done in 11 healthy women at 34 to 35 weeks' gestation, the time when the plasma E_3 concentration begins to rise rapidly and becomes a useful index of fetoplacental function. Studies were done under controlled conditions of posture and dietary in-

(1–12) Am. J. Obstet. Gynecol. 135:791–798, Nov. 15, 1979.

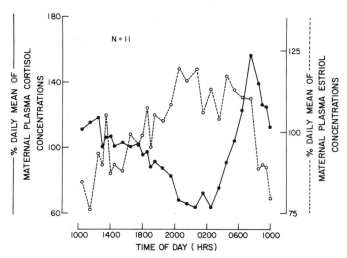

Fig 1–2.—There was an inverse relationship between mean maternal plasma F *(solid lines with dark circles)* and E_3 concentrations *(dashed lines with open circles)* over 24-hour periods. (Courtesy of Patrick, J., et al.: Am. J. Obstet. Gynecol. 135:791–798, Nov. 15, 1979.)

take. The infants were normal and had an average birth weight of 3,478 gm.

The mean maternal plasma F concentration was 273 ng/ml, and a significant circadian rhythm was noted. The mean maternal plasma E_3 concentration was 6.2 ng/ml, and this also showed a significant circadian rhythm. The relationship between F and E_3 concentrations is shown in Figure 1–2. Maternal plasma E_1 concentrations showed transient increases for 60 to 90 minutes after meals. When postprandial values were excluded, E_1 concentrations fell from a peak of 8.6 ng/ml at 10 to 11:30 A.M. to a trough of 5.7 ng/ml at 4:30 to 6:30 A.M. The mean maternal E_2 concentration was 17.05 ng/ml. When data were normalized, maternal E_2 concentrations at 12:30 P.M. were 18.7% greater than the concentration at 12:30 A.M., but no significant circadian change was noted in analyzing uncorrected data.

There is an inverse relationship between maternal F and E_3 concentrations, consistent with a maternal effect on fetal adrenal function. Circadian rhythms in F, E_1, E_2, and E_3 concentrations must be taken into account in clinical studies of these hormones during pregnancy.

▶ [This study demonstrates a circadian rhythm in plasma free estriol levels in late pregnancy, with highest values in the evening and lowest values in the morning hours. The pattern is virtually opposite to that of cortisol, suggesting that the fetal adrenal precursors of estriol (ie, dehydroepiandrosterone sulfate) are suppressed by maternal cortisol elevations crossing the placenta. Estrone, and to a lesser extent estradiol, levels more nearly paralleled cortisol, which would be consistent with a substantial origin of these steroids from the maternal adrenal.

In another study, this same investigative group (Am. J. Obstet. Gynecol. 136:325, 1980) found an absence of circadian rhythm in estriol levels at term, suggesting influences in addition to the maternal adrenal during late gestation.] ◀

Plasma Estriol in Evaluation of Third-Trimester Gestational Age. Recent reports have indicated that an identifiable serum unconjugated estriol surge at 36 weeks' gestation could be used to determine gestational age in late third-trimester pregnancies, when clinical and sonographic studies are notably unreliable. Timothy R. B. Johnson, Jr., Alan A. Compton, Lorraine S. Kirkish, Mary Ellen A. Bozynski, Mel L. Barclay, and Daisy S. McCann[1-13] evaluated this possibility in women considered to be about 30 to 33 weeks' pregnant when first seen. Plasma unconjugated estriol concentration was determined with ^{125}I-estriol radioimmunoassay kit.

Analysis of the findings in 32 cases confirmed a progressive rise in estriol concentrations toward term, but it showed no significant surge at 36 weeks' gestation. Surge points, however, could be identified statistically at various gestational ages in 78% of subjects, the average being 36 ± 2.1 weeks. All but 1 of 25 surges were grossly identifiable by visual inspection of graphic data. True gestational age was predicted to within 1 week in only half the cases. If a 2-week range was allowed, the method was only 66% accurate. One gestation was underestimated by 3 weeks.

Most women have a plasma estriol surge at about 36 weeks' gestation, but this cannot be documented consistently enough to be used as a marker of fetal age. The effect is not necessarily closely associated with fetal physiologic and functional maturity and is less reliable than other methods available for following problem pregnancies in the third trimester.

▶ [Previous authors have described an abrupt increase in serum unconjugated estriol level at about 36 weeks' gestation, presumably reflecting a surge in corticotropic activity in mother or fetus, or both, and have suggested that it may be sufficiently constant to provide an index of pregnancy duration. In this study, unconjugated estriol levels did indeed increase abruptly in 78% of patients sampled weekly, but the timing of the surge ranged from 30 to 39 weeks, hardly consistent or constant enough to be of clinical use.] ◀

Intra-amniotic or Intravenous Injection of Dehydroepiandrosterone Sulfate in Midgestation: Effect on Prolactin Level in Maternal Serum and Amniotic Fluid.

Prolactin is the chief secretory product of the maternal pituitary gland during pregnancy, presumably through increased circulating estrogen levels. Olavi Ylikorkala, Antti Keuppila, and Lasse Viinikka[1-14] (Univ. of Oulu) determined whether an elevation in serum estrogens after intravenous administration of dehydroepiandrosterone sulfate (DHEA-S) influences the midgestational levels of prolactin in maternal serum or amniotic fluid. Thirty-two women admitted for midtrimester abortion at 12 to 20 weeks' pregnancy were studied. The mean gestational period was 14.7 weeks. A dose of 100–200 mg DHEA-S was given intra-amniotically to 13 women and intravenously to 10, whereas 9 served as controls. The groups were comparable in gestational age.

Prolactin levels in serum rose significantly 2 to 6 hours after the intra-amniotic administration of 100 mg DHEA-S, and 4 to 6 hours after the 200-mg dose. Intravenous injection of DHEA-S increased the mean prolactin level 2 to 6 hours after administration. No consistent

(1–13) Obstet. Gynecol. 55:621–624, May 1980.
(1–14) J. Clin. Endocrinol. Metab. 49:452–455, September 1979.

changes in amniotic-fluid prolactin were observed after intra-amniotic administration of DHEA-S. Amniotic fluid and maternal serum prolactin levels correlated weakly.

Intra-amniotic or intravenous administration of DHEA-S led to increases in serum prolactin in nearly all subjects in this study. The prolactin response is most likely secondary to an elevation in serum estrogens. Preliminary findings indicate that the maternal circulation is not the chief source of amniotic fluid prolactin.

▶ [In this study, intravenous or intra-amniotic DHEA-S in midpregnancy raised prolactin levels in maternal serum but not in amniotic fluid (where they are normally much higher). Presumably, DHEA-S was aromatized to estrogen, which then stimulated prolactin release from the maternal pituitary but not from whatever is the source of amniotic fluid prolactin. The latter is not known, but decidua is thought to be a likely candidate (see 1980 YEAR BOOK OF OBSTETRICS AND GYNECOLOGY, p. 33).] ◀

Role of Fetal Adrenal Glands: Contribution to Etiology and Mechanism of Fetal Pulmonary Maturation. The role of the fetal adrenals in intrauterine lung maturation has not been clearly defined. Dan Peleg, Jack A. Goldman, and Ezra Elian[1-15] (Tel Aviv Univ.) assessed maturation of the fetal lungs in 3 anencephalic monsters and 2 microcephalic infants. The foam test and the lecithin-sphingomyelin (L-S) ratio were used as measures of fetal pulmonary maturation. Tests were done on amniotic fluid. Fetal pulmonary maturation was lacking in the anencephalics, but definite signs of lung maturation were observed in the micrencephalic infants. All 3 anencephalics lacked lung maturation by the foam test and the L-S ratio, although 1 pregnancy was definitely prolonged and no infant was premature. In the case of prolonged gestation, maternal corticosteroid administration was followed by an increase in active material related to surface tension.

The fetal adrenal appears to have an important role in fetal lung maturation. Fetuses with hypoplastic or hypofunctional adrenals have difficulty in reaching lung maturity. Only glucocorticoid administration will lead to maturation of their lungs. The findings support the view that the fetal adrenals and their proper function are the basis of fetal lung maturation.

▶ [These experiments of nature are consistent with the view that fetal adrenal function is important in maturation of the fetal lung. Anencephalic, but not microcephalic, fetuses had immature L-S ratios. Maternal betamethasone therapy increased the L-S ratio over three days from 0.7 to 1.9 in a case of anencephaly. This neonate had normal lung alveoli at autopsy.] ◀

Total and Free Testosterone During Pregnancy. Plasma testosterone concentrations are significantly elevated during pregnancy. Barbara L. Bammann, Carolyn B. Coulam, and Nai-Siang Jiang[1-16] (Mayo Clinic and Found.) attempted to determine whether this can be explained entirely by an increase in sex hormone-binding globulin (SHBG) or by an increase in testosterone production. Free testosterone levels were measured by equilibrium dialysis in 45 women at various stages of pregnancy and in 1,670 nonpregnant, normally menstruating women.

(1–15) Gynecol. Obstet. Invest. 9:325–330, 1978.
(1–16) Am. J. Obstet. Gynecol. 137:293–298, June 1, 1980.

Total testosterone concentration showed a variable increase throughout pregnancy. Only 3 of 61 determinations yielded values within the normal nonpregnant range, and 2 of these women subsequently aborted. The mean value after week 28 was 416 ng/dl, ninefold greater than in nonpregnant women. Free testosterone values were elevated after week 28 of pregnancy. The mean percentage free testosterone was 0.67%, compared with 2.12% in controls. Fetal free testosterone values were higher than maternal levels in all 5 deliveries studied. No differences in testosterone values were found between mothers with female and those with male fetuses.

The production rate of testosterone is probably increased later in pregnancy, but the source of this production is unknown. The fetus may be the source of the maternal testosterone elevations. Fetal gonadal testosterone as the source would be consistent with the increased production observed in the third trimester. The need for an increase in testosterone production is of interest in view of the known anabolic actions of this hormone.

▶ [This study demonstrates quite nicely that most of the increase in maternal total testosterone levels in pregnancy reflects the protein-bound portion, although there is a significant (twofold to threefold) elevation in free hormone levels during the third trimester. Noting that free testosterone in the fetus exceeded that of the mother in all four cases in which it was assessed (but with no sex difference), the authors suggest the fetus as a source of increased testosterone production in late pregnancy.] ◀

Placental Luteinizing Hormone Releasing Factor and Its Synthesis. Luteinizing hormone releasing factor (LRF) is synthesized and stored in the hypothalamus. It acts on the pituitary gland to stimulate the release of luteinizing hormone and follicle-stimulating hormone. Placental LRF (pLRF) is also found in the cytotrophoblast, but not in the syncytiotrophoblast, of the placental villi. G. S. Khodr and T. M. Siler-Khodr[1-17] (Univ. of Texas) provide evidence of the in vitro synthesis of pLRF by the term placenta.

Tritiated leucine was incorporated by the human placenta in vitro into a peptide that was biochemically, immunologically, and biologically identical to LRF. The percentage of tritiated leucine incorporated into pLRF was constant during the first 5 days, then increased significantly on days 6 to 8. When compared to the immunoreactive pLRF released into the culture medium, a similar pattern was noted from days 2 to 8. A constant specific activity was observed for pLRF released from days 2 to 8. Thus, after day 1 of culture, the rate of release reflected the rate of synthesis.

The specific activity of the labeled pLRF increased 100-fold from day 1 to day 2 and attained a maximum constant specific activity of 2.84 μCi/μg of pLRF thereafter. This suggests that the pLRF released on day 1 was predominantly endogenous and the pLRF released thereafter was primarily newly synthesized.

The amino acid sequence, chemical nature, and biologic significance of the pLRF synthesized by the placenta remain to be determined.

▶ [Synthesis of luteinizing hormone releasing factor by the cytotrophoblast has been

---

(1–17) Science 207:315–317, Jan. 18, 1980.

demonstrated. This placental luteinizing hormone releasing factor is thought to be involved in the control of human chorionic gonadotropin secretion.] ◄

Brachial and Femoral Blood Pressures During the Prenatal Period were investigated by Gertie F. Marx, F. J. Husain, and H. F. Shiau[1-18] (Albert Einstein College of Medicine, New York). During the latter part of pregnancy, the enlarged uterus of the supine woman can compress the inferior vena cava and partially obstruct the lower aorta. Arm and leg blood pressure measurements were used to ascertain early evidence of aortocaval compression and to determine any relationship it has to the development of preeclampsia.

In 202 young primigravidas, brachial and femoral arterial pressures were taken in the supine and left lateral positions during the second and third trimesters. Roll-over tests were performed in 78 patients between 28 and 32 weeks of gestation. An increase of 20 mm Hg or greater was considered to be a positive response.

Reproducible decreases in brachial or femoral systolic pressures, or both, greater than 10 mm Hg in the supine position occurred on at least one occasion in 156 patients. Signs and symptoms of the supine hypotensive syndrome developed in 20 women with both brachial and femoral blood pressure decreases. The earliest evidence of femoral pressure decline was seen at 19 weeks of gestation. The incidence rose progressively with a peak between 28 and 32 weeks of gestation. Declines in brachial pressure were noted only after 28 weeks.

Preeclampsia occurred in 25 (12%) women. There was no difference in the incidence of supine hypotensive manifestations between those who are subsequently preeclamptic and those without gestational hypertension.

Roll-over tests were positive in 45 (58%) of the 78 patients tested. Preeclampsia developed in one third of these, whereas preeclampsia occurred in only two patients having a negative roll-over test.

This study indicates that position-related declines occur more frequently in leg pressure than in arm pressure during pregnancy and that the leg pressure declines are demonstrable earlier in gestation.

► [It is generally recognized that the supine position in late pregnancy leads to vena caval occlusion (ie, the "inferior vena cava syndrome"). Less appreciated is that aortic compression occurs as well. In fact, the findings reported here that pressure drops of the femoral artery occurred more frequently than those of the brachial artery suggests that aortic compression is more common than vena caval compression. However, it may be that the compensatory mechanisms of increased vascular resistance and heart rate operate to "mask" the hemodynamic effects of vena caval compression in some patients.] ◄

Factors Controlling Plasma Renin and Aldosterone During Pregnancy. The striking rise in renin and aldosterone secretion noted during pregnancy probably is not due to functional volume depletion or increased shunting of blood in the uterine circulation. William H. Bay and Thomas F. Ferris[1-19] (Ohio State Univ.) examined plasma renin activity (PRA) and plasma aldosterone (PA) responses to altered sodium intake in normotensive women in the third trimester of pregnancy, who had no history of renal or cardiovascular dis-

(1–18) Am. J. Obstet. Gynecol. 136:11–13, Jan. 1, 1980.
(1–19) Hypertension 1:410–415, July–Aug., 1979.

ease. A diet containing 10 or 300 mEq sodium and 100 mEq potassium was given. Nonpregnant women also were evaluated. Plasma renin activity and PA were estimated by radioimmunoassays.

Pregnant women had higher supine PRA values than controls, and both PRA and PA increased on standing. Both PRA and PA were increased in both groups on the low-sodium diet, and urinary aldosterone excretion also increased. Pregnant women retained 170 mEq sodium with the high-sodium diet, with a 1.2-kg weight gain. No weight gain occurred in control subjects. Both PRA and PA were much higher in study subjects after six days. Urinary prostaglandin E levels were higher in pregnant women than in controls on an unrestricted sodium intake.

These findings indicate that, although renin and aldosterone secretion respond to altered sodium intake in pregnancy, the increased renin secretion of pregnancy may be secondary to the increase in prostaglandin synthesis that occurs. Conceivably, increased sensitivity to angiotensin with development of toxemia represents a decrease in prostaglandin E synthesis, with a resulting imbalance of the renin-angiotensin-PGE axis. Serial measurements of urinary prostaglandin E throughout pregnancy are needed to determine whether changes in angiotensin sensitivity with toxemia can be correlated with prostaglandin E excretion.

▶ [The renin-angiotensin system undergoes increased activation during pregnancy but something seems to blunt the hypertensive effect, permitting stimulation of aldosterone secretion to continue and thus promoting the increased sodium retention needed during gestation. Prostaglandins are thought to be the "something" that cause angiotensin insensitivity. What is new about this study is the suggestion that prostaglandin E may also be responsible for the gestational increase in renin secretion.] ◀

Adrenergic Innervation of Human Uterus: Disappearance of Transmitter and Transmitter-Forming Enzymes During Pregnancy. The human uterus is well supplied with adrenergic nerves, but the physiologic role of this innervation remains unclear. The uterine norepinephrine transmitter is extensively reduced as pregnancy advances. Gunnar Thorbert, Per Alm, Anders B. Björklund, Christer Owman, and Nils-Otto Sjöberg[1-20] (Univ. of Lund) investigated the human uterine adrenergic innervation in pregnant and nonpregnant women by using fluorescence microscopy, chemical measurements of the uterine norepinephrine transmitter and quantitative determination of tyrosine hydroxylase and dopa decarboxylase activity. Myometrial tissue from the ventral isthmus was taken from 6 parous menstruating women aged 42 to 51 years, 2 patients undergoing therapeutic abortion and 6 patients at 39 to 41 weeks of gestation who underwent cesarean section. All of the women were healthy.

A moderate to large number of fluorescent nerves was found in the nonpregnant uterus. The number of nerves and the intensity of fluorescence were reduced in the second trimester; almost none were seen at term. A sharp fall in the tissue norepinephrine level occurred in the second trimester; an even more marked reduction was noted at term, when the uterine norepinephrine concentration was only about

(1–20) Am. J. Obstet. Gynecol. 135:223–226, Sept. 15, 1979.

2% of that in nonpregnant samples. Tyrosine hydroxylase activity also declined with advancing pregnancy, at term being 13% of the nonpregnant value. Similar changes occurred in dopa decarboxylase activity, which at term was 14% of the nonpregnant level. No significant differences were noted in choline acetyltransferase activity.

The adrenergic nerves of the human uterus undergo substantial changes during pregnancy, probably reflecting entirely different conditions for a sympathetic influence on the myometrium in the last two trimesters. The quantitative relation between the cholinergic nerves and the mass of uterine smooth musculature is unchanged during pregnancy.

▶ [The authors of this study suggest that there is an absolute, not just relative, decrease in adrenergic nerve terminals in the human uterus during pregnancy. The assumption is that this derangement of nerve function may be important in the maintenance of uterine quiescence during pregnancy.] ◀

In Vitro Production of Prostanoids by the Human Cervix During Pregnancy: Preliminary Observations. The ovine cervix can produce prostanoids both in vitro and in vivo, and delivery appears to be associated with increased prostaglandin E production. There are data that indicate a direct local action of prostaglandin E on human cervical tissue. D. A. Ellwood, M. D. Mitchell, Anne B. M. Anderson, and A. C. Turnbull[1-21] (Univ. of Oxford) examined the ability of the pregnant human cervix to produce prostanoids with the use of an in vitro superfusion technique. Tissues were obtained from 7 patients having hysterectomy at various stages of pregnancy. Four had operations at 7–12 weeks' pregnancy and 3 had hysterectomy after cesarean section delivery in the last trimester.

Tissues from the patients sampled in the first trimester of pregnancy produced prostaglandins E and F, 13,14-dihydro-15-oxo-prostaglandin F, and 6-oxo-prostaglandin $F_{1\alpha}$. Production of thromboxane B_2 was minimal. Preliminary assessment of tissues taken in the last trimester indicated that the cervix may exhibit increased prostanoid production during active dilatation.

The pregnant human cervix can produce prostaglandins during in vitro superfusion. There is some indication that the human cervix has an increased rate of prostanoid synthesis during active dilatation, but the data must be viewed with caution as all cases were associated with abnormal uterine bleeding. Prostanoids produced by the human cervix may act locally within the cervix during pregnancy and parturition. An improved understanding of the mechanism of cervical softening may aid research into improved methods for inducing labor.

▶ [Prostaglandin E_2 has been used as a "cervical ripener" in women. This study demonstrates that the human pregnant or recently pregnant cervix produces prostaglandins in vitro. Whether this has biologic relevance concerning changes in the cervix in late pregnancy is unknown.] ◀

Twenty-Four-Hour Creatinine Clearance During Third Trimester of Normal Pregnancy was studied by J. M. Davison, W. Dunlop, and M. Ezimokhai[1-22] (Newcastle upon Tyne) in 10 healthy

(1–21) Br. J. Obstet. Gynaecol. 87:210–214, March 1980.
(1–22) Ibid., pp. 106–109, February 1980.

women to determine changes in the 24-hour creatinine clearance rate and the relationship of these changes to the assessment of glomerular filtration rates. Creatinine clearance rates were determined in each subject one time between 25 and 28 weeks' gestation, at weekly intervals from 32 weeks until delivery, and finally on one occasion between 8 and 12 weeks post partum.

There was a downward trend in the clearance rate of each subject throughout the last 6 weeks of pregnancy. A significant difference was found between values obtained at 6 weeks and 1 week before delivery by using paired Student's t test, but linear regression analysis failed to show a uniform change across subjects. Mean values in the last 3 weeks of pregnancy did not differ significantly from the nonpregnant mean. The change in the creatinine clearance rate did not appear to be caused by either the 24-hour creatinine excretion value or the plasma creatinine level acting independently (Fig 1–3).

The results suggest a mean decrease of 16% in 24-hour creatinine clearance rates during the third trimester of pregnancy, a reduction well beyond the limits of laboratory error and day-to-day variability. To what extent 24-hour creatinine clearance values represent true glomerular filtration rates has always been controversial, but its clinical validity in pregnancy has generally been accepted. Because creatinine is not only filtered at the glomerulus but is also secreted in

Fig 1–3.—Twenty-four–hour creatinine clearance and excretion and plasma creatinine concentration in 10 healthy women. (Courtesy of Davison, J. M., et al.: Br. J. Obstet. Gynaecol. 87:106–109, February 1980.)

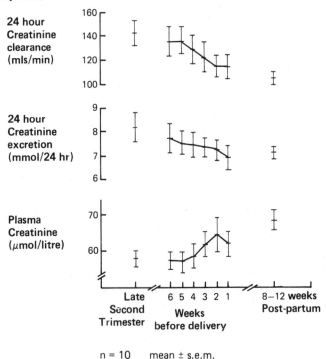

the proximal tubule, it is unclear whether these findings indicate a genuine reduction in glomerular filtration rate or an alteration in the renal handling of creatinine.

▶ [This article nicely demonstrates that the creatinine clearance in outpatient pregnant women decreases in late pregnancy to levels comparable with those of the nonpregnant state.] ◀

Urodynamic Studies in Normal Pregnancy and in Puerperium. Pregnancy and childbirth predispose to such urinary tract disorders as stress incontinence and urine retention. Serafim Iosif, Ingemar Ingemarsson, and Ulf Ulmsten[1-23] used a new pressure-recording instrument to perform urethral pressure profile measurements and urethrocystometry simultaneously in 14 primiparas, 3 of whom had had 1 abortion. Studies were done at weeks 12 to 16 of gestation, at week 38, and 5 to 7 days after vaginal delivery. Average time of delivery was 40.5 weeks, and average duration of labor was 9 hours. Average birth weight was 3,700 gm.

The average absolute length of the urethra increased from 36.3 mm at 12 to 16 weeks to 43 mm at 38 weeks' gestation and decreased to 32 mm 1 week after delivery. The average functional urethral length rose from 30.3 to 35.1 mm at 38 weeks and decreased to 27.6 mm 1 week after delivery. Mean maximum urethral pressure rose markedly, from 70 cm water at 12 to 16 weeks to 93 cm at the end of pregnancy, and fell to 69 cm water after delivery. Average bladder pressure also increased substantially, from 9 to 20 cm water toward the end of pregnancy, returning to 9 cm water after delivery. Average urethral closure pressure rose from 61 to 73 cm water at the end of pregnancy. Closure pressure was positive under cough provocation in all patients at all intervals.

The elasticity of all urinary passages appears to be increased during pregnancy. An average increase of 12 cm water in closure pressure of the urethra occurred during pregnancy in these subjects, indicating overcompensation of continence ability. It will be of interest to determine the extent to which these measurements may deviate in stress-incontinent women during pregnancy or in women who acquire symptoms of stress incontinence during pregnancy.

▶ [This study documents pregnancy changes in function of the lower urinary tract. Urethral length increased, with respect to both absolute and functional length. Maximal urethral pressure increased (by an average of 23 cm H_2O) whereas bladder pressure rose to a lesser extent (11 cm H_2O); thus, urethral closure pressure tended to increase with gestation. These two effects—urethral length and closure pressure—would both tend to promote continence. None of the subjects studied complained of incontinence and it would be interesting to compare these results with those in gravidas with this symptom, which the authors say is in progress. Moreover, all of the subjects were in their first term pregnancy, and comparison with a group of women who had previously delivered might prove interesting.] ◀

Effects of Pregnancy and Contraceptive Steroids on Gallbladder Function. Cholesterol cholelithiasis is more common among women than men. The difference begins in puberty, is present throughout the childbearing years, and is believed to be increased by pregnancy. Little information is available about gallbladder function,

(1–23) Am. J. Obstet. Gynecol. 137:696–700, July 15, 1980.

especially during pregnancy. Dan Z. Braverman, Michael L. Johnson, and Fred Kern, Jr.[1-24] (Univ. of Colorado) used real-time ultrasonography to study gallbladder function in 11 nonpregnant women (controls), 33 pregnant women, and 17 women using oral contraceptives. Of the 33 pregnant women, 8 were in the first, 13 in the second, and 12 in the third trimester.

Gallbladder volume was measured in the fasting state and serially for 90 minutes after a standard liquid meal. Ingestion of the meal initiated a gallbladder contraction which lasted for 20 to 45 minutes. During the first few minutes there was a relatively large decrease in volume, which diminished as the gallbladder became smaller. The gallbladder did not empty completely in any patient, and often appeared to refill partially after maximum emptying.

In women at 14 or more weeks of gestation, every index of gallbladder function differed significantly from those observed in early pregnancy. Gallbladder volume during fasting was more than twice as large in women in the late stages of pregnancy (15 to 36 ml) than in controls (4 to 24 ml). During the first trimester, gallbladder volume was comparable to that in nonpregnant women.

In women whose gestations were over 13 weeks, the rate of emptying was significantly slower than in nonpregnant women; also, the maximum percent emptied was significantly lower. In the first trimester the rate of emptying was significantly slower than in controls, but not as slow as in later pregnancy. The maximum percent emptied in the first trimester was lower than in controls, but not significantly.

The residual gallbladder volume after maximum emptying was twice as great in the last two trimesters as compared to controls. There was no significant increase in residual volume during the first trimester.

All measures of gallbladder function were the same in women taking oral contraceptives as in controls.

Incomplete emptying of the gallbladder in late pregnancy leaves a large residual volume which may cause retention of cholesterol crystals, a prerequisite for cholesterol-gallstone formation. These findings are consistent with the view that pregnancy increases the risk of cholesterol gallstones. However, the increased incidence of gallstones associated with the use of contraceptive steroids does not involve abnormal gallbladder kinetics.

▶ [Pregnancy and the pill are both thought to be predisposing factors to the development of gallstones. These altered hormonal states are associated with changes in blood and bile lipid profiles and, in the case of pregnancy, with altered gallbladder function as well. This ultrasound study nicely demonstrates increased fasting and residual gallbladder volumes in late pregnancy and a decreased rate of emptying in response to the ingestion of a test meal.] ◀

Carbohydrate Metabolism in Women with a Twin Pregnancy. Pregnancy is associated with alterations in carbohydrate metabolism. W. N. Spellacy, W. C. Buhi, and S. A. Birk[1-25] (Univ. of Florida) un-

(1-24) N. Engl. J. Med. 302:362–364, Feb. 14, 1980.
(1-25) Obstet. Gynecol. 55:688–691, June 1980.

dertook to determine whether twin pregnancies have more significant alterations in carbohydrate metabolism than singleton pregnancies at the same gestational period. Forty-eight women in the second half of gestation were studied. The 24 with twin pregnancies took over 250 gm of carbohydrate for 3 days before evaluation and fasted overnight before receiving 25 gm of glucose intravenously. The two groups were similar in age, parity, weight, and gestational age. Plasma placental lactogen levels were significantly higher in the women with twin gestations.

Fasting and 5- and 15-minute blood glucose values were significantly lower in women with twin pregnancies. Glucose disappearance rates were insignificantly lower in the twin than in the singleton group. Plasma insulin values rose significantly after glucose injection in both groups, but concentrations were lower in the twin pregnancy group. Only the difference in 15-minute values was significant.

The findings suggest that twin gestations are not at an unusually high risk of clinical hyperglycemia. Routine glucose tolerance testing in twin pregnancies does not appear to be justified. Placental lactogen appears not to be the major pregnancy factor causing the insulin resistance of pregnancy. Studies of factors such as placental steroids and their effects on peripheral insulin receptors are being conducted to clarify the insulin resistance of pregnancy.

▶ [Since human placental lactogen generally has been considered to be an important factor in the insulin resistance seen in late pregnancy and since placental lactogen levels are high in twin pregnancies, one might predict that patients carrying twins would respond to a glucose challenge with increased secretion of insulin and higher plasma levels in an attempt to override the effects of placental lactogen. Nice try, but no cigar, according to this study! Patients carrying twins had lower blood glucose *and* insulin levels than did patients with singleton pregnancies. Back to the drawing board!] ◀

Significance of Amniotic Fluid Glucose in Late Pregnancy. R. D. Marin and W. Hood[1-26] measured amniotic fluid glucose in normal pregnancies and in those complicated by fetal growth retardation, compared the relative merits of serum human placental lactogen (hPL) and amniotic fluid glucose in assessing fetal growth retardation, and studied the permeability of the fetal membranes to glucose as a function of gestational age.

In this study, glucose levels were estimated in more than 150 amniotic fluid samples and were found to fall with advancing gestational age (Fig 1–4). Significantly lower levels were found in postterm pregnancies and in association with fetal growth retardation. Seventeen patients had hPL values below the 5th percentile; 11 of these were delivered of low birth weight infants. An amniotic fluid glucose value of less than 0.8 mmol/L predicted a low birth weight infant in 10 of the 11 patients. Of 47 patients in whom both serum hPL and amniotic fluid glucose were measured, 13 had low birth weight infants. Serum hPL was positively correlated with the outcome in 83% of these cases, and amniotic fluid glucose was positively correlated in 96%. Thus, amniotic fluid glucose estimations were superior to serum hPL mea-

(1–26)   Aust. N.Z. J. Obstet. Gynaecol. 19:91–94, May 1979.

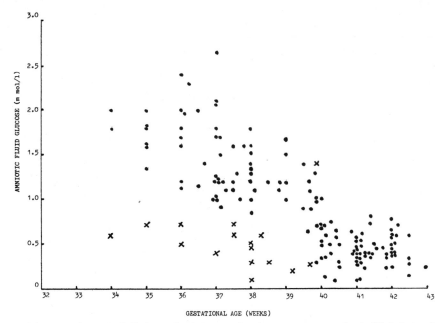

Fig 1–4.—Amniotic fluid glucose levels in normal and postterm pregnancies *(solid circles)* and in those complicated by fetal growth retardation *(X)*. (Courtesy of Marin, R. D., and Hood, W.: Aust. N.Z. J. Obstet. Gynaecol. 19:91–94, May 1979.)

surements in distinguishing between normal pregnancies and those complicated by intrauterine growth retardation. In vitro perfusion studies showed that the permeability of the membranes to glucose decreased with advancing gestational age, suggesting that this route is less important than fetoamniotic exchange in determining the level of amniotic fluid glucose in late pregnancy.

▶ [This report confirms earlier studies indicating that amniotic fluid glucose levels decline progressively during late pregnancy and that lower than normal levels are found with fetal growth retardation. Further, in vitro investigations imply a diminution of the rate of glucose transfer across the chorioamnion as the mechanism. However, other studies have suggested that amniotic fluid glucose in late gestation is probably more directly of fetal than of maternal origin.] ◀

2. Medical Complications of Pregnancy

Severe Rheumatic Cardiac Disease and Pregnancy: Ultimate Prognosis. Many clinicians believe that pregnancy irreversibly depletes the cardiac reserve of a woman with cardiac disease, thereby shortening her life expectancy. Leon C. Chesley[2-1] (SUNY, Downstate Med. Center) followed through 1975 all of the 134 women diagnosed from 1931 to 1943 as having "functionally severe" rheumatic cardiac disease and surviving pregnancy. In 1975, 9 patients were still alive.

All patients satisfied one or more of the following criteria: history of cardiac decompensation, except during acute rheumatic carditis; cardiac functional Class III or IV at time of conception; atrial fibrillation; or cardiac decompensation in pregnancy. All had mitral stenosis, and 17 also had aortic lesions.

The average length of follow-up, 14.9 years, reflects a high mortality: 50% of the patients died in the first 11 years. The average annual death rate was 62.8/1000.

Analysis of the mortality shows that the women died at an exponential rate. The "half-life" of the entire series is 11 years. On the average, 6.3% of the survivors to any given year died in that year.

Women who did and did not have subsequent pregnancies were compared. A time bias exists in favor of women who lived long enough to have another pregnancy; this is circumvented by a statistical bias tabulated against women having later pregnancies. The two groups are comparable in average age at entry into the study and distribution of age groups in which the patient-years were lived.

Five subgroups of signs and symptoms were associated with the highest annual death rates in the first 5 years after delivery. Except for the criterion of atrial fibrillation, each of the subgroups is proportionately represented in the women having had later pregnancies. Thus, it appears that women who had later pregnancies had no less impairment of cardiac function than those who had no additional pregnancies.

Among 22 sterilized women, the annual death rates in the first and second 5 years, as well as in the entire follow-up period, were only slightly lower. Sterilizations appeared to approach random distribution.

The remote mortality rates and later pregnancies were correlated. The group with later pregnancies had a relative excess of deaths in the first year due to five deaths occurring during later pregnancies. Immediate maternal death precludes any assessment of long-term effects of pregnancy. Provided that a women survives the hazard of

---

(2–1) Am. J. Obstet. Gynecol. 136:552–558, Mar. 1, 1980.

pregnancy itself, there is no evidence for a delayed or remote effect on her life expectancy.

The 55 women with only cardiac decompensation in pregnancy had a lower average annual death rate than other women in the series. Less severe conditions may be included in this subgroup. In an analysis excluding these patients, no evidence was found for a delayed adverse effect of pregnancy on survival. Similarly, even in those patients with the most severe cardiac disease, no remote adverse effects of pregnancy were demonstrated.

▶ [Leon Chesley periodically updates the long-term follow-up of women with certain complications of pregnancy—notably, eclampsia and rheumatic heart disease—at the Margaret Hague Maternity Hospital during the 1930s. The reports are always marked by thoroughness, care, and perceptiveness. This one reports 100% follow-up of 134 women with severe rheumatic heart disease, of whom only 9 were still alive at the time of writing. Its most important message is that pregnancy does not seem to worsen the long-term prognosis of this disease in women who survive pregnancy.] ◀

Effect of Maternal Cardiac Disease and Digoxin Administration on Labor, Fetal Weight, and Maturity at Birth. P. C. Ho, T. Y. Chen, and Vivian Wong[2-2] (Univ. of Hong Kong) compared 122 patients with cardiac disease and 250 controls with respect to the course of pregnancy and infant condition. The groups did not differ significantly in duration of pregnancy for nulliparas, duration of the first stage of labor, or infant Apgar scores 1 minute after delivery. Multiparas with heart disease had significantly earlier spontaneous onset of labor than control multiparas. Birth weights were significantly lower in the multiparous cardiac group. Birth weights in the nulliparous cardiac group were insignificantly lower than in controls. Significantly more cardiac patients than controls had infants light for dates (18% versus 8.4%). New York Heart Association functional class 3 and class 4 cardiac patients tended to have earlier deliveries and lighter infants, but these effects were not significant.

Patients with heart disease have an increased tendency to deliver infants light for dates. Digoxin therapy had no effect on duration of pregnancy or labor in this study. The controlling factor is probably the severity of heart disease. Infants of patients with cardiac disease were not depressed at birth, but follow-up appears to be worthwhile in view of the possibility of future manifestations of cerebral damage.

▶ [The principal finding of this study is that women with cardiac disease (predominantly rheumatic and functional classes 1 and 2) tend to have infants small for gestational age. The tendency is a slight one; 18% of infants were below the 10th percentile of birth weight for gestation age. It is well known that fetal growth is impaired with maternal cyanotic heart disease, but only 1 of 122 subjects had this condition.] ◀

Maternal and Fetal Sequelae of Anticoagulation During Pregnancy. Judith G. Hall, Richard M. Pauli, and Kathleen M. Wilson[2-3] (Univ. of Washington) reviewed reports of pregnancies in which coumarin derivatives or heparin were given. Apparently, either class of anticoagulant carries substantial risks. The minimal criteria for warfarin embryopathy are exposure to coumarin derivatives in the first trimester and the presence of nasal hypoplasia or stippled epiphyses.

(2-2) Aust. N.Z. J. Obstet. Gynaecol. 20:24–27, February 1980.
(2-3) Am. J. Med. 68:122–140, January 1980

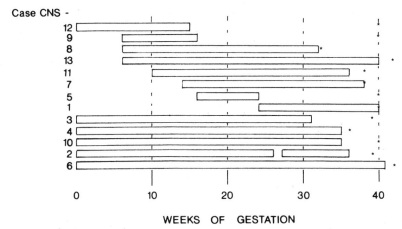

Fig 2–1.—Exposure to coumarin derivatives shown by weeks of gestation in 13 infants in whom central nervous system abnormalities were attributable to exposure to coumarin derivatives. Each bar represents exposure in an individual infant. Asterisks indicate time of birth in gestational weeks. There is apparently not any one critical period of exposure, although all infants represented here were exposed in the second or third trimesters. (Courtesy of Hall, J. G., et al.: Am. J. Med. 68:122–140, January 1980.)

The central nervous system (CNS) and eye abnormalities probably are due to exposure in later pregnancy. Mental retardation also is associated with exposure in the last two trimesters as well as the first trimester. The occurrence of CNS abnormalities is related to exposure to coumarin drugs in Figure 2–1.

The outcome of pregnancies involving exposure to coumarin drugs or heparin is given in the table. Of 418 reported pregnancies in which coumarin derivatives were used, one-sixth resulted in abnormal live-born infants and another sixth in abortion or stillbirth. Central nervous system abnormalities and specific embryopathy were encountered, as well as the expected hemorrhagic complications. The use of heparin in pregnancy does not appear to result in a significantly better outcome. One eighth of the infants in 135 reported cases were stillborn and one fifth were premature; one third of the latter infants died. At most, two thirds of infants were apparently normal.

Both heparin and coumarin derivatives, given during pregnancy, carry substantial risks to both mother and fetus. Prevention of preg-

SUMMARY OF FETAL AND NEONATAL OUTCOME AFTER
ANTICOAGULANT USE IN PREGNANCY

| | Per Cent of Pregnancies | |
	Coumarins	Heparin
Liveborn		
Subsequent infant death	2.4	7.4
Persistent sequelae	10.4	0.7
Premature, otherwise 'normal'	1.9	14.1
Spontaneous abortions	8.6	1.5
Stillbirths	7.7	12.6

nancy is, in general, advised. If a woman conceives, or if medical indications for anticoagulation arise during pregnancy, therapeutic abortion should be offered. Prenatal diagnosis by roentgenologic study may be possible. The overall likelihood of a relatively normal outcome is only about two-thirds when either coumarin drugs or heparin are utilized. Perhaps a way of abrogating the adverse effects of anticoagulant drugs will be found.

▶ [Adverse perinatal consequences of anticoagulation in pregnancy can be due to the underlying maternal process necessitating angicoagulation (usually the presence of a prosthetic cardiac valve or thromboembolism), to the indirect fetal effects of maternal hemorrhagic complications, or to the direct effects of the anticoagulant on the fetus. Because heparin does not cross the placenta, the third mechanism is restricted to coumarin derivatives. Although fetal death from hemorrhage and nasal hypoplasia secondary to first-trimester exposure are generally well-known risks of warfarin therapy, this thorough review points out the additional slight risk of central nervous system or eye abnormalities in exposed fetuses. Furthermore, this exposure apparently need not be in the first trimester. It is speculated that brain deformations may occur secondary to hemorrhage and subsequent scarring.

A case report of maternal "heparin osteoporosis" with spinal fractures appeared in the 1980 YEAR BOOK (p. 72). It seems there is no easy solution to the problem of indicated anticoagulation during pregnancy. Certainly, nonpregnant patients on anticoagulants should receive careful contraceptive counseling.] ◄

Hypertension During Pregnancy With and Without Specific Treatment; Development of Children at Age Four Years. Margaret K. Ounsted, Valerie A. Moar, Francis J. Good, and C. W. G. Redman[2-4] (John Radcliffe Hosp.) have followed 168 children born to hypertensive mothers.

In a controlled trial, pregnant women who were hypertensive before the 28th week of gestation were randomly allocated to treatment with methyldopa or no treatment. The children from these pregnancies (86 from treated mothers; 82 from untreated mothers) have been reexamined at age 4 and their development compared with a random sample from the same hospital (107 children). Their health, height, weight, and the incidence of sight, hearing, and speech problems did not differ. None had gross neurologic abnormalities.

Boys in the treated hypertensive group had significantly smaller head circumference than those in the untreated group or random sample, but there was no correlation between head size and developmental score. The reduction in head circumference was not related to the total amount or duration of methyldopa received during pregnancy, and this effect was confined to children of women in whom treatment was started between 16 and 20 weeks of gestation.

On average, children in the random sample were the most advanced when assessed by a global score of development. There were no significant differences between treated and untreated hypertensive groups with respect to total score or score on any of the subcategories tested, although individual scores tended to be higher in the treated subjects.

These findings suggest that maternal hypertension is associated with slight developmental delay in early childhood and that treat-

(2–4) Br. J. Obstet. Gynaecol. 87:19–24, January 1980.

ment of the pregnant hypertensive woman with methyldopa may reduce this effect.

▶ [The controversy concerning the use of antihypertensive drugs in patients with moderate chronic hypertension in pregnancy is not settled by this report. The pro-drug folks can take comfort from the trend toward higher developmental scores in the treated group compared with the untreated group (not statistically significant). The antidrug folks can point to the significantly smaller head circumferences in boys at four years of age in the treated group. "Better" developmental scores were related to the absence of hypertension (both treated and untreated) and to higher social class.] ◀

Effect of Dihydralazine on the Fetus in the Treatment of Maternal Hypertension. The use of intravenous dihydralazine to reduce maternal blood pressure in cases of severe hypertension in late pregnancy has caused fetal heart rate changes in some patients. G. J. Vink, J. Moodley, and R. H. Philpott[2-5] (Durban, South Africa) examined the effects of maternal dihydralazine therapy on the fetus in a prospective study of 33 patients with diastolic blood pressures of 110 mm Hg or more after two hours' bed rest in the lateral position. All were more than 30 weeks pregnant. A 12.5-mg dose of dihydralazine was given intravenously in 16 ml of normal saline over a period of 4 minutes.

The blood pressure fell to therapeutic levels in 30 of 33 patients after dihydralazine administration. Pressure reductions occurred within 5 minutes of drug administration and lasted 1 hour. Marked tachycardia of more than 100 beats per minute was present in all patients, and 10 reported headache and flushing. Fetal heart rate decelerations were seen in 19 patients (group A) and no change in fetal heart rate patterns was seen in 14 (group B). Thirteen infants in group A were growth retarded, compared to only 1 in group B. Two patients showed an apparent increase in uterine activity. Three stillbirths occurred in group A. One was associated with abruptio placentae and 1 with spina bifida occulta. Further doses of dihydralazine and reserpine had been used in the third case, without fetal monitoring. No perinatal deaths occurred in group B.

Continuous fetal heart rate monitoring during dihydralazine administration for maternal hypertension can help identify the compromised fetus. Dihydralazine therapy is not recommended if the fetus of a hypertensive patient is identified as growth retarded.

▶ [Abrupt reduction of blood pressure was associated with fetal heart rate decelerations in these hypertensive patients. It is interesting, although not really surprising, that the fetal heart rate changes were most likely to occur in growth-retarded fetuses. The growth retardation in these cases apparently reflected inadequate uterine blood flow. A further decrease in uterine blood flow resulted from the antihypertensive drug treatment, and cardiotocographic signs of fetal distress appeared. Patients with preeclampsia were not considered separately from those with chronic hypertension. They probably should have been.] ◀

Systemic Lupus Erythematosus in Pregnancy. Systemic lupus erythematosus (SLE) has a propensity for women in the reproductive years and presents problems of varying complexity during pregnancy. Lawrence D. Devoe and Roger L. Taylor[2-6] (Univ. of Chicago) reviewed

(2–5) Obstet. Gynecol. 55:519–522, April 1980.
(2–6) Am. J. Obstet. Gynecol. 135:473–479, Oct. 15, 1979.

experience with 13 pregnancies in 8 patients with SLE who were seen from 1973 to 1978. Mean age at diagnosis of SLE was 19.3 years, and average prepregnancy duration of disease was 5.5 years. All patients but 1 conceived during a clinical remission. Only 3 women had exacerbations during pregnancy or post partum. There were 3 induced abortions. No maternal deaths occurred. Exacerbation was usually signaled by declining complement levels and less often by rising antinuclear immunofluorescence titers or positive anti-DNA antibody tests.

All patients but 1 entered pregnancy on prednisone therapy. One patient received azathioprine also. Hydrocortisone 21-sodium succinate (Solu-Cortef) was administered at delivery or induced abortion. Most patients had a satisfactory clinical course, but 2 had a postpartum exacerbation. The corrected perinatal wastage rate was 30%. Three of 8 pregnancies that reached viability ended in premature delivery. Two of the 5 infants delivered at term were considered to be growth retarded. The only neonatal death was due to *Escherichia coli* meningitis. No infant had signs of lupus erythematosus, cardiac or central nervous system abnormalities, or adrenal insufficiency. All surviving offspring have done well.

Induced abortion confers little clinical benefit on the course of SLE and should be reserved for cases complicated by cardiac or renal disease. Fetal outcome is still adversely affected by SLE. Intrauterine exposure to immunosuppressive agents is an inadequately studied source of potential risk to offspring of women with SLE. Systemic lupus erythematosus is a high-risk condition for pregnancy.

▶ [This report confirms much of what has been known previously about systemic lupus erythematosus complicating pregnancy: the prognostic importance of renal involvement and duration of remission, the risk of puerperal exacerbation, and a number of adverse effects on the fetus (spontaneous abortion, premature birth, and fetal growth retardation). New information of potentially great significance is the data on serial serologic changes. The levels of C_3 and C_4 seemed to decline with exacerbation or even before, presumably reflecting consumption by formation of antigen-antibody complexes, suggesting that careful monitoring of these complement levels might permit early identification and intervention (eg, increased steroid dosage). Levels of antinuclear factor and anti-DNA, which typically rise with exacerbation, were less helpful, which probably reflects the fact that these indices relate to more chronic changes.] ◀

Pancreatitis, Pregnancy, and Gallstones. A specific association between acute pancreatitis and pregnancy has long been suggested. A. J. McKay, J. O'Neill, and C. W. Imrie[2-7] (Royal Infirm., Glasgow) report their 17-year experience with acute pancreatitis. Of 519 patients with acute pancreatitis, 282 were women, 40 younger than age 30 years. In 20 (50%) the disease developed in association with pregnancy.

Six cases were reviewed retrospectively and 14 were treated during the prospective study. In 19 patients, diagnosis was based on clinical presentation and laboratory values; 1 patient had diagnosis at laparotomy. Onset of the acute disease occurred during pregnancy in 7 patients, in the postpartum period in 12, and at 8 weeks after abortion in 1. Treatment of pregnant patients was similar to that of non-

(2–7) Br. J. Obstet. Gynaecol. 87:47–50, January 1980.

pregnant patients, except that conventional radiology was not used in the former group.

Gallstones were demonstrated in 18 of the 20 patients. The pancreatitis was associated with type I hyperlipoproteinemia in 1 patient and with alcohol abuse in another. Of those with biliary disease, 17 underwent cholecystectomy with or without exploration of the common bile duct. None of these patients has experienced a further attack of acute pancreatitis.

Pancreatitis occurred during the first, second, and third pregnancies in 2 patients each and in the fourth pregnancy in 1.

In 2 patients the attack occurred during the first trimester, in 1 during the second trimester, and in four during the last trimester. There were no maternal deaths, but 1 fetal death and 1 neonatal death occurred. In both cases, the woman had surgery during the third trimester. One patient with type I hyperlipoproteinemia had drainage of an acutely inflamed pancreas; she aborted the fetus postoperatively. The other patient was thought to have appendicitis, but was found to have acute pancreatitis at operation. Her infant was full term, but died due to respiratory distress syndrome at 1 week of age.

There were 12 patients whose pancreatitis developed in the postpartum period. Of these, 6 attacks followed the first pregnancy, 5 followed the second, and 1 followed the fourth.

Gallstones are found in most patients of childbearing age with acute pancreatitis, but other etiologic factors (eg, alcohol abuse or virus) must be excluded.

Management should be conservative, with surgery reserved for the patient who continues to deteriorate. In the occasional patient who has pancreatitis during the first trimester, gallstones can be detected with ultrasonography, with surgery performed during the second trimester, if necessary.

▶ [The take-home lesson here is that 18 of 20 patients with acute pancreatitis associated with pregnancy had gallstones. The treatment of the acute episode is supportive; ultrasound provides a safe and effective means of diagnosing the associated cholelithiasis.] ◀

Prophylactic Transfusions of Normal Red Blood Cells During Pregnancies Complicated by Sickle Cell Hemoglobinopathies. F. Gary Cunningham and Jack A. Pritchard[2-8] (Univ. of Texas Southwestern Med. School), with the technical assistance of Ruble Mason and Gwendolyn Chase, administered transfusions of normal donor red blood cells prophylactically to women with sickle cell anemia, sickle cell-hemoglobin C disease or sickle cell–β-thalassemia during 37 pregnancies. In vitro labeling of the red blood cells with ^{51}Cr was used to estimate the amount of donor cells needed to reduce circulating red blood cells containing hemoglobin S to 50% or less. Severely anemic women either received multiple units over 2 to 3 days or were given furosemide intravenously and then red blood cells over 4 to 6 hours. If the hematocrit was close to normal, partial exchange transfusion was carried out. Packed red blood cells were infused whenever cells

(2–8) Am. J. Obstet. Gynecol. 135:994–1003, Dec. 1, 1979.

that sickled in sodium metabisulfite solution rose to about 60% or the hematocrit fell below 25.

Fourteen women with sickle cell anemia were given transfusions in 16 pregnancies, receiving an average of 13 treatments over 23 weeks of pregnancy. Fourteen liveborn infants survived. One was growth retarded. Meconium staining of amniotic fluid was seen in 4 cases. Nineteen women with sickle cell-hemoglobin C disease were given transfusions an average of 15 times over 18 weeks. Only 1 woman exhibited morbidity related to this condition. All infants were healthy, but 5 weighed under 2,501 gm at birth. Two larger infants were growth retarded. Two women with sickle cell–β-thalassemia received an average of 10 units over 14 weeks, with successful outcomes. Transfusion reactions included fever and myalgia-like discomfort. Difficulty in cross-matching occurred in 1 case. Two women with sickle cell anemia had profound suppression of red blood cell production. One infant had mild hemolysis.

Prophylactic transfusions of red blood cells are of value for pregnant women with sickle cell hemoglobinopathy. Careful monitoring of fetal well-being is necessary. Subsequent pregnancies should be discouraged.

▶ [Few, if any, medical complications of pregnancy pose as grave risks for mother and fetus as do sickle hemoglobinopathies. There has been much interest in recent years in transfusion therapy—either repeated "suppressive" transfusions or exchange transfusions—as a means of temporary treatment during gestation. This article reports the Dallas experience, in which the aims were to maintain the hematocrit above 25% and the proportion of hemoglobin S-erythrocytes below 60%, usually by intermittent transfusion but occasionally (when the hematocrit was relatively high) by partial exchange transfusion. No maternal deaths occurred and maternal morbidity was lowered; perinatal outcome was also improved, although fetal growth retardation and evidence of fetal distress persisted.] ◀

Prenatal and Postnatal Growth and Development in Sickle Cell Anemia. It is generally thought that homozygous sickle cell disease impairs physical growth during childhood, but previous studies have been cross-sectional in design, raising important methodological questions. Michael S. Kramer, Yolanda Rooks, LaRue A. Washington, and Howard A. Pearson[2-9] followed a cohort of children with hemoglobin SS from birth through ages 3 to 6 years. Postnatal effects were examined in 10 infants who were aged 33 months or more at follow-up. These children and their matched controls were aged 35 to 70 months at evaluation.

None of 14 black newborn infants studied was premature, and no significant differences from normal were found in birth weight or length or Apgar scores. Significant deficits in height, weight, skinfold thickness, and bone age were observed at follow-up. Head circumference and muscle mass were similar to those of controls. Most of the growth variables tended toward increasing deficits over time. Measures of cognitive development showed no significant differences between sickle cell patients and control children and no evidence of a trend toward deficits in affected children over time.

There is definite evidence of impaired body growth and skeletal

(2–9) J. Pediatr. 96:857–860, May 1980.

maturation in children with sickle cell disease. Cognitive development appears to be normal, but larger samples are needed to confirm this. Further study is also needed to determine the course of the growth defects observed.

▶ [Maternal SS hemoglobinopathy quite regularly produces fetal growth retardation by virtue of the chronic hypoxic state associated with the disease. This report indicates that sickle cell anemia in the infant, by contrast, is not associated with any impairment of fetal growth, although postnatal growth over the first 3 to 6 years of life was retarded.] ◀

Fetal Platelet Counts in Obstetric Management of Immunologic Thrombocytopenic Purpura (ITP) were investigated by James R. Scott, Dwight P. Cruikshank, Neil K. Kochenour, Roy M. Pitkin, and James C. Warenski.[2-10] Fetal scalp blood was obtained prior to or early in the course of labor in 12 patients with ITP to determine the optimal method of delivery. In 5 patients labor began spontaneously and amniotomy and scalp sampling were done as soon as cervical dilation reached 2 to 3 cm. In 7 subjects at full term, who had a similar degree of cervical dilation before labor, amniotomy was done for elective induction and fetal scalp blood was obtained immediately thereafter.

Selection of the method of delivery was based on the platelet count in the fetal scalp blood sample. Three fetuses had platelet counts below 50,000/cu mm in scalp blood and were delivered by cesarean section immediately. The other 9 fetuses had platelet counts above 50,000/cu mm and labor was allowed to continue. Cesarean section delivery was used for 1 fetus with cephalopelvic disproportion, whereas the remaining 8 were delivered vaginally.

Only the 3 infants with low platelet counts, who were delivered abdominally, acquired neonatal thrombocytopenia. Although neonatal bleeding problems developed in all 3, none showed intracranial hemorrhage. The fetal scalp platelet count accurately predicted whether or not the neonate would become thrombocytopenic. The potential danger of bleeding from the scalp puncture site in a fetus with thrombocytopenia did not occur when pressure was carefully applied with a gauze sponge through two subsequent uterine contractions.

Fig 2–2.—Proposed management of deliveries in ITP pregnancy. (Courtesy of Scott, J. R., et al.: Am. J. Obstet. Gynecol. 136:495–499, Feb. 15, 1980.)

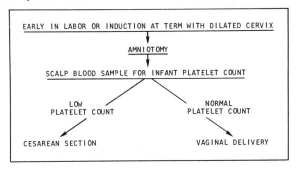

(2–10) Am. J. Obstet. Gynecol. 136:495–499, Feb. 15, 1980.

In the management of pregnancy complicated by ITP, amniotomy should be done as soon as conditions permit fetal blood sampling, either at the time of induction of labor or early in the course of spontaneous labor. Fetal blood should then be obtained and a platelet count performed. If the count is above 50,000/cu mm, vaginal delivery should be anticipated, whereas fetuses with lower platelet counts should be delivered by cesarean section as soon as possible (Fig 2–2). Fetal blood sampling appears to be more accurate than the maternal platelet count.

▶ [This paper describes our management of delivery of patients with immunologic thrombocytopenic purpura at the University of Iowa, utilizing fetal platelet counts. The approach is summarized in Figure 2–2. The cutoff point for definition of fetal thrombocytopenia is 50,000 per cu mm based on information from the literature indicating that significant neonatal bleeding is rare above this level.

The question of whether intracranial hemorrhage occurs during "normal" labor when the fetus is thrombocytopenic is controversial. Read on.] ◀

Intracranial Hemorrhage In Utero as a Complication of Isoimmune Thrombocytopenia. Isoimmune thrombocytopenia is a known cause of bleeding in the newborn infant, including central nervous system hemorrhage, and cesarean section has been suggested for infants at risk. Edwin L. Zalneraitis, Richard S. K. Young, and Kalpathy S. Krishnamoorthy[2-11] (Harvard Med. School) describe two infants who had intracranial hemorrhage in utero and would not have been benefited by operative delivery. Both had perinatal hemorrhage in the presence of extremely low platelet counts, which responded dramatically to transfusion of maternal platelets. There had been a poor response to random donor platelets and an intermediate response to a combination of random donor platelets and exchange transfusion. Both patients were promptly treated but had congenital hydrocephalus and required ventriculoperitoneal shunts.

The risk of intracranial hemorrhage in the face of established isoimmune thrombocytopenia is substantial. Vaginal delivery and other perinatal stresses increase the risk of intracranial bleeding in this setting. These two patients were not known to be at risk of isoimmune platelet destruction, and both probably had prior in utero central nervous system insults. Both had enlarged heads with separated sutures at birth. It would seem to be prudent to continue to deliver all infants at known risk of isoimmune thrombocytopenia by cesarean section. This alone, however, will not eliminate the risk of hemorrhagic central nervous system complications in infants with this condition.

▶ [In these two cases of isoimmune thrombocytopenia (a condition in which the mother produces antibodies gainst the fetus' platelets) the computerized axial tomography scan findings indicated that intracranial hemorrhage had occurred *prior to* labor. Thus, cesarean section would not have prevented the complication.] ◀

Diabetes Subsequent to Birth of a Large Baby: A 16-Year Prospective Study. John B. O'Sullivan and Clare M. Mahan[2-12] (Boston Univ. Med. Center) reviewed data collected over 16 years to determine the predictive capabilities of large birth weight infants for sub-

(2–11) J. Pediatr. 95:611–614, October 1979.
(2–12) J. Chronic Dis. 33:37–45, 1980.

sequent diabetes in the mother. Data were obtained in the Boston Gestational Diabetes Study, a prospective study of 615 potentially diabetic women and 328 controls with normal glucose tolerance, documented in an index pregnancy in 1954–1960. Data collection was terminated in 1970. Data from 308 untreated potential diabetics were available for analysis. Infants weighing 9 lb or more were considered large, regardless of dates.

Diabetes on follow-up was not related to birth weight of the offspring of the index pregnancy for either the potentially diabetic women or negative controls. Incidence curves were not significantly different in the two cohorts. Lack of significance of birth weight as a predictor of subsequent diabetes was confirmed in a multifactor context through analyses using the logistic risk model. The relative risk of decompensated diabetes was 2.8 for potentially diabetic women who bore large infants in the index pregnancy, compared to those who bore infants of normal size. Over 16 years, there was an estimated 35% rate of progression to decompensation among women who bore large infants, compared to an 18% rate for mothers of normal-sized infants. Parity and a history of having borne a large or premature infant did not enhance predictive capabilities for decompensated diabetes.

Although large-infant births are definitely increased in diabetic women, the prevalence of diabetes in the population is relatively low; large birth weights are more likely to occur for constitutional or other reasons than diabetes. The glycemic factor was controlled in the present analysis. The birth of a large infant to a potentially diabetic woman has strong prognostic value which is not explained by such factors as weight, family history of diabetes, blood glucose during the index pregnancy, or age, after adjustment for duration of follow-up.

▶ [These results seem contrary to current clinical dogma in that they imply that giving birth to a large infant is not a good indicator of the risk of developing diabetes subsequently. Among those women who did develop diabetes, however, a previous large infant was associated with increased severity of the disease. Does this mean that birth weights should not be used to select patients for diabetes screening?] ◀

Feasibility of Maintaining Normal Glucose Profiles in Insulin-Dependent Pregnant Diabetic Women. There is little doubt about the need for optimal control of diabetes during pregnancy. Lois Jovanovic, Charles M. Peterson, Brij B. Saxena, M. Yusoff Dawood, and Christopher D. Saudek[2-13] (New York Hosp.-Cornell Univ. Med. Center) attempted to determine whether optimal metabolic levels of glucose can be maintained in ambulatory pregnant diabetic subjects using self-monitored determinations of glucose and hemoglobin A_{1c} levels.

Ten pregnant insulin-dependent diabetics participated in the study. The mean age was 27.5 years, and the mean duration of diabetes was 7.1 years. The goals were a fasting plasma glucose level of 60–70 mg/dl, a mean plasma glucose level over 24 hours of 80–87 mg/dl, and a postprandial glucose level not exceeding 140 mg/dl. The initial insulin dose was 0.7 units/kg. A 30-kcal-kg diet with 40% carbohydrate

(2–13) Am. J. Med. 68:105–112, January 1980.

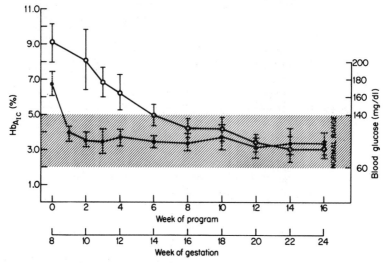

Fig 2–3.—Time course for normalization of HbA$_{1c}$ and blood glucose for 10 insulin-dependent women. *Open circles,* mean HbA$_{1c}$ ± 1 SD; each point based on HbA$_{1c}$ determination obtained from all 10 patients at 2-week intervals. *Solid circles,* mean blood glucose ± 1 SD; each point based on 8 to 10 glucose determinations a day for preceding 2 weeks for all 10 patients. First point (week 0) determined from plasma glucose values obtained in hospital during 24-hour glucose profile. *Hatched area,* normal range for HbA$_{1c}$ and blood glucose in third trimester. (Courtesy of Javanovic, L., et al.: Am. J. Med. 68:105–112, January 1980.)

was prescribed. Patients were seen weekly in the clinic. Fingerstick blood glucose determinations were made before breakfast and dinner, and 1 hour after each meal.

The course of normalization of blood glucose and hemoglobin A$_{1c}$ levels is shown in Figure 2–3. Patients averaged one symptomatic hypoglycemic episode a week for the first two weeks, but blood glucose levels never fell below 50 mg/dl. Only 1 patient required glucose

INFANT STATUS AT BIRTH

Case No.	Gestational Time (wk)	Infant Birth Weight (g)	APGAR 5 Min.	Mean Blood Glucose 1st 6 Hours After Birth	Hematocrit (%)	Calcium (mg/dl)	Bilirubin (mg/dl)
1	39	3,100	10	60	50	10.7	2.0
2	39.5	3,000	10	56	54	9.5	2.6
3	40	3,100	10	76	60.0	10.0	4.0
4	38	3,000	10	75	56	10.8	8.0
5	38	2,590	10	60	54	10.2	2.8
6	37.5	3,200	10	80	50	10.1	4.0
7	40	3,150	10	78	49	9.6	5.2
8	40	2,990	10	60	47	9.6	2.0
9	37	2,850	10	70	46	10.0	2.4
10	39	2,990	10	68	47	9.5	1.0
Mean	38.8	2,988	10	68.1	51.3	10.0	3.4
SD	1.11	959.4	—	12.65	4.53	0.47	2.02

White Class	Gestation Time (wk)	Birth Weight (g) Mean	Range
B	36.7	3,380	2,615–4,100
C	35.7	3,220	2,340–4,105
D	36.1	3,150	2,330–3,970
F	35.5	2,490	1,204–3,395

on one occasion. Serum estradiol levels, initially subnormal, returned toward normal within 2 weeks. Prolactin levels did not become normal until 5 weeks after the normalization of glucose levels, paralleling normalization of the hemoglobin A_{1c}. Delivery occurred at a mean of 39 weeks' gestation. Mean birth weight was normal for gestational age, and all the infants were well and not hypoglycemic (table).

Normoglycemia can be achieved and maintained for prolonged periods in pregnant diabetic outpatients through the use of patient-monitored glucose determinations. It now is feasible to design large-scale trials to define optimal control for pregnant diabetic women, in order to assure the best outcome.

▶ [Achieving excellent diabetic control is easier to talk about (or to write about!) than it is to do. Though the number of subjects is small, this report is exciting. Using a reflectance meter at home, these patients determined their blood glucose levels several times a day and adjusted their insulin dosages as needed. Excellent control resulted and the neonatal results are impressive. Although we rely on frequent blood glucose determinations in our management of pregnant diabetics, we do not have personal experience with this type of patient self-monitoring. The technique certainly looks promising.

The importance of strict diabetic control was emphasized by Haukkamaa and associates (Obstet. Gynecol. 55:596, 1980), who reported only 1 perinatal death in a series of 94 diabetic pregnancies, 45 of them insulin dependent. The management was in accordance with modern principles, and any of several features (frequent hospitalization, biochemical and biophysical monitoring, amniocentesis, or luck) might have been responsible for the low frequency of morbidity and mortality, but the authors felt that tight control was the most important.

In a related study, Cruikshank and colleagues (J. Clin. Endocrinol. Metab. 50:264, 1980) found that diabetics have lower parathyroid hormone and magnesium levels throughout pregnancy than do nondiabetics. Somewhat curiously, these effects bore no relationship to level of diabetic control.] ◀

Subcutaneous Continuous Insulin Infusion and Control of Blood Glucose Concentration in Diabetics in Third Trimester of Pregnancy. Improved control of maternal blood glucose concentrations appears to be important in minimizing perinatal mortality in pregnant diabetics, but mortality and morbidity remain elevated in this setting. Blood glucose concentrations can be improved by subcutaneous continuous insulin infusion in nonpregnant diabetics. Jonathan M. Potter, John P. D. Reckless, and Derek R. Cullen[2-14] (Hallamshire Hosp., Sheffield, England) evaluated this approach in 8 pregnant diabetics in the third trimester. Six were established insulin-dependent diabetics before pregnancy, whereas 2 had diabetes requiring insulin at the start of the third trimester. The former patients were managed on a twice-daily insulin regimen during the first two trimesters. Twenty-four-hour glucose profiles were obtained after strict inpatient control on a conventional insulin regimen and after the start of continuous infusion, which was maintained for 5 to 55 days. The basal infusion rate was adjusted to produce fasting glucose concentrations of about 90 mg/dl, with an increased infusion rate over mealtimes. A Pye Dynamic MS 16 syringe driver was used for the insulin infusion and was carried in a holster.

Patients were able to alter the rate of infusion at mealtime and

(2–14) Br. Med. J. 1:1099–1101, Apr. 26, 1980.

recharge the syringe with insulin without difficulty. They were mobile and could bathe and sleep without hindrance. Five patients were able to go home on weekends. Basal infusion rates ranged from 0.66 to 1.5 units per hour and augmented rates from 8 to 47 units per hour. More insulin was required at breakfast than at other mealtimes. Mean 24-hour blood glucose concentrations were similar on continuous infusion and intermittent insulin injection. Fasting concentrations tended to be higher on continuous infusion, but the lower concentrations on intermittent therapy were associated with nocturnal hypoglycemia in some patients. A trend to less daytime variation in blood glucose concentrations on continuous infusion was evident.

The infusion system was found to be practical and reliable and to produce less diurnal variation in blood glucose concentrations. Further development of this system could result in appreciably improved diabetic control and better management of diabetics in the third trimester of pregnancy.

Management of the Pregnant Diabetic: Home or Hospital, With or Without Glucose Meters? Good control of maternal diabetes is an important determinant of successful pregnancy. Interest has increased in self-monitoring of blood glucose concentration by diabetics at home. S. M. Stubbs, J. M. Brudenell, D. A. Pyke, P. J. Watkins, W. A. Stubbs, and K. G. M. M. Alberti[2-15] compared blood glucose concentration and metabolic control in conventionally managed patients and those monitoring their blood glucose concentrations with a meter. Seven insulin-dependent diabetics were assigned to glucose self-monitoring at home; they used Dextrostix and an Eyetone meter. Six others had glucose determinations made every 2 weeks at clinic visits. Mean ages were 26 and 29 years, respectively, and mean durations of diabetes were 13 and 11 years, respectively. Eight normal women at 32 to 36 weeks' gestation were also evaluated.

All patients delivered normal infants. Cot death of an infant in the nonmeter diabetic group later occurred. No significant differences in mean diurnal blood glucose values were found in the meter, nonmeter, and control groups. There were no major differences in mean blood glucose, lactate or alanine values during the day among diabetics at home, those in the hospital, or normal pregnant women. Blood glucose levels concentrations in hospitalized diabetics were higher in the morning and after dinner than in patients at home. Small differences in blood alanine and lactate values were observed at various times of day.

Patients at home maintained somewhat better blood glucose control than did hospitalized patients in this study, for reasons that are unclear. The policy of admitting all patients at 32 weeks' gestation is being reevaluated. Early admission is still recommended if social or medical circumstances are unsatisfactory. Glucose self-monitoring has a role, especially in early pregnancy, for patients whose control is inadequate. It can also be a useul part of patient education, partic-

(2–15) Lancet 1:1122–1124, 1980.

ularly in pregnancy. Conventional methods alone, however, can be just as effective in some patients.

▶ [The consensus is that careful blood glucose control improves the perinatal outcome in pregnancies complicated by diabetes mellitus. How should this careful control be achieved? In the report by Potter and co-workers, continuous subcutaneous insulin infusion did not significantly improve blood sugar levels; however, the 8 patients were in excellent control to start with. Twice each week, four blood glucose determinations were performed at home; the patients received split doses of various insulin preparations each day. Because the continuously infused insulin was given subcutaneously, not intravenously, and because the rate of infusion was changed in response to spot blood glucose values (continuous glucose monitoring was not performed), the failure to see a difference with the pump is not surprising.

Stubbs et al. also studied a small number of diabetic patients in good control. Use of a glucose meter 2 days a week at home did not result in blood glucose control statistically significantly better than did careful traditional management. In fairness, however, the mean diurnal blood glucose was slightly (13 mg/dl) lower in the meter group. Control was better at home than in the hospital; differences in the amount of physical activity are probably partially responsible. We are certain to read more reports that evaluate the role of the reflectance meter in the home as a means of improving blood glucose control in the pregnant patient with diabetes.] ◀

Appraisal of "Rigid" Blood Glucose Control During Pregnancy in the Overtly Diabetic Woman. Considerable importance has been attached to "rigid" control of maternal glycemia in diabetic pregnancies. Kenneth J. Leveno, John C. Hauth, Larry C. Gilstrap III, and Peggy J. Whalley[2-16] (Univ. of Texas Southwestern Med. School) assessed the degree of control achieved in the third trimester in 120 overtly diabetic women hospitalized on a high-risk pregnancy ward for class B through class F diabetes. Rigid control was defined as a mean preprandial plasma glucose concentration below 115 mg/dl. A diet of 30 to 35 calories per kg was prescribed, and oral hypoglycemic agents were discontinued. After initial hospitalization for 3 to 7 days, the patients were followed weekly, and diet and insulin adjustments were made on the basis of fasting plasma glucose values. The patients were rehospitalized at 32 to 34 weeks' gestation.

The mean preprandial glucose concentration during the final hospitalization was 150.1 mg/dl. Only 14% of patients achieved rigid blood glucose control, and mean preprandial glucose concentrations exceeded 172 mg/dl in 20% of subjects. The perinatal salvage rate exceeded 95%. No significant association was found between perinatal deaths and maternal plasma glucose values, although the 1 possibly avoidable fetal death was associated with a preprandial glucose concentration of 205 mg/dl. Neonatal morbidity also showed no association with the degree of maternal hyperglycemia. Glucose concentration control did not influence the rate of macrosomia. Malformations occurred in 11 of the 121 infants. Pregnancy-induced hypertension was associated with a mean preprandial glucose concentration exceeding 172 mg/dl.

Practical, realistically achievable glucose concentration control, liberal hospitalization, careful monitoring of pregnancy, and intensive neonatal care where necessary have resulted in a perinatal salvage

(2–16) Am. J. Obstet. Gynecol. 135:853–862, Dec. 1, 1979.

rate exceeding 95% in overtly diabetic pregnancies. Although maternal hyperglycemia exceeding a mean preprandial glucose concentration of 172 mg/dl should be avoided, rigid control appears to be unnecessary for a successful perinatal outcome.

▶ [Tight blood glucose regulation has come to be regarded as the most important aspect of care of the diabetic pregnancy. This report seems to cast doubt on its value. Terminal antepartum care of diabetics at Parkland Hospital tends to emphasize the clinical, as opposed to the biophysical (heart rate monitoring) or biochemical (estriol), aspects. What this study demonstrates is that with such an approach, a very respectable perinatal mortality (42/1,000) can be achieved. Moreover, because the blood glucose level bore no clear relation to perinatal morbidity or mortality, the "modern" emphasis on metabolic normalization may not be so important after all. However, the time of blood sampling was preprandial and it is possible, though perhaps not likely, that some patients in group I (<115 mg/dl) might have had marked hyperglycemia postprandially. In addition, important details of management are lacking. It is implied that delivery occurred around 37 weeks' gestation and by cesarean section in most patients; could a "beneficial" effect of euglycemia have been overidden by these influences?] ◀

Hemoglobin A$_{1c}$ in Normal and Diabetic Pregnancy. Hemoglobin A$_{1c}$ (HbA$_{1c}$) is a minor variant of hemoglobin A with a single glucose moiety covalently bound to the N-terminal valine of the β-chain. Levels of HbA$_{1c}$ relate directly to the blood glucose concentration in nonpregnant women and increase during pregnancy. Some have observed a correlation of HbA$_{1c}$ values with infant birth weight. Joseph M. Miller, Jr., M. Carlyle Crenshaw, Jr., and Selman I. Welt[2-17] (Duke Univ.) examined the clinical usefulness of HbA$_{1c}$ measurements to screen for the presence and degree of control of diabetes in pregnancy and to predict infant birth weight and outcome of pregnancy. Patients who had class A, B, C, or D diabetes were compared with pregnant women who had normal glucose tolerance tests and no family history of diabetes or glycosuria.

No significant difference in HbA$_{1c}$ values was found between subjects with normal and those with abnormal glucose tolerance test results. Normal pregnant women had an average third-trimester HbA$_{1c}$ level of 6.0%, compared to 6.4% for 27 class A diabetics and 6.7% for 15 insulin-dependent diabetics. The differences were not significant. Little correlation was found between third-trimester HbA$_{1c}$ values and infant birth weights. No correlation between infants large for gestational age and elevated HbA$_{1c}$ values was found. Glucose control correlated with HbA$_{1c}$ values in 11 insulin-requiring pregnant women with diabetes.

Values for HbA$_{1c}$ are correlated with gross parameters of glucose control in later pregnancy in insulin-requiring diabetics, but the values do not predict birth weight or the presence of chemical diabetes. The greatest usefulness of the HbA$_{1c}$ value may be its correlation with standard blood glucose and urine findings to evaluate metabolic control in insulin-requiring women with diabetes in pregnancy.

Glycosylated Hemoglobins in Normal Pregnancy and Gestational Diabetes Mellitus. Glycosylated hemoglobins (HbA$_1$) are minor variants of hemoglobin characterized by attachment of a carbo-

(2–17) JAMA 242:2785–2786, Dec. 21, 1979.

hydrated moiety to the *N*-terminal amino acid of the β-chain. The HbA₁ accurately reflects the degree of diabetic control in nonpregnant persons. Hossam E. Fadel, Stephen D. Hammond, Thomas A. Huff, and Rollie J. Harp[2-18] (Med. College of Georgia, Augusta) measured HbA₁ using a microcolumn technique in 23 nonpregnant women, 53 normal pregnant women, and 22 pregnant class A diabetics. The HbA₁ was determined in aliquots of fasting venous blood obtained in the course of oral glucose tolerance testing.

A significant increase in HbA₁ was found in the diabetic group. The average was 7.0% in this group, 6.1% in the nonpregnant women, and 5.8% in the normal pregnant women. Levels of HbA₁ did not correlate with maternal age, gravidity, or gestational age. No racial difference in HbA₁ was observed, and there was no difference between primigravidas and multigravidas. The HbA₁ levels did not correlate with birth weight ratios in either normal pregnancies or in the diabetic group. This probably was due to the long interval between HbA₁ determination and delivery, which averaged 9.9 weeks.

Levels of glycosylated hemoglobin in this study reflected primarily second-trimester plasma glucose levels. In class A diabetic patients, HbA₁ levels did not reflect the effects of management after abnormal oral glucose tolerance was discovered. Strict management is expected to result in normoglycemia and a reduction in birth weight. It remains to be determined whether such management will also result in a decrease in HbA₁ levels.

▶ [This article and the preceding one are considerably less enthusiastic than earlier publications (see 1979 YEAR BOOK, p. 65) about the *clinical* use of glycosylated hemoglobin measurements. In the study by Miller and associates, HbA₁c levels had no correlation with either diagnosis of diabetics or frequency of macrosomia, although there was some relation to adequacy of control in insulin-requiring diabetics. In the report of Fadel and colleagues, HbA₁ levels were also not related to birth weight ratios, which the authors think may be due to the relatively long interval between sampling and delivery. Moreover, although we previously suggested that HbA₁ levels might identify diabetics in the puerperium (1980 YEAR BOOK, p. 63) it appears that the considerable overlap between the values of normal controls and diabetics may limit the usefulness of HbA₁ as a diagnostic screen, even though differences exist between mean values for diabetics and normal controls.] ◀

Maternal Outcome in Class H Diabetes Mellitus. Class H diabetes of pregnancy is defined as diabetes of any duration and age of onset accompanied by ischemic heart disease. Only 3 of 11 women with this diagnosis have survived pregnancy. Sheryl L. Silfen, Ronald J. Wapner, and Steven G. Gabbe[2-19] (Philadelphia) describe a fourth class H diabetic woman who survived pregnancy.

Primigravida, 23, had a diagnosis of diabetes at age 13 years and had been started on insulin at age 17, but she had used insulin intermittently and failed to follow her diet. Her mother, also diabetic, died at age 51 of myocardial infarction. Examination at 12 weeks' gestation showed scattered fundic microaneurysms and hemorrhages and hypertensive changes. Blood pressure was 140/85 mm Hg. Chest pain had occurred on exertion for over 2 months, and similar episodes had occurred 10 months before. An ECG at 15 weeks showed an anteroseptal infarction of uncertain age. An echocardiogram

(2–18) Obstet. Gynecol. 54:322–326, September 1979.
(2–19) Ibid., 55:749–751, June 1980.

54 / OBSTETRICS

showed normal ventricular function, and cardiac enzyme values were normal. Chest pain did not recur after discharge. The lecithin-sphingomyelin ratio at 36 weeks' gestation was 3.5. Elective cesarean section was carried out, with delivery of a 2,690-gm girl with normal Apgar scores. The ECG was unchanged postoperatively. No insulin was necessary after delivery, despite a small wound abscess. The patient was well 7 months after delivery. She refused tubal ligation.

Myocardial infarction, a rare complication of pregnancy, has been associated with a maternal mortality of 30%. Diabetes need not be of long duration in pregnant patients who develop ischemic heart disease. Therapeutic abortion and sterilization should be considered in stable class H patients. Infarction occurring early in pregnancy should be managed conservatively, because therapeutic abortion also presents a serious risk. There is no evidence that the risk of death is increased once the patient has survived a myocardial infarction. Management of class H diabetic pregnancies must include meticulous blood sugar regulation. Adequate pain relief in labor is important. Hypotension is dangerous. Maternal risk can be reduced by constant intrapartum monitoring of ventricular filling pressures and rapid treatment of arrhythmias and heart failure.

▶ [Class H diabetes can occur in young women whose diabetes is not of long duration. The authors' suggestion that a baseline ECG be obtained in the pregnant patient with diabetes is a good one. Close attention should also be paid to symptoms that may suggest cardiac disease.] ◀

Serial Ultrasonography to Assess Evolving Fetal Macrosomia: Studies in 23 Pregnant Diabetic Women. Although large infants tend to occur more often in class A to class C diabetics than in those with longer-standing and more severe diabetes, fetal macrosomia is not predictable. Its early intrauterine diagnosis would be helpful because of associations with various perinatal risks, as birth trauma, asphyxia, or delivery by cesarean section. Edward S. Ogata, Rudy Sabbagha, Boyd E. Metzger, Richard L. Phelps, Richard Depp, and Norbert Freinkel[2-20] (Northwestern Univ.) attempted to detect evolving diabetic macrosomia by serial ultrasonographic assessments of biparietal diameter (BPD) and abdominal circumference. Prospective studies were done in 23 class A to class C diabetic women from 20 weeks' gestation onward. Each patient was examined at least three times in the latter half of pregnancy.

All women were delivered of term infants that were well neonatally. Values of BPD were within the normal range for fetuses of nondiabetic women at all stages. Only 13 fetuses had normal abdominal circumference values; 10 had values more than 2 SD above the normal mean for nondiabetics at 28 to 32 weeks' gestation. These infants weighed more than the others at birth and had significantly more subcutaneous fat, as estimated by skin-fold measurements. Their body lengths and head circumferences also tended to be increased, but the differences were not significant at the 5% level. Insulin concentrations in amniotic fluid at 34 to 36 weeks' gestation were significantly greater in fetuses with accelerated somatic growth than in the

(2-20) JAMA 243:2405-2408, June 20, 1980.

others (28.5 vs. 13.9 μU/ml, respectively). Glucose levels in amniotic fluid did not differ significantly.

Ultrasound may identify disparate rates of growth in different fetal structures during late gestation and may prove useful for detecting macrosomia in utero. Abnormalities can be detected as early as 28 weeks' gestation, and serial differential ultrasonography may aid the evaluation of attempts to arrest evolving macrosomia by tighter regulation of maternal diabetes.

▶ [In this study, fetal head growth in cases of maternal diabetes remained normal up to at least 38 weeks' gestation whereas abdominal circumference began to grow excessively in the early third trimester in approximately half of the cases. Moreover, large abdomens correlated with high amniotic fluid insulin levels and increased subcutaneous fat. These findings are predictable, because head size reflects brain growth, which should not be influenced by insulin levels, whereas girth reflects the size of the liver and subcutaneous tissues, which should grow more with hyperinsulinism. From a clinical viewpoint, this approach holds promise of providing a means of identifying macrosomia early enough for one to intervene with tighter metabolic control or at least to become alert to the dangers of birth trauma.] ◀

Infant of the Diabetic Mother: Correlation of Increased Cord C-Peptide Levels With Macrosomia and Hypoglycemia. Macrosomia, postnatal hypoglycemia, and hyaline membrane disease are major complications occurring in infants of diabetic mothers and may be related to a fetal hyperinsulinemic state. The measurement of serum C-peptide levels in infants by radioimmunoassay is confounded by the presence of cross-reacting fetal proinsulin, which is bound to maternal insulin antibodies. Ilene R. Sosenko, John L. Kitzmiller, Sherry W. Loo, Petra Blix, Arthur H. Rubenstein and Kenneth H. Gabbay[2-21] have used an assay for C-peptide that eliminates interference by antibody-bound proinsulin. Studied were 79 infants of diabetic mothers and 62 infants of nondiabetic mothers. Only 5% of the diabetic mothers did not require insulin during pregnancy. Serum C-peptide was measured by radioimmunoassay in umbilical cord blood

RELATION OF CORD SERUM C-PEPTIDE LEVELS TO HYPOGLYCEMIA AND MACROSOMIA IN INFANTS OF DIABETIC MOTHERS

FEATURE	NO. OF INFANTS	MEAN C PEPTIDE	P VALUE
		$ng/ml \pm SEM$	
No hypoglycemia	35	3.91±0.69	<0.025
Hypoglycemia*	37	7.37±1.23	
No macrosomia	43	4.18±0.60	<0.05
Macrosomia†	31	7.51±1.46	
Hypoglycemia only	16	4.13±0.74	<0.01
Hypoglycemia and macrosomia	21	9.84±1.95	
			<0.001
Macrosomia only	10	2.61±0.55	

*Serum glucose <30 mg/dl (<1.7 mmol/L) in first 6 hours of life.
†Birth weight >90th percentile for gestational age.

(2–21) N. Engl. J. Med. 301:859–862, Oct. 18, 1979.

after precipitation of the antibody-proinsulin complex with polyethylene glycol.

Diabetic mothers had significantly lower serum C-peptide levels than control mothers at the time of delivery, whereas their infants had significantly higher cord serum levels than did control infants. Cord glucose levels were similar. Cord C-peptide levels increased with increasing severity of maternal diabetes. Study infants had significantly elevated C-peptide levels before 34 weeks' gestational age, and no further increase was apparent. Levels are related to postnatal hypoglycemia and macrosomia (table). A significant relationship with both occurrences was apparent, but no significant relationship was found for hyaline membrane disease.

Increased cord C-peptide levels are associated with more severe maternal diabetes and with the occurrence of macrosomia and hypoglycemia in the neonatal period. A more aggressive approach to producing physiologic blood glucose levels in diabetic pregnant women may prevent some complications found in their infants.

▶ [Measuring C-peptide in cord blood obviates the problem, caused by maternal anti-insulin antibodies, inherent in trying to measure cord blood insulin levels directly. These results are generally what one would predict and are consistent with the Pedersen hypothesis (maternal hyperglycemia → fetal hyperglycemia → fetal hyperinsulinemia → macrosomia and neonatal hypoglycemia).] ◀

▶ ↓ The following article considers amniotic fluid C-peptide levels. Read on. ◀

Amniotic Fluid C-Peptide in Normal and Insulin-Dependent Diabetic Pregnancies. Plasma C-peptide measurements are now used to assess islet secretion despite the presence of circulating insulin antibodies. G. Tchobroutsky, I. Heard, C. Tchobroutsky, and E. Eschwege[2-22] examined possible relations between concentrations of glucose, insulin, and C-peptide in amniotic fluid and certain clinical variables in 28 normal and 46 insulin-dependent diabetic pregnant women. The diabetics had received insulin therapy for a mean of 7.5 years. Amniocenteses were done to estimate fetal pulmonary maturity before elective cesarean section or in women with incomplete anti-D antibodies.

Insulin-binding antibody was detected in only one sample from a diabetic pregnancy. Amniotic fluid glucose, insulin and C-peptide concentrations were higher in diabetics than in controls. The difference was barely significant for C-peptide. Correlation between the insulin and the C-peptide concentrations was greater in normal subjects than in the diabetics. Birth weight correlated positively with C-peptide concentrations in diabetics, but glucose and insulin concentrations in amniotic fluid did not correlate with birth weight. None of the variables was related to an immature or mature lecithin-sphingomyelin ratio.

Amniotic fluid insulin and C-peptide concentrations correlate closely in non-insulin-treated diabetic women, and the cheaper commercial kits for insulin may be preferable. In insulin-treated diabetics, however, amniotic fluid C-peptide radioimmunoassay is more re-

---

(2–22) Diabetologia 18:289–292, April 1980.

liable than the insulin radioimmunoassay. The findings do not support the suggestion that high insulin concentrations may inhibit pulmonary surfactant synthesis and contribute to respiratory distress syndrome in infants of diabetic mothers.

▶ [In this study, amniotic fluid insulin levels in diabetics did not correlate significantly with birth weight either independently or in relation to gestational age but C-peptide concentrations did, presumably reflecting urinary secretion.] ◀

Echocardiographic Abnormalities in Infants of Diabetic Mothers. Increased cardiac weight and myocardial hypertrophy have been found in live-born infants of diabetic mothers (IDM), and some infants have congestive heart failure and a peculiar form of subaortic stenosis resembling the idiopathic hypertrophic subaortic stenosis seen in adults. Sharon Mace, Stephen S. Hirschfeld, Thomas Riggs, Avroy A. Fanaroff, and Irwin R. Merkatz[2-23] (Cleveland), with the technical assistance of Wendy Franklin, undertook a prospective echocardiographic study of 34 consecutive infants born to mothers with overt diabetes mellitus or gestational diabetes. Forty-three control infants also were evaluated. Sixteen study infants were preterm. Mean gestational age was 38 weeks. Twenty-three infants were considered large for gestational age. Twelve control infants were preterm, and 15 were large for gestational age.

Infants of diabetic mothers had thickening of the cardiac walls, most markedly in the interventricular septum, which was greater than expected from their birth weights. The septum was thickest in infants in congestive heart failure, and left ventricular contractility was increased in this group. A disproportionate septal thickening was reflected by an interventricular septum–left ventricle wall ratio of greater than 2.0. Changes were less marked in infants in respiratory distress. The major abnormality in asymptomatic infants was a thickened interventricular septum. In several IDMs the ratio of right ventricular preejection period to right ventricular ejection time was greater than normal for age.

Infants presenting with heart failure had the most marked myocardial hypertrophy in this series. Four of 7 had evidence of obstruction to left ventricular outflow. Cardiac hypertrophy usually was of little consequence in IDM with respiratory distress and those with no clinical symptoms. It is not clear how poor maternal diabetic control can result in myocardial hypertrophy in the fetus. Any IDM with heart failure should have echocardiography to diagnose left ventricular outflow obstruction, since digitalis therapy is contraindicated. Rigid control of maternal diabetes appears to reduce the incidence of myocardial abnormalities in these infants.

▶ [This interesting report notes an increased frequency of cardiac hypertrophy, involving the left and right ventricular walls as well as the interventricular septum, among infants born to diabetic women. An apparent association with poor maternal diabetic control suggests that the finding may reflect excessive myocardial glycogen deposition from fetal hyperglycemia-hyperinsulinism. However, a substantial proportion (6 of 34) of the infants had echocardiographic indications of subaortic stenosis, so at least the left ventricular changes, and possibly the septal changes, could be secondary to

(2–23) J. Pediatr. 95:1013–1019, December 1979.

mechanical outflow obstruction. The authors emphasize that echocardiographic studies are vital in those infants with cardiac failure because digitalis is contraindicated in
the presence of outflow obstruction since it aggravates the condition by enhancing
myocardial contractility; propranolol is the treatment of choice.

In a related study, Gutgesell and associates (Circulation 61:441, 1980) also found a
high incidence of hypertrophic cardiomyopathy (left ventricular outflow obstruction,
right ventricular wall thickness, and interventricular septal hypertrophy) among infants
of diabetic mothers, which the authors speculated was a manifestation of generalized
organomegaly.] ◄

**Prevention of Chronic HBsAg Carrier State in Infants of
HBsAg-Positive Mothers by Hepatitis B Immunoglobulin.**
Transmission of hepatitis B virus from mother to infant has occurred
when the mother was a chronic hepatitis B surface antigen (HBsAg)
carrier or had acute hepatitis B during pregnancy, especially in the
third trimester. Henk W. Reesink, Eveline E. Reerink-Brongers, Bep
J. Th. Lafeber-Schut, Jo Kalshoven-Benschop, and Henk G. J. Brum-
melhuis[2-24] (Amsterdam) attempted to determine whether hepatitis B
immunoglobulin, given monthly to newborn infants of HBsAg-positive mothers, can prevent these infants from acquiring neonatal hepatitis B or becoming chronic HBsAg carriers. Of 44 children of 40
chronic carriers who were followed up prospectively, 21 received 0.5
ml/kg of hepatitis B immunoglobulin within 48 hours after birth, and
then 0.16 ml/kg every month for 6 months.

After follow-up for 6 to 9 months, 5 of 20 untreated children and
none of 21 treated children were HBsAg positive, a significant difference. Four of 6 untreated children with mothers who were positive
for e antigen (HBeAg) became HBsAg positive, as did 1 of 11 with
anti-HBe-positive mothers. None of 16 treated children who were followed up for 9 to 36 months were found to have HBsAg. The mothers
of 5 of these children were HBeAg positive, and 4 of these children
had anti-HBs. Two of 3 children whose hepatitis B immunoglobulin
treatment began 4 to 5 days after birth became HBsAg positive. Five
children became chronic HBsAg carriers.

Treatment of infants of HBsAg-positive mothers with hepatitis B
immunoglobulin within 48 hours after birth and then monthly for 6
months can prevent a chronic HBsAg carrier state. It is unlikely that
transplacental infection with hepatitis B virus occurs in children of
HBsAg-positive mothers. All infants of HBeAg-positive carriers, as
well as infants born to women who have had acute hepatitis B in the
third trimester of pregnancy, should receive hepatitis B immunoglobulin injections. All pregnant women should be studied for the presence of serum HBsAg; if the test is positive, these women should also
be tested for HBeAg and anti-HBe.

► [Babies delivered of mothers with acute hepatitis B infection in pregnancy should
receive hepatitis B immune globulin (HBIg). This report suggests that monthly injections should be given for 6 months and that the first injection should be given within
48 hours. Two of 3 children not treated until the 4th or 5th day became HbeAg positive.
The importance of HBeAg as a risk factor for vertical transmission is again illustrated
(cf. 1979 YEAR BOOK, p. 196). The authors suggest routine antepartum screening for
HbsAg and administration of HBIg to the offspring of positive women. More informa-

(2–24) Lancet 2:436–438, Sept. 1, 1979.

tion is needed concerning the prevalence of HBeAg and the risk of vertical transmission in various populations before this suggestion is generally applied.] ◄

Chronic Persistent Hepatitis and Pregnancy. Chronic persistent hepatitis (CPH) and chronic active hepatitis are among the most common forms of chronic hepatitis in young women. Donald S. Infled, Harold I. Borkowf, and Rajiv R. Varma[2-25] (Med. College of Wisconsin) reviewed experience with seven women having ten pregnancies during the course of CPH. They had no other major systemic disease and were followed up for at least 2 years during 1972–1978. The duration of CPH ranged from 3 to 8 years. The diagnosis was made from the liver biopsy findings or elevation of the serum aminotransferases for at least 2 years. The patients had mild to moderate fatigue, reduced exercise tolerance and vague abdominal complaints. None had cutaneous signs of chronic liver disease.

Four fetuses were aborted for nonmedical reasons. Six women had normal full-term vaginal deliveries. Pregnancy had no apparent effect on the liver disease in any patient. Serum aspartate transaminase levels did not change significantly. No patient progressed to chronic active hepatitis or cirrhosis. The course of the pregnancies also was unremarkable. There were no obstetric complications. The neonates were healthy and developmentally normal. All the patients when not pregnant had maintained regular menses after the diagnosis of liver disease.

Pregnancy in CPH appears to be safe for both the mother and fetus. Careful observation of these patients remains necessary, since the natural history of CPH is not fully known. Cirrhosis and portal hypertension are significant factors associated with maternal and fetal complications, and the course of CPH may not always be benign.

► [Chronic active hepatitis (CAH) and cirrhosis in pregnancy are both associated with adverse maternal and perinatal outcome. The prognosis is apparently better with chronic persistent hepatitis (CPH). Chronic persistent hepatitis is distinguished from CAH on the basis of the histology of the liver biopsy. When a patient with previous hepatitis and persistently elevated transaminase levels is contemplating pregnancy, the distinction between CAH and CPH would seem to be important.] ◄

Diagnostic Evaluation of Syphilis During Pregnancy. James E. Jones, Jr., and Robert E. Harris[2-26] (Lackland Air Force Base, Texas) prospectively studied the incidence and significance of neurosyphilis in pregnant patients seen in a 5-year period. Most were well nourished, cooperative, young (average age, 23 years), white, and of low parity. All were screened with a Venereal Disease Research Laboratories (VDRL) test at the initial obstetric visit and, when possible, at 36 weeks' gestation as well. Those with a positive VDRL test and a positive fluorescent treponemal antibody absorption (FTA-ABS) test were evaluated for asymptomatic neurosyphilis by cerebrospinal fluid FTA-ABS testing. Initially, the undiluted cerebrospinal fluid was screened; if reactivity was detected, the fluid was diluted in sorbent to extract nonspecific reactive antibodies other than pallidum to treponema.

(2–25) Gastroenterology 77:524–527, September 1979.
(2–26) Obstet. Gynecol. 54:611–614, November 1979.

SEROLOGIC EVALUATIONS FOR 8,343 PATIENTS
WHO DELIVERED

	Total tested	No. positive
Serum		
VDRL	8343	28
FTA-ABS	28	21*
CSF		
VDRL and FTA-ABS	16†	3

VDRL, Venereal Disease Research Laboratories; *FTA-ABS,* fluorescent treponemal antibody absorption; *CSF,* cerebrospinal fluid.
*One patient had documented systemic lupus erythematosus, and tests were biologically false positive.
†Only untreated patients with positive FTA-ABS.

Of the 8,343 women screened, 20 (0.24%) had positive VDRL and FTA-ABS tests. All 20 were asymptomatic. Of the 16 patients who were untreated prior to cerebrospinal fluid analysis, 3 (19%) had positive FTA-ABS tests (table).

Of the 20 patients with serologic evidence of syphilis, 2 delivered elsewhere. Birth weight of the remaining 18 infants ranged from 2,895 gm to 3,912 gm; gestational age ranged from 35 to 42 weeks. No infant had physical signs of congenital syphilis, but 1 with elevated IgM-specific FTA-ABS in serum and cerebrospinal fluid had respiratory distress and radiographic evidence of congenital syphilitic pneumonia. Nine of the 18 neonates had positive VDRL tests; 6 of the 9 had positive FTA-ABS tests, and 3 of the 6 also had positive cerebrospinal fluid serology. One of these 3 was born to a mother with no evidence of neurosyphilis, but the other 2 were born to mothers with positive cerebrospinal fluid serology. Two with positive FTA-ABS tests had elevated values of serum and cerebrospinal fluid IgM-specific FTA-ABS.

Although only 0.24% of these pregnant women had syphilis, 19% of untreated and asymptomatic patients with serologic evidence of syphilis had tertiary disease and, despite maternal therapy, 11% of infants born to mothers with syphilis had reactive serum and cerebrospinal fluid involvement. Thus, serologic examination of the cerebrospinal fluid should be included in the evaluation of all pregnant women with positive serum VDRL and FTA-ABS tests. Pregnant patients with syphilis should be treated with penicillin and undergo monthly quantitative serologic testing. Those who show a rise in titer of four dilutions should be retreated.

▶ [The fact that 3 of 16 cerebrospinal fluids tested were positive underscores the need for cerebrospinal fluid testing in pregnant patients with newly diagnosed syphilis. We were surprised by this 19% rate of asymptomatic neurosyphilis. Details as to when in pregnancy these patients were treated are lacking, but some of the neonates had IgM antibody, suggesting in utero infection rather than transfer of maternal antibody. One penicillin-allergic patient treated with cephaloridine delivered a baby with congenital syphilitic pneumonia and central nervous system involvement. The policy on our service is to obtain a VDRL on the first antepartum visit and again at 36 weeks' gestation.] ◀

Prospective Study of Primary Cytomegalovirus Infection in Pregnant Women. P. D. Griffiths, A. Campbell-Benzie, and R. B. Heath[2-27] (St. Bartholomew's Hosp., London) examined serum from 5,575 women, who had antepartum care from 1975 to 1979, to obtain further information on primary maternal cytomegalovirus (CMV) infection and its effects on the fetus. Serum specimens were screened at a dilution of 1:8 for complement-fixing CMV antibodies. The virus was isolated from urine specimens with use of human embryo lung cell cultures.

The overall rate of seropositivity for CMV was 57.2% in this series. Seropositivity increased with age. Of 1,608 seronegative women, 14 (0.87%) had primary infection during pregnancy. Only 1 had symptoms attributable to CMV infection. Eight primary infections could have occurred in either the second or the third trimester; only 3 were localized to the second and 3 to the third trimester. Virus was cultured from the urine of 3 of 9 infants. In 2 cord serum specimens, CMV-specific IgM antibody was detected. Congenital infection was documented in 3 of 12 infants. All 14 infants born to mothers with primary CMV infection appeared to be normal at birth. One has developed a hearing defect and another has become microcephalic. Twelve women had primary rubella during the study, 7 during a large epidemic. Seven cases of rubella infection were suspected clinically. Only 1 of 7 cord serum specimens contained specific IgM antibody. All 10 infants appeared to be normal at birth, with no signs of congenital rubella infection.

Cytomegalovirus infection was as frequent as rubella infection in this series. Apart from those years in which extensive epidemics of rubella occur, many more pregnant women are infected with CMV than with rubella virus. The ability of CMV to cross the placenta in successive pregnancies casts theoretical doubt on the potential efficacy of the prototype vaccines currently being evaluated. Much more needs to be learned of the natural history of congenital CMV infection before attempts at intervention by vaccination or termination of pregnancy can be considered.

▶ [This report serves to remind us that primary CMV infection in the pregnant woman is usually asymptomatic and that an apparently normal neonate delivered of such a patient may later manifest neurologic impairment. About half of the patients in the study population lacked antibody to CMV. Approximately 1% of these women acquired infection during pregnancy and 25% of their infants had evidence of congenital infection. Certain surveys in the United States have shown a higher prevalence of congenital infection. Although CMV infection in pregnancy can cause problems, there are no easy obstetric solutions. A vaccine is not available and the fact that CMV can cross the placenta in successive pregnancies casts doubt as to its ultimate value. The natural history of antepartum CMV infection has not been sufficiently well defined to permit the practitioner to easily answer the questions patients have.] ◀

False Positive Amniotic Fluid Cytology in Parturient With Active Genital Herpes Infection at Term. Herpesvirus hominis (HVH) infection of the newborn is a serious, often fatal disease refractory to known therapeutic measures. The major source of exposure is delivery through an infected genital tract. Elective cesarean

(2–27) Br. J. Obstet. Gynaecol. 87:308–314, April 1980.

section is recommended as a prophylactic measure in patients with evidence of active infection at term. Transplacental spread of virus has been demonstrated in animals. Most laboratories require two to 11 days to confirm HVH infection, but cytologic screening of stained amniotic fluid smears can be done in a few hours.

Barry S. B. Block and David M. Goodner[2-28] (Temple Univ.) report a case in which, despite the presence of typical cellular herpetic changes, viral culture was negative, invalidating the cytologic findings as presumptive evidence of HVH infection.

Woman, 29, in her third pregnancy, had had two unexplained second-trimester spontaneous losses without antecedent premature labor. Findings of cervical incompetence were noted at 14 weeks' gestation, when a Shirodkar operation was performed. Vesicular vulvar lesions were confirmed as herpetic at 37 weeks. Amniocentesis was performed at 38 weeks' gestation. The fetal epithelial cells exhibited cytopathologic changes typical of herpetic infection, but viral culture was reported as negative a week later. A 3,240-gm infant was delivered by elective cesarean section 2 days before the estimated date of confinement. The mother and infant were strictly isolated for 10 days. Multiple viral cultures of amniotic fluid and the infant's urine, throat and cerebrospinal fluid were negative. The infant was well at age 3 months.

It appears that viral isolation by culture or immunofluorescence from the amniotic fluid is necessary before vaginal delivery is selected over prophylactic cesarean section. Any pregnant patient who presents with HVH infection should be followed by viral isolation methods. Vaginal delivery is recommended at term if the virus has not been isolated for 4 to 6 weeks. If evidence of infection persists at 37 weeks' gestation, amniocentesis should be performed and cesarean section delivery considered until viral isolation from the fluid is completed, regardless of the cytologic findings.

▶ [This case report makes a good point. Cytologic changes typical of herpetic infection were found in the amniotic fluid specimen, yet multiple viral cultures of both amniotic fluid and baby were negative. Therefore, the authors suggest that one should not regard a positive amniotic fluid cytology report as the final word. These patients should not be denied cesarean section when it is appropriate, unless the amniotic fluid viral culture also indicates that the fetus is already infected. Possible explanations for the misleading cytologic findings are not provided.] ◀

▶ ↓ That amniotic fluid infection does not necessarily mean fetal infection is indicated by the following article. Read on. ◀

Herpes Simplex in Amniotic Fluid of Unaffected Fetus. Neonatal herpesvirus infection is associated with a high morbidity and mortality. The infection may be transmitted through placental transfer from the cervix after membrane rupture or by contact with an infected birth canal during delivery. Ioannis A. Zervoudakis, Frederick Siverman, Lawrence B. Senterfit, Michael J. Strongin, Stanley Read, and Lars L. Cederqvist[2-29] (New York Hosp.-Cornell Med. Center) report the findings in a healthy infant born to a mother with a 7-year history of herpes progenitalis. The infant was apparently unaffected despite viral isolation from the amniotic fluid on the day of delivery.

(2–28) Obstet. Gynecol. 54:658–660, November 1979.
(2–29) Ibid., 55(Suppl.):16S–17S, March 1980.

Woman, aged 32, had herpes simplex virus isolated from the cervix at 31 weeks' gestation in her first pregnancy. At 40 weeks, a healthy infant was delivered by cesarean section. During the second pregnancy, herpes simplex was isolated from the endocervix at 36 and 37 weeks of gestation. When amniocentesis was performed at 39 weeks for assessment of fetal lung maturity, herpes simplex was isolated from the amniotic fluid specimen. A female infant was delivered by cesarean section on the same day; the child had no clinical evidence of infection at birth or during the following 18 months. Immunoglobulin concentrations in the cord serum and amniotic fluid did not indicate intrauterine infection.

This case illustrates that the presence of herpes simplex virus in the amniotic fluid does not necessarily indicate overt fetal infection. Maternal antibodies to the virus may have been transferred to the fetus transplacentally as IgG. Similar titers of antibodies against herpes simplex were found in the maternal serum and cord blood. The maternal antibodies may have protected the fetus from infection.

▶ [It has previously been suggested that if herpesvirus is cultured from the amniotic fluid the fetus is already infected and nothing is to be gained by cesarean section. "It ain't necessarily so" according to this case report. The authors suggest that the fetus may have been protected by maternal antibody transferred through the placenta. The virus probably gained access to the amniotic fluid from the cervix through intact membranes. How often the fetus is spared overt infection in the face of infected amniotic fluid is unknown, but, as was demonstrated here, it can occur. Whether cesarean section provides any "protection" in these cases is a separate matter (ie, it may be that further exposure to the virus in the birth canal over that already received in utero does not increase the chance of infection). Growth of the virus from the amniotic fluid probably means that cesarean section is not required, but it does not necessarily mean that the neonate will suffer from overt congenital herpesvirus infection.] ◀

Failure of Penicillin to Eradicate Group B Streptococcal Colonization in the Pregnant Woman: Couple Study. Susan E. Gardner, Martha D. Yow, Leroy J. Leeds, Peter K. Thompson, Edward O. Mason, Jr., and Dorothy J. Clark[2-30] (Baylor College of Medicine) evaluated oral penicillin prophylaxis for eradication of group B streptococci (GBS) from the parturient in a series of 327 married women from a private obstetric practice who had rectal and vaginal cultures taken in the third trimester of pregnancy. Of these, 21% were culture positive at one or both sites. Forty couples comprised the study population, and 19 control women from the same practice were matched with the study subjects for age, marital status, and socioeconomic status. Study subjects, including the spouses, received penicillin or

COMPARISON OF GBS CULTURE RESULTS IN PENICILLIN-TREATED AND UNTREATED PREGNANT WOMEN

	Treated women	*Nontreated women*
Number enrolled third trimester	40	19
Number positive (percentage), time of delivery	27 (67%)	12 (63%)

(2–30) Am. J. Obstet. Gynecol. 135:1062–1065, Dec. 15, 1979.

erythromycin orally in a dosage of 250 mg daily for 12 to 14 days. Cultures were repeated 3 weeks after completion of therapy.

All women and 63% of their spouses were colonized at the outset. On follow-up, 70% of study women were still colonized in one or both sites. Serotype concordance was shown in all cases but 1. Of the 37 men in whom cultures were repeated, 40% were still colonized with GBS. Two thirds of study women were colonized at delivery, all but 2 with the original serotype. Over half the 27 men evaluated were colonized. Four of 29 women who were colonized after completion of therapy spontaneously became culture negative by the time of delivery. The findings are summarized in the table.

Oral penicillin therapy did not significantly alter the GBS colonization status of pregnant women at delivery in this study. Possibly another antibiotic with a different mode of action might be more effective. Intrapartum antibiotic therapy of the mother holds more promise as a reliable means of interrupting GBS transmission.

▶ [Group B streptococcal infection is an unusual but very serious neonatal problem, and the concept of eradication of the maternal carrier state has theoretical appeal. Unfortunately, in this case the theory is not borne out in practice, as indicated in several studies, of which this is the most recent. Simultaneous penicillin treatment of both husband and wife was generally ineffective, for about two thirds of culture-positive women still had colonization of streptococci 3 weeks after treatment and again at delivery.] ◀

Group B Streptococcal Colonization of Pregnant Women and Their Neonates: Epidemiologic Study and Controlled Trial of Prophylactic Treatment of the Newborn. Early-onset group B streptococcal (GBS) infection is an important cause of neonatal mortality, and contamination of the neonate is secondary to the presence of GBS in the maternal genital tract. Previous trials aimed at preventing infection in the newborn by eradicating GBS from the mother have given inconclusive results. P. Gerard, M. Verghote-D'Hulst, A. Bachy, and G. Duhaut[2-31] (Charleroi, Belgium) evaluated immediate antimicrobial therapy in newborn infants of GBS-positive mothers after encountering 2 cases of neonatal GBS sepsis, 1 fatal. Bacteriologic samples were obtained from infants of known GBS-positive mothers immediately after birth. A controlled study was carried out of penicillin G therapy given in intramuscular doses of 50,000 to 100,000 units per kg daily for the first week after delivery.

Of 1,115 women who had vaginal cultures in the last trimester, 6.8% carried GBS in their genital tracts. The rate of colonization was greater in primigravidas. Of 68 infants of GBS-positive mothers studied, 43% had at least one site that yielded GBS when samples were taken from the external auditory canal, gastric aspirate, and fetal side of the placenta. Preterm delivery and low birth weight tended to be more frequent in infants of GBS-positive mothers. Twenty-nine of 67 infants were treated immediately; 13 were later found to be colonized by GBS. All were free from infectious symptoms. Sixteen of 38 infants treated later were contaminated; they were usually treated at ages 24 to 48 hours. None of these had signs of GBS infection. No

(2–31) Acta Paediatr. Scand. 68:819–823, November 1979.

systemic GBS disease occurred during the study. No side effects of antibiotic therapy were observed.

Immediate treatment of infants of GBS-positive mothers with penicillin appears to have no definite advantage over delayed therapy. It appears to be useful to screen pregnant women for GBS and to consider their infants at high risk if abnormal perinatal events, such as prematurity or prolonged membrane rupture, occur.

▶ [The number of babies colonized by GBS in this study (29) was too small to assess the value of early penicillin treatment. Only about 2% of colonized babies develop early-onset invasive disease. What to do about the group B streptococci problem is not at all clear (1980 YEAR BOOK, pp. 222–223). Another avenue is explored in the following two articles.] ◀

Natural History of Group B Streptococcal Colonization in the Pregnant Woman and Her Offspring: II. Determination of Serum Antibody to Capsular Polysaccharide From Type III, Group B *Streptococcus*. Extremely low concentrations of antibody to capsular polysaccharide of type III, group B *Streptococcus* in the serum of pregnant women have been significantly related to invasive disease due to this organism in the offspring. Carol J. Baker, Bette J. Webb, Dennis L. Kasper, Martha D. Yow, and Craig W. Beachler[2-32] made serial observations on serum from 93 pregnant women and on cord serum from their infants. Antibody against capsular polysaccharide from type III, group B *Streptococcus* was determined by a radioactive antigen-binding assay.

No significant difference in antibody concentrations was found during gestation in 25 patients providing serum from early pregnancy and within a month of delivery or post partum. The median serum concentration in 70 noncolonized women was 0.65 µg/ml, compared with 5.53 µg/ml for 12 patients who were colonized with type III, group B streptococci. Nine women colonized by other types or strains of group B streptococci had a median antibody concentration of 0.55 µg/ml. A significant correlation was found between antibody concentrations in maternal-cord pairs of serum specimens.

Antibody detected in the serum of these pregnant women was primarily of the IgG class. The reasons for the presence of high antibody concentrations in some women are unclear. Further study is needed of the mechanism by which genital colonization with type III or possibly other serotypes of group B streptococci is related to high serum concentrations of antibody to the capsular antigens of these bacteria.

▶ [The major problem in understanding the pathophysiology of group B streptococcal infection is the wide discrepancy between vaginal carriage rates (as high as 10% or 20% in some series) and the attack rates, which could conceivably reflect variation in maternal antibody response. This study of antibody levels to the capsular polysaccharide of the organism indicates that maternal levels are unaffected by pregnancy. Thus, if antibody studies should prove to be useful in identifying an "at-risk" group (ie, high titers indicate protection, and low titers indicate risk), studies in early gestation should have validity later. Moreover, maternal and cord levels were found to correlate significantly ($r = 0.71$), implying placental transfer of the antibody.] ◀

▶ ↓ The following article suggests that maternal antibody levels do not provide the entire answer. ◀

(2–32) Am. J. Obstet. Gynecol. 137:39–42, May 1, 1980.

Prevalence of Type-Specific Group B Streptococcal Antibody in Pregnant Women. Immunity to group B streptococci (GBS) appears to be mediated by antibody-dependent phagocytosis, and low levels of maternal serum antibody are associated with susceptibility to GBS infection in the newborn infant. An indirect immunofluorescent antibody test for type-specific IgG antibody against the five serotypes of GBS has recently been developed. Lawrence C. Vogel, Kenneth M. Boyer, Cecile A. Gadzala, and Samuel P. Gotoff[2-33] (Michael Reese Hosp.) measured IgG antibody against the four major serotypes of GBS by indirect immunofluorescence in the serum of 200 consecutive pregnant women seen at an urban teaching hospital. The subjects were predominantly black and of lower socioeconomic status. Mean age was 22 years, and mean number of previous pregnancies was 2.7. Studies also were done in 108 women colonized with GBS and in 54 mothers of neonates with invasive GBS infection.

Antibody against types Ia, Ib, II, and III was found in serum from 53, 103, 164, and 89 of the 200 consecutive subjects, respectively. Only 19 subjects had antibody against all four GBS types. Colonized and noncolonized women differed significantly in antibody prevalence only when type Ia was present. Neither of the mothers of infants with type Ia infection had antibody to Ia in undiluted serum. Eight of 40 serum specimens from mothers of infants with GBS type III infection contained detectable type-specific antibody; this was significantly less than the prevalence of antibody in noncolonized women. Titers of antibody protective of chick embryos against lethal challenge with GBS were strikingly low in all groups of women.

Susceptibility to GBS infection appears to be common to most newborn infants. The absence of humoral immunity cannot explain the wide discrepancy between the rates of asymptomatic colonization and of invasive neonatal infection. Other host and microbial factors must be important in the pathogenesis of neonatal GBS sepsis.

▶ [Some have suggested that the low incidence of early-onset invasive GBS infection in the face of neonatal colonization (approximately 2%) may be due to passively acquired maternal antibody against group B streptococci protecting the newborn. This report suggests otherwise. Only 9% of pregnant women had antibody against all four GBS types. Furthermore, in the authors' test system, fewer than 10% of women had antibody levels that were considered "protective" against any of the types. The disparity between neonatal colonization and infection rates cannot, therefore, be accounted for by the maternal antibody status.] ◀

(2–33) J. Pediatr. 96:1047–1051, June 1980.

3. Obstetric Complications

Delivery at 40 Years of Age and Over. E. Caspi and Y. Lif-shitz[3-1] reviewed the outcome of 494 deliveries during 1965–1974 in women aged 40 and older. Most were grand multiparas. A control group of 298 grand multiparas under age 40 was randomly selected. Deliveries in women aged 40 and older constituted 1.7% of all deliveries in 1965–1974. The incidence of deliveries in this age group declined from 2.1% in 1965 to 1.2% in 1974.

Hypertensive disorders and diabetes were more frequent in the study group than in both the control group and the general obstetric population under age 40. Placenta previa, uterine inertia, ruptured uterus, retained placenta, and early postpartum hemorrhage also were more frequent in the study group. There were no maternal deaths. The cesarean section rate was 9.7%, compared with 3.7% in the grand multipara control group and 4% in the general population. The high cesarean section rate in the study group was related to age rather than multiparity. The rate for primiparas over age 40 was 53.8%. The incidence of low birth weight infants was 7%, compared with 3.3% in the control group. Low 1-minute Apgar scores were $1^{1}/_{2}$-fold more frequent in the study group than in the control group and fivefold more frequent than in the general obstetric population. Perinatal mortality at over 28 weeks' gestation was nearly $2^{1}/_{2}$-fold higher than in the control group and threefold higher than in the general population. Congenital malformations occurred in 4.5% of study infants and in 2.3% of control infants. Down's syndrome was found in 1.4% of study infants.

The major causes of increased perinatal mortality in this over-40 age group were hypertensive disorders of pregnancy, congenital malformations, and respiratory distress syndrome associated with prematurity. Maternal and fetal complications may be reduced by earlier and more intensive prenatal care, modern obstetric monitoring during labor, ultrasound diagnostic methods, the more liberal use of cesarean section, and neonatal intensive care.

▶ [Though this paper contains nothing new or startling about the elderly gravida, it does confirm what has been shown in earlier studies—increased frequency of hypertensive disease, diabetes, labor problems, antepartum and postpartum bleeding, and congenital malformations. The decline in perinatal mortality over the 10-year period of review—10.4% in the first year to 0% in the last—is impressive. The authors attribute it to "important advances in obstetrics and perinatology" during the period. No comment is made as to the frequency of prenatal genetic studies in Israel in 1965–1974, but amniocentesis could also be responsible for the drop in perinatal mortality, as well as for a decreasing incidence of deliveries to older women.] ◄

Perinatal Mortality by Birth Order Within Cohorts Based on Sibship Size was analyzed by Leiv S. Bakketeig (Univ. of Trond-

(3–1) Isr. J. Med. Sci. 15:418–421, May 1979.

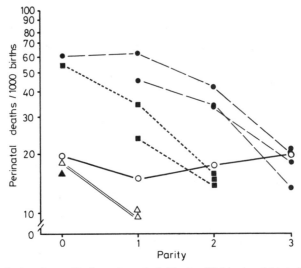

Fig 3–1.—Perinatal mortality by parity and sibship size. Sibship size of 4 is indicated by solid circles; of 3, by solid squares; of 2, by open triangles; of 1, by solid triangle; and all four sibship sizes combined, by open circles. (Courtesy of Bakketeig, L. S., and Hoffman, H. J.: Br. Med. J. 2:693–696, Sept. 22, 1979.)

heim) and Howard J. Hoffman[3-2] (Natl. Inst. of Health). Cross-sectional surveys of perinatal mortality yield a U-shaped curve when plotted against parity, implying that fourth and subsequent infants are at increased risk. Study of a large, population-based longitudinal data set has now shown this result to be an artifact. Analysis was made of data on 294,534 mothers who gave birth to 1 or more of their first 4 single babies from 1967 to 1973. A total of 417,086 births were available for study. Perinatal mortality fell with increasing parity (Fig 3–1). Within cohorts of mothers based on attained sibship size, perinatal mortality decreased with increasing parity and increased with sibship size.

These associations, which are not noticeably affected by maternal age, seem in part to operate through a relation among parity, sibship size, and birth weight. Maternal age does appear to have an appreciable influence on perinatal mortality of the first infant. The findings show the importance of examining the effects of age and parity in longitudinal samples of women and with the analysis based on sibships. This approach could be applied to various epidemiologic observations using measures of pregnancy outcome other than perinatal mortality. By use of cohort analysis, previously unrecognized associations with maternal age or parity might be discovered.

▶ [This study nicely demonstrates that one must be very careful in viewing the relationship between demographic characteristics and perinatal mortality. A cross-sectional analysis of these data indicates that perinatal mortality increases after the second baby. The longitudinal analysis shows that, although perinatal mortality increases with sibship size, within cohorts of mothers based on attained sibship size the perinatal mortality decreases with increasing parity. The cross-sectional analysis misses this important point.] ◀

(3–2) Br. Med. J. 2:693–696, Sept. 22, 1979.

Outcome of Pregnancies Complicated by Early Vaginal Bleeding. S. J. Funderburk, D. Guthrie, and D. Meldrum[3-3] (Univ. of California, Los Angeles) analyzed obstetric and neonatal data from 259 patients with first- or second-trimester vaginal bleeding to measure perinatal risk and to determine whether prior maternal illness or complications of prior pregnancies added to that risk.

As shown in the table, there was a significant association between early vaginal bleeding and complications of pregnancy. Fetal anomalies were slightly though not significantly increased. Pregnancy outcome appeared to be associated with the severity of early bleeding, because suboptimal outcome occurred in 63 of 210 patients (30%) who experienced heavy bleeding compared with 8 of 42 patients (19%) who experienced light bleeding. The risk of early bleeding was increased by a history of previous abortions, premature births, or perinatal deaths, and was diminished by a history of previous full-term births.

Suboptimal pregnancy outcome occurred in 77 of 259 pregnancies (29.7%) with early bleeding compared with 3,809 of 25,118 (15.2%) concurrent deliveries without reported early pregnancy bleeding. The combined risk remained approximately doubled even for primigravidae and for women without prior illness or pregnancy complications. The highest combined risk, 61.5%, was for women with at least two prior abortions, premature births, or perinatal deaths, and no prior term births.

Early gestational vaginal bleeding is one predictor of possible suboptimal pregnancy outcome.

▶ [This report concerns the controversial issue of subsequent pregnancy performance in patients with vaginal bleeding in early pregnancy. Unfortunately, it does not provide final answers. The reported prevalence in this chart review study is 1%, which seems much too low and suggests biased reporting. Bleeding in the second trimester is not distinguished from that in the first trimester and probably should be (one would predict that second-trimester bleeding would be more apt to reflect a placental abnormality that might lead to premature labor than would first-trimester vaginal bleeding that had stopped and was not associated with spontaneous abortion). The outcomes

PERINATAL VARIBLES ASSOCIATED WITH EARLY BLEEDING

Per cent of pregnancies affected

Pregnancy outcome	No early bleeding	Early bleeding	Chi square
	(25,118)*	(259)*	
Low birth weight	6·91	17·37	p <0·0001
Very low birth weight	1·33	8·88	p <0·0001
Low gestational age	5·41	12·74	p <0·0001
Breech delivery	2·53	8·49	p <0·0001
Perinatal death	2·00	7·72	p <0·0001
Asphyxia	2·27	6·95	p <0·0001
Placental infarct	0·73	2·70	p <0·01
Small-for-dates term infant	2·72	5·02	p <0·05
Fetal anomaly	1·63	2·70	NS†

*Total cases.
†Not significant.

(3–3) Br. J. Obstet. Gynaecol. 87:100–105, February 1980.

reported in the table are disturbing, but we do not think they provide much help when we attempt to answer questions posed by individual patients with bleeding in early pregnancy.] ◄

An Unexpectedly High Rate of Ectopic Pregnancy Following Induction of Ovulation With Human Pituitary and Chorionic Gonadotropin. J. C. McBain, J. H. Evans (Royal Women's Hosp., Melbourne), R. J. Pepperell, H. P. Robinson, Margery A. Smith, and J. B. Brown[3-4] (Univ. of Melbourne) found six tubal ectopic pregnancies among 193 pregnancies after induced ovulation with human pituitary gonadotropin (hPG) and human chorionic gonadotropin (hCG). This ectopic pregnancy rate of 3.1% is higher than quoted incidences in the general population and occurred in the absence of pelvic inflammatory disease. Urinary estrogen levels were measured during and after induction of ovulation and pregnanediol levels, after induced ovulation.

There was an association between ectopic pregnancy and elevated urinary estrogen excretion in the periovulatory phases of the induced ovulatory cycles. The estrogen values from four patients were in the upper range, and a value exceeding 200 μg/day on the day after hCG administration was associated with a 10% chance of ectopic pregnancy. The urinary pregnanediol values were similarly analyzed and were within the middle range, with the exception of one patient who had an intrauterine triplet pregnancy accompanying the ectopic pregnancy.

It has been reported elsewhere that ovarian hyperstimulation enhances the pregnancy rates with gonadotropin therapy, but results of this study suggest that there is also an associated increase in the ectopic pregnancy rate, which should be considered in the management of patients who become pregnant as a result of gonadotropin therapy, particularly if there is biochemical evidence of overstimulation of the ovaries.

Another patient has been observed recently with ectopic pregnancy after induction of ovulation with hPG; total urinary estrogen excretion on the day after gonadotropin administration was 279 μg/day. This increases the risk of ectopic pregnancy in this series to 12.5% when estrogen excretion exceeds 200 μg/day on the day after administration.

► [Tubal pregnancies were unusually common in this series of patients treated with gonadotropins and seemed especially likely to occur when periovulatory estrogen excretion was high. The authors suggest possible estrogen effects on tubal transport or multiple ovulations as explanations.] ◄

Complications of Cerclage. Cervical incompetence is an infrequent cause of fetal loss. Reported results of cervical cerclage have almost always been good, and few complications have been described. J. G. Aarnoudse and H. J. Huisjes[3-5] (Univ. of Groningen) reviewed the results of 55 cerclage operations, done in 52 pregnancies of 40 patients from 1971 to 1976, when there were 5,278 deliveries at the authors' department. The women had had 97 previous pregnancies,

(3-4) Br. J. Obstet. Gynaecol. 87:5-9, January 1980.
(3-5) Acta Obstet. Gynecol. Scand. 58:255-257, 1979.

with 80 spontaneous abortions and premature deliveries, 20 occurring before 16 weeks' gestation. Only 17 children had survived. Cervical incompetence was suspected from the obstetric history in 38 pregnancies. Fourteen operations were done for symptoms of developing cervical incompetence, such as a watery vaginal discharge and a feeling of pressure in the vagina. The mean period of gestation at the time of cervical suturing in this group was 26 weeks. Previous cervical injury was a possible factor in 6 cases.

Twenty-one pregnancies (40%) ended after a gestation exceeding 260 days. Cerclage failed in the other 31 cases, including three sets of twins and one of triplets. Premature membrane rupture occurred in 12 failed cases, a slipping suture in 7, uterine infection in 4, and untreatable premature labor in 6. Two fetuses died in utero. In 2 cases there was no obvious cause for failure.

The pregnancy outcome is clearly improved after cervical cerclage in cases of cervical incompetence, but complications are frequent, and careful patient selection is necessary. Treatment of preexisting cervical infection may reduce the number of complications. Frequent inspection of the cervix after cerclage is advised to detect slipping off of the suture at an early stage, when resuture is still possible.

▶ [Because the diagnosis of cervical incompetence is usually not crystal clear, indications for cerclage and hence the prevalence of cerclage procedures vary from service to service. The 1% treatment rate reported here is higher than our own. There is no question that recognition of this entity and the development of procedures designed to treat it represent genuine advances in obstetric care, but once again we are reminded of the complications that can occur; 73% of the pregnancies resulted in viable offspring, but intrauterine infection and prematurely ruptured membranes were not rare. One third of the surviving newborns were born prematurely.] ◀

Cervical Cerclage: Twenty Years' Experience with 40 pregnancies in 32 patients with cervical incompetence (an incidence of one in 775 deliveries) is presented by William A. Peters III, Siva Thiagarajah, and Guy H. Harbert, Jr.[3-6] (Univ. of Virginia). Ten patients had a history of factors predisposing to cervical incompetence such as obstetric or surgical trauma to the cervix; 22 had no such history, although ten had either a second trimester spontaneous abortion or a diagnosis of incompetent cervix established during their first pregnancy. All 40 pregnancies were managed with primary Shirodkar or McDonald cervical cerclage.

Of 25 pregnancies in which asymptomatic cervical changes were present at the time of suture placement (diagnosis based on history and follow-up), 23 (92%) produced surviving infants and 17 reached 36 weeks' gestation. Of 10 pregnancies in which second trimester symptoms such as mucoid discharge and fullness in the vagina led to examination and diagnosis, four (40%) resulted in surviving infants and only three reached 36 weeks of gestation. Of five pregnancies managed with a Shirodkar cerclage in place from a previous pregnancy, four progressed to 36 weeks' gestation and produced healthy infants by elective repeat cesarean section; one ended in abortion following suture removal because the suture cut through the cervix in the second trimester.

(3–6) South. Med. J. 72:933–937, August 1979.

MAJOR MATERNAL COMPLICATIONS

Complication	Age	Parity	Gestational Age at Cerclage	Presentation	Findings	Therapy	Fetal Outcome	Maternal Outcome
(A) Uterine rupture								
Case 1 (1960)	20	$G_5P_3A_1$	30 weeks, Shirodkar	In active labor at 36 weeks	Delivery through posterior wall rupture	Abdominal hysterectomy	Viable 2,250 gm infant	Uneventful recovery
Case 2 (1962)	22	$G_6P_2A_3$	Shirodkar from previous pregnancy	Previous C-section. Active labor at 37 weeks	Complete dehiscence of uterine incision	Cesarean, hysterectomy	Viable 3,100 gm infant	Uneventful recovery
Case 3 (1963)	28	$G_4P_0A_3$	21 weeks, Shirodkar	Admitted at 33 weeks for management of toxemia	Elective cesarean at 38 weeks. Occult rupture of lower segment.	Rupture repaired. Reexplored 36 hours later due to development of a hematoma. Bleeders ligated.	Viable 2,800 gm infant	Uneventful recovery
(B) Chorioamnionitis								
Case 1 (1974)	24	$G_4P_1A_2$	22 weeks, McDonald	Rupture of membranes one day after cerclage	Chorioamnionitis	Removal of of suture, antibiotics, induction of labor.	Nonviable fetus	Uneventful recovery
Case 2 (1976)	20	$G_1P_0A_1$	19 weeks, McDonald	Rupture of membranes at 32 weeks	Febrile 24 hours after rupture of membranes. Chorioamnionitis.	Suture removal, antibiotics, induction of labor.	Viable 1,930 gm infant	Uneventful recovery

Of the 16 women who had pregnancies which did not reach 36 weeks' gestation, ten had the cerclage removed because of premature contractions and six because of premature rupture of the membranes. None of the three patients with cervical dilation greater than 3 cm, and only one of seven with membranes bulging beyond the cervix at the time of surgery, reached 36 weeks' gestation. Only two of eight patients operated on after 26 weeks' gestation progressed to 36 weeks. Major maternal complications (table) occurred in five (12.5%) of the 40 pregnancies.

Although some authors advocate suture placement based solely upon past obstetric history, the mere presence of the suture may cause premature labor and more serious complications. Thus, patients with suggestive histories should be examined weekly, with cerclage withheld unless appropriate changes occur in cervical length or dilation. The 92% fetal survival in patients treated before becoming symptomatic, vs. the 40% survival in those receiving cerclage only after symptoms developed, documents the importance of the previous obstetric history and of early diagnosis and treatment.

The McDonald and Shirodkar procedures are equally effective in preventing premature delivery. The former method is preferred because of the simple technique, minimal blood loss, and likelihood of vaginal delivery after suture removal. In subsequent pregnancies, repeat cerclages are done at 12 to 14 weeks' gestation. Number 5 braided silk sutures are preferred to no. 2 sutures. Sutures are removed at about 36 weeks to allow vaginal delivery. Cerclage is removed promptly if membrane rupture or persistent uterine contractions occur. Cerclage is contraindicated when close follow-up is unavailable.

▶ [This report also reminds us that although cervical cerclage procedures are relatively simple to perform they can be associated with severe subsequent complications. Uterine rupture can result after apparently mild uterine contractions. Patients with sutures in place should be instructed to come in whenever they think they might be starting labor. Although inhibition of labor can be considered in this situation, most times the removal of the stitch is probably the safest way to go.] ◀

Impaired Reproductive Performance in DES-Exposed Women. Although the incidence of malignancy in females exposed in utero to diethylstilbestrol (DES) is lower than originally anticipated, concern over anatomical abnormalities of the cervix and vagina is increasing. Merle J. Berger and Donald Peter Goldstein[3-7] (Harvard Med. School) sought to learn whether these abnormalities might significantly alter reproductive performance. Sixty-nine patients with characteristic cervical and vaginal abnormalities who might conceive were evaluated. Age range was 18 to 32 years. Fifty-five subjects were planning a family. The period of risk of conception ranged from 6 months to 8 years.

Forty-six patients had 80 pregnancies, but 14 of them elected therapeutic abortions. The other 32 patients conceived 62 times, resulting in 36 pregnancy failures (58.1%) and 26 live births. All successes were in 16 patients. Cervical cerclage was necessary in 8 successful

(3–7) Obstet. Gynecol. 55:25–27, January 1980.

OUTCOME OF 62 PREGNANCIES IN 32 DES-EXPOSED WOMEN

Trimester	Outcome	No. pregnant	Percent
1	Spontaneous abortion	19	30.6
	Ectopic pregnancy	3	4.8
2	Spontaneous abortion	11	17.7
3	Premature delivery	8*	12.9
	Term delivery	21†	33.9

*Includes 3 neonatal deaths.
†Includes 8 patients with cerclage.

pregnancies because of demonstrated cervical incompetence. The outcome of the pregnancies is summarized in the table. The abnormalities observed in the 25 patients who underwent hysterosalpingography ranged from minimal to severe.

It appears that DES-exposed women have impaired reproductive function. Many have difficulty conceiving, but the major problem appears to be related to increased fetal wastage. Losses in each trimester are significantly more frequent than might be expected in the general population and are probably more frequent than expected even in a sample of patients with reproductive problems. Further studies of reproductive performance in large numbers of DES-exposed women are needed.

▶ [The authors of this retrospective study appreciate that biases exist and that extrapolation of these findings to all DES-exposed women is not possible. For example, all patients included here had vaginal and cervical lesions associated with in utero DES exposure and some patients were referred to the authors only following adverse obstetric outcomes. Nevertheless, even considering these limitations, the reported results are dismal. Second-trimester loss and premature labor were serious problems. We have seen several DES-exposed women with similar outcomes. The most important chapter of the DES story may well concern not the rare clear cell carcinomas, but the frequent poor obstetric outcomes.

In a related study, Brian and colleagues of the Mayo Clinic (Mayo Clin. Proc. 55:89, 1980) examined the question of an association between intrauterine DES exposure and subsequent breast cancer. No relation was found.] ◀

▶ ↓The following three articles also focus on the obstetric performance of DES-exposed women. The picture is not bright. ◀

Upper Genital Tract Changes and Pregnancy Outcome in Offspring Exposed In Utero to Diethylstilbestrol. Raymond H. Kaufman, Ervin Adam, Gary L. Binder, and Elizabeth Gerthoffer[3-8] (St. Luke's Episcopal Hosp., Houston) reviewed the physical and hysterosalpingographic findings in 267 women exposed in utero to diethylstilbestrol (DES) and the outcome of pregnancy in 93 of them. A total of 223 subjects had documented evidence of in utero exposure to DES. Medication was begun before 13 weeks' gestation in 134 of these cases. Mean age of the study group was 23.6 years. Hysterosalpingograms from 34 unexposed women were used for comparison.

(3–8) Am. J. Obstet. Gynecol. 137:299–308, June 1, 1980.

TABLE 1.—TYPES OF HYSTEROSALPINGOGRAPHY (HSG) FINDINGS

HSG findings

No. of women	Structural changes	Normal findings	T-shaped	Small cavity	Con-striction	T shape plus small cavity	T shape plus con-striction	Small cavity plus con-striction	T shape plus small cavity plus constriction	Other abnor-mality	Total of abnormal findings
118	Present	17	12	15	3	34	7	7	16	7	101 (86%)
149	Absent	65	24	10	4	23	4	3	9	7	84 (56%)
267		82 (31%)	36 (19%)	25 (13%)	7 (4%)	57 (31%)	11 (6%)	10 (5%)	25 (13%)	14 (8%)	185 (69%)

TABLE 2.—OUTCOME OF 144 PREGNANCIES IN 93 WOMEN
EXPOSED TO DES IN UTERO

HSG	Total No. of pregnancies	Elective abortion	Ectopic pregnancies	Spontaneous abortions Trimester First	Second	Total	Premature deliveries	Term deliveries	Total No. of live births
Abnormal	78	12	5 (8%)	16 (26%)	8 (13%)	24 (39%)	14 (38%)*	23 (34%)	37
Normal	66	13	2 (4%)	6 (21%)	6 (12%)	12 (23%)	8 (20%)*	31 (58%)	39
Total	144	25	7 (6%)	22 (20%))	14 (12%)	36 (32%)	22 (29%)*	54 (45%)	76

*Percent of live births.

The hysterosalpingographic findings are summarized in Table 1. Abnormalities were present in 69% of exposed women. The most common was a T-shaped uterus with a small cavity, which was present in 31%. Structural changes of the cervix were present in 44% of subjects and were associated with abnormal hysterosalpingographic findings. Over 80% of the 179 women with vaginal epithelial changes had abnormal x-ray findings. Total dosage of DES was not related to rate of upper genital tract abnormalities. The outcome of pregnancies is shown in Table 2. Spontaneous abortions were not significantly more frequent in exposed women with abnormal x-ray findings than in exposed women with normal x-ray films. Term pregnancies were less frequent in exposed women with abnormal x-ray findings, and ectopic pregnancies and premature deliveries were more frequent in exposed women who underwent hysterosalpingography than in unexposed subjects.

It is important to determine what can be done to improve the pregnancy outcome in women exposed in utero to DES. The possibility of ectopic pregnancy must be kept constantly in mind. Routine cervical cerclage is not recommended, but this procedure may well be of some value in prolonging pregnancies in women with a single past mid-trimester abortion or premature delivery.

▶ [An old adage goes, "A difference, to be a difference, must make a difference." In this article, Kaufman and his colleagues present evidence that the upper genital tract changes with intrauterine DES exposure Kaufman first described several years ago *probably* make a difference in reproductive performance. Patients with abnormal hysterosalpingographic findings (usually a small and/or T-shaped endometrial cavity) had had more ectopic pregnancies, spontaneous abortions, and premature deliveries than normal women, although the difference for the outcomes individually was not statistically significant. When adverse outcomes were lumped together and the opposite side of the coin—term birth—examined, the goal of statistical significance was reached. A problem in interpretation of these data arises because of the correlation of upper and lower (ie, cervical and vaginal) abnormalities, making it uncertain as to whether the increase in adverse outcome reflects uterine or cervical pathology.

Very similar results were found by Cousins and associates (Obstet. Gynecol. 56:70, 1980). Women exposed to DES in utero, in comparison with matched controls, had significantly more premature deliveries and perinatal deaths; difficulties with conception and complications in early pregnancy did not differ.] ◄

Comparison of Pregnancy Experience in DES-Exposed and DES-Unexposed Daughters. Arthur L. Herbst, Marian M. Hubby, Richard R. Blough, and Freidoon Azizi[3-9] (Univ. of Chicago) compared the reproductive histories of 226 diethylstilbestrol (DES)-exposed and 203 unexposed daughters whose mothers had participated in a double-blind study in 1951 to 1952. Initial gynecologic evaluation at about age 23 years showed nonmalignant vaginal epithelial changes in 67% of exposed subjects and in 4% of unexposed subjects. About 40% of exposed subjects had transverse ridges of the vagina and cervix. In no daughter has vaginal or cervical clear cell adenocarcinoma developed to date. Doses of DES had been raised during pregnancy from 5 to 150 mg daily, starting at a mean of 12 weeks' gestation. Subjects were aged 25 to 28 years at the time of evaluation.

Irregular menses were slightly more frequent in the exposed than in the unexposed group (10% vs. 4%). Nineteen exposed subjects and four unexposed subjects had primary infertility. Of those at risk, 86% of unexposed and 67% of exposed subjects had conceived. The outcome of first pregnancies is summarized in the table. Full-term live births were more common in the unexposed group, and premature live births and nonviable births in the exposed group. Only 55% of subjects with cervicovaginal ridges had live births in their first pregnancies, compared with 88% of those without ridges. Five exposed subjects who had cervical cerclage after a premature stillbirth or miscarriage have subsequently delivered live infants.

Frequent prenatal evaluation appears indicated for DES-exposed subjects who are pregnant, especially for the first time. Four exposed

OUTCOME OF FIRST PREGNANCY			
	Exposed N = 89		Unexposed N = 118
Elective abortion	18		28
Current pregnancy	7		6
Completed pregnancy	64		84
Full-term live birth	30	(47%)	71 (85%)
Premature live birth	14	(22%)	6* (7%)
Premature nonviable	4 ⎫		1 ⎫
Miscarriage	12 ⎬ (31%)		6 ⎬ (8%)
Ectopic pregnancy	4 ⎭		0 ⎭
			$P \ll 0.0005$†

*Includes one twin birth.
†Comparison for distribution of the three outcomes as grouped.

(3–9) J. Reprod. Med. 24:62–69, February 1980.

and no unexposed subjects in this series had ectopic pregnancies. The cervix should be periodically evaluated throughout pregnancy. Cervical cerclage should be done if there is evidence of cervical dilation or incompetence, or if the usual obstetric indications exist. Routine cerclage is not indicated, because most exposed women have had live infants.

Fertility and Outcome of Pregnancy in Women Exposed In Utero to Diethylstilbestrol. Ann B. Barnes, Theodore Colton, Jerome Gundersen, Kenneth L. Noller, Barbara C. Tilley, Thomas Strama, Duane E. Townsend, Paul Hatab, and Peter C. O'Brien[3-10] examined fertility and the outcome of pregnancy in women participating in the National Cooperative Diethylstilbestrol Adenosis Project. In all, 618 individuals having prenatal exposure to diethylstilbestrol (DES) were matched with sisters or controls for subject and maternal ages.

Fertility, measured in terms of pregnancies achieved, did not differ in the DES-exposed and control groups. However, an increased risk of unfavorable outcome of pregnancy was associated with DES exposure (table). The relative risk of any unfavorable outcome was 1.69. The strongest dose-response relationship was found for premature births. Of 220 DES-exposed women with outcomes other than induced abortion, 36 had structural defects of the cervix and upper vagina. The anomalies included partial cervical hoods, complete cervical collars, cervical pseudopolyps, absence of the pars vaginalis, transverse septa, and hypoplastic cervices.

Diethylstilbestrol-exposed women are normally able to conceive, but they are at increased risk of an unfavorable pregnancy outcome, although most of these pregnancies result in a live birth. Careful monitoring of these pregnancies is warranted. This may include pelvic examination and two or more ultrasound examinations. Prophy-

NUMBERS AND PERCENTAGES OF WOMEN EXPOSED TO DES AND OF
CONTROL SUBJECTS WHO HAD UNFAVORABLE OUTCOMES OF
PREGNANCY, AND RELATIVE RISKS OF UNFAVORABLE OUTCOMES
WITH DES EXPOSURE

OUTCOME	EXPOSED TO DES (220)*	CONTROLS (224)*	RELATIVE RISK	P VALUE	95 PER CENT CONFIDENCE LIMITS ON RELATIVE RISK
Any unfavorable outcome	83 (37.7)	50 (22.3)	1.69	<0.001	1.20–2.18
Miscarriage	57 (25.9)	36 (16.1)	1.61	0.008	1.11–2.34
Ectopic pregnancy	8 (3.6)	3 (1.3)	2.77	ns†	0.73–10.46
Stillbirth	8 (3.6)	3 (1.3)	2.77	ns	0.73–10.46
Premature birth	17 (7.7)	10 (4.5)	1.71	ns	0.80–3.65
Never had a full-term live birth	42 (19.1)	11 (4.9)	3.90	<0.001	2.06–7.37

*Figures in parentheses denote percentages.
†Not significant (P > 0.10).

(3–10)   N. Engl. J. Med. 302:609–613, Mar. 13, 1980.

lactic surgical intervention (eg, cerclage) is not warranted unless classic indications are present.

▶ [Two more looks at the reproductive performance of women exposed to DES in utero are provided by the article and the preceding one. Whereas fertility is not affected, miscarriage and premature delivery are more common in the DES-exposed group. In our view, patients with a DES-exposure history should have frequent antepartum visits at which the state of the cervix is assessed, because cervical incompetence seems to be the problem.] ◀

Pregnancy Following Conization of the Cervix: Complications Related to Cone Size. Gladwyn Leiman, Neville A. Harrison, and Abraham Rubin[3-11] (Univ. of the Witwatersrand) undertook a retrospective study of 88 pregnancies in 77 patients who had cervical conization to relate the outcome of pregnancy to cone size. Cone specimens measuring more than 2 cm in height or 4 cc in volume were considered large cones. The mean patient age was 30 years; preconization parity averaged 3.2. The interval from conization to conception ranged from 1 month to 5 years. The final diagnosis was carcinoma in situ in 49 cases and severe dysplasia in 25. Three patients had early stromal invasion but refused further treatment because they wished to conceive.

Pregnancy outcome is related to cone volume in the table. The rate of spontaneous abortion was 22.7%, and second-trimester abortion was related to large cone size, using either cone volume or height as a parameter. Prematurity was documented in 14.8% of the cases. The rate was significantly increased in subjects with large cones. The only 2 patients in whom cerclage was performed were delivered of premature infants. The cesarean section rate was 12.5%. Six cesarean sections were done for cervical fibrosis and failure of dilatation in labor. Small cones appeared to predispose to stenosis. The rate of stillbirths was 2.3% and showed no relation to prior conization. The term normal vaginal delivery rate was inversely proportional to cone size.

This study indicates a poor pregnancy outcome after cervical conization. Large cones are associated with a high risk of midtrimester abortion and prematurity, and small cones are associated with cervical dystocia. Elective cerclage appears indicated with a large cone size. Colposcopically directed cone biopsies should involve removal of the minimum amount of cervical tissue consistent with eradication of the intraepithelial lesion.

▶ [While these results—a positive relationship between the cone size and the frequencies of second-trimester abortion and premature labor in subsequent pregnancy—are exactly what would be predicted, things do not always work out so neatly. We were

PREGNANCY OUTCOME RELATED TO CONE VOLUME

Cone volume (cc)	Ectopic pregnancy	Spontaneous abortion Trimester 1	Spontaneous abortion Trimester 2	Premature delivery	Cesarean section	Stillbirth	Term vaginal delivery	Total
<4	1 3.2%	4 12.9%	2 6.5%	1 3.2%	5 16.1%	2 6.5%	16 51.6%	31 100%
>4	— —	3 13.7%	4 18.2%	7 31.7%	3 13.7%	— —	5 22.7%	22 100%

(3–11) Am. J. Obstet. Gynecol. 136:14–18, Jan. 1, 1980.

curious as to why a statistical analysis was not done. By our evaluation (ie, chi-square test), the differences in premature delivery with large and small cones is statistically significant (P < 0.05), but not with respect to second-trimester abortion or cesarean section.

A technique for assessing that the size of the cone is the minimal amount necessary to remove abnormal tissue was described by Veridiano and Tancer (J. Reprod. Med. 24:212, 1980). The conization was done under colposcopic guidance in the operating room in 108 patients with a diagnosis of carcinoma in situ by previous "satisfactory" colposcopy who wished to retain fertility. On follow-up ranging from 4 to 48 months, only 1 patient had recurrent carcinoma in situ and 2 others had mild dysplasia.] ◄

Outcome of Pregnancy After Cone Biopsy of the Cervix: Case-Control Study. High rates of spontaneous abortion and premature labor have previously been reported in women having a cone biopsy. Jane M. Jones, P. Sweetnam, and B. M. Hibbard[3-12] (Welsh Natl. School of Medicine) examined the outcome of singleton pregnancies proceeding beyond 28 weeks' gestation in 66 women who previously had a cervical cone biopsy. Fifty-five had first pregnancies after the biopsy, and 10 had second pregnancies; 1 had a third pregnancy. Each index patient was matched with 4 controls for maternal age, parity, and social class. The index patients were among 76 who had had 91 pregnancies after a cone biopsy. Spontaneous abortion had occurred in 14% of the pregnancies, and 12% were terminated.

There were 11 spontaneous (17%) and 1 (1.5%) induced preterm labors and deliveries after cone biopsy, compared with 3% and 2%, respectively, among 264 controls. Both differences were significant. The risk of spontaneous preterm delivery was greater in the second than in the first pregnancy after cone biopsy. Birth weights below 2,500 gm were significantly more frequent in the index group. Mean duration of labor was 8.5 hours in the cone biopsy group and 6.3 hours in the control group. Labor exceeded 12 hours in 20% of index cases and 10.2% of control cases. Labor lasted less than 2 hours in 5 index patients and 15 controls.

In this series, preterm delivery and low birth weight were more frequent and the duration of labor was longer in patients with cone biopsy of the cervix than in controls. Patients who have had a cervical cone biopsy should seek medical advice early and be supervised closely throughout pregnancy.

► [Previous surveys have suggested that cervical conization impairs the outcome in subsequent pregnancies, but this controlled study is the most convincing to date. The most important effect was on the ability to carry to term, with the incidence of spontaneous premature labor and low birth weight increased by 6 and 3 times, respectively, in postconization patients over controls. The only other statistically significant difference was a modest prolongation of the length of labor. Though pregnancy risks are clearly increased by previous cone biopsy, the overall outcome is not too bad (eg, 82% carried to term). Fortunately, problems of this type should diminish markedly with the widespread use of colposcopy.

Other recent studies are more optimistic concerning the effects of previous conization on pregnancy. Read on.] ◄

Pregnancy Complications Following Conization of the Uterine Cervix.—*Part I.*—It is expected that the increase in screening for malignant cervical disease will result in an increase in conizations

(3–12) Br. J. Obstet. Gynaecol. 86:913–916, December 1979.

done on fertile women, some of whom will conceive. Tom Weber and Erik Obel[3-13] (Univ. of Copenhagen) reviewed twenty studies concerning fertility and the course of pregnancy after conization. Rates of conception after conization range from 20% to 84%, and the total rate of conception ranges from 14% to 78%. Reported rates of early "spontaneous" abortion range from 1% to 56%; the authors' estimate is below 9%. Ectopic pregnancy has been reported after 1.2% of conizations. Late abortion has been reported in 2% to 11% of patients. Prematurity rates have ranged from 1% to 17%. Rates of up to 8% for cesarean section have been reported.

No studies have adequately described their patient material, and most have not attempted to establish control groups. Studies of the effects of conization should be based on a comparison of pregnancies before and after conization or a comparison between pregnancies in women with a previous conization and those in a control group of women who have not undergone conization. It cannot be concluded at present that conization leads to reduced fertility or an increase in spontaneous abortions or perinatal mortality. An increased prematurity rate is still a possibility.

▶ [The effects of previous conization of the cervix on fertility and pregnancy complications have been both stressed and minimized by various "authorities." That there are no easy answers is underscored by this comprehensive literature review. Few studies have had control groups, and the appropriateness of those controls is open to question. Many medical, demographic, and "life-style" factors in patients undergoing conization certainly are different from those in the general population. In studying the subsequent reproductive risks of conization, one should carefully choose noncone control groups. Even with the careful selection of controls, definitive answers will be hard to come by.] ◀

Part II.—Weber and Obel[3-14] examined the effects of conization on the course of pregnancy and on fertility in 44 women who had a total of 66 pregnancies after conization. Seventeen had had one or more pregnancies between conization and the pregnancy in question. Comparison was with an age-matched group of women who did not have conization, and also a group matched for both age and parity. There were more smokers among women who had conization, but in other respects the groups were comparable. They were similar in social status and educational level. A tendency toward an increased rate of induced abortions was noted in the study group, but the difference was not significant.

No difference in rate of prematurity was noted between the groups. The course of future pregnancies is outlined in the table. There were no significant differences in spontaneous and induced abortions, prematurity, or cesarean section between women who had conization and control women. The second stage of labor was prolonged in the former women. Fertility, judged from the time elapsed between the start of intercourse without contraception to the current pregnancy, was comparable in the two groups.

More data are necessary for definitive conclusions to be drawn, but

(3–13) Acta Obstet. Gynecol. Scand. 58:259–263, 1979.
(3–14) Ibid., pp. 347–351.

NUMBER OF SPONTANEOUS ABORTIONS, INDUCED ABORTIONS, LOW BIRTH WEIGHT INFANTS, AND
CESAREAN SECTIONS IN CONIZED AND NONCONIZED WOMEN COMPARED ACCORDING
.TO DESCRIBED METHODS

Method No.	Early abortion (before 13. week) No.	p-value	Induced abortion No.	p-value	Late abortion (after 12. week) No.	p-value	Premature delivery (ery < 2501 g) No.	p-value	Caesarean section/ No. of deliveries no.	p-value
1. Conized women Age-matched group					3/44 1/44	0.31	5/41 1/41	0.09	8/41 5/43	0.32
2. 1.st preg. foll. coniz. Age-matched controls					2/27 1/27	0.50	1/25 1/26	0.75		
3. 1.st preg. foll coniz. Age-and parity-matched group					3/34 0/43	0.08	1/31 1/43	0.67		
4. 1.st preg. foll. coniz. Age-matched group	6/44 3/44	0.24	3/44 1/44	0.31	3/34 1/40	0.25	1/31 1/39	0.69		

the present study did not show increased risks of spontaneous abortion or prematurity in women who had cervical conization. No reduction in fertility was demonstrated in these women.

▶ [As noted above, there are no ideal control groups for this sort of study. The authors have chosen different sets of controls and, although the numbers are not large, the reported results are generally reassuring. Colposcopy has diminished the need for cone biopsy, but when cone biopsy should be done (eg, when the squamocolumnar junction cannot be seen or, in our view, when the directed biopsy reads carcinoma in situ or severe dysplasia), it can be carried out without excessive hand-wringing concerning subsequent reproductive performance.] ◀

Pregnancy and Delivery After Conization of the Cervix. Conization is adequate treatment for cervical dysplasia and carcinoma in situ, but amputation of the cervix increases complications related to pregnancy and labor and causes changes in menstruation. M. Grönroos, P. Liukko, P. Kilkku, and R. Punnonen[3-15] (Univ. of Turku) reviewed the findings in 249 patients, among 327 who had conization of the cervix during 1968–1974, who replied to a questionnaire regarding pregnancies after conization. Eighty-nine subjects had had a total of 112 pregnancies. Before conization, 12 patients had had one or two spontaneous abortions and 7 had undergone legal abortion. Dysplasia was diagnosed in 87% of patients, carcinoma in situ in 8%, and cervicitis in 5%.

After conization, 10 patients had spontaneous abortions, 20 had legal abortions, and 2 had ectopic pregnancies. Of 8 patients who had spontaneous abortions in the first trimester, 5 later had a normal-weight infant. Sixty-nine patients had 80 deliveries. One infant weighed less than 1,501 gm, and 10 infants weighed 1,501 to 2,500 gm at birth. Fourteen patients noted spotting lasting a few days during pregnancy. Only a few complications of labor were observed, and there were no precipitate labors. Two cesarean sections were done. Little effect of conization on menstrual pain was apparent.

Conization had only minimal effect on pregnancies and none on deliveries in this survey. More than 90% of newborns were full term and without anomalies. The rate of spontaneous abortion did not dif-

(3–15)   Acta Obstet. Gynecol. Scand. 58:477–480, 1979.

fer from normal. Conization can be recommended as both a diagnostic and therapeutic procedure where fertility is to be preserved.

▶ [Previous cervical conization was not found to affect pregnancy outcome adversely in this study.] ◀

Cholestatic Jaundice of Pregnancy: New Perspectives. Cholestatic jaundice of pregnancy has traditionally been considered a benign maternal condition that has no ill effects on the fetus and requires no special surveillance during pregnancy. Brian R. I. Wilson and Albert D. Haverkamp[3-16] (Denver Genl. Hosp.) reviewed nine cases of cholestatic jaundice seen in a six-month period in 1977, among 1,317 deliveries. One antepartum death and two premature labors occurred. Seven of the nine infants had meconium staining in the amniotic fluid. The symptoms of this condition are primarily pruritus and jaundice. No hepatosplenomegaly or other signs of liver disease are present, but laboratory evidence of liver derangement may be obtained.

Patients diagnosed as having cholestatic jaundice of pregnancy should be followed in high-risk clinics where fetal well-being can be monitored by nonstress tests. Cholestyramine is quite effective in controlling pruritus, but it does not always relieve symptoms in patients with cholestasis of pregnancy. Patients may require phenobarbital as well. This drug increases excretion of bile salts and bile acids and potentiates the effects of cholestyramine.

▶ [Nothing really new is presented here, although it is important that we be reminded that cholestasis of pregnancy may not be benign as far as the fetus is concerned. The increased fetal risks previously recognized in Scandanavia and Chile as being associated with this condition have now been noted in the United States as well. Fetal surveillance in late pregnancy is indicated.] ◀

Genetic Control of Severe Preeclampsia. The causes of severe preeclampsia and eclampsia remain unknown, though several immunogenetic hypotheses have been advanced. Recent reports indicate an unusual distribution of HLA types both in women who have had severe preeclampsia and their husbands. D. W. Cooper and W. A. Liston[3-17] carried out genetic analyses of published and new data on the familial occurrence of severe preeclampsia in primigravid women. Data were collected on primigravidas seen in the Aberdeen Maternity Hospital in 1968–1972, during which time the incidence of severe preeclampsia was 5.3%.

The condition apparently may be largely a mendelian recessive state. Data on severe preeclampsia in the relatives of women who have had eclampsia support the maternal genotype hypothesis. Similar data in which the index cases were women with severe preeclampsia are, however, more compatible with the fetal genotype hypothesis. The fetal genotype hypothesis may be correct for most cases, whereas other genes may have to be present in the maternal genome for eclampsia to result. The maternal genotype hypothesis may be correct, but not all bearers of the recessive homozygous genotype may

(3–16) Obstet. Gynecol. 54:650–652, November 1979.
(3–17) J. Med. Genet. 16:409–416, December 1979.

have the condition in their first pregnancy; that is, penetrance may not be complete.

Data on the incidence of severe preeclampsia in relatives of index cases compared to that in their in-laws are now needed. This would allow a choice between the two hypotheses if one or the other were correct, or would assess the contributions of each if an interaction between genotypes were involved. Recurrent severe preeclampsia appears to have the same genetic basis as the more common primigravid type. Mild nonproteinuric preeclampsia, however, usually seems to be inherited independently of the severe form. It may prove possible to prevent severe preeclampsia by prior immunization with the relevant paternal antigens.

▶ [This is an intriguing speculation about an immunogenetic basis of preeclampsia, using family study data from Aberdeen and from Leon Chesley. If the tendency for the disease is inherited as an autosomal recessive trait, as suggested, the involved genotype can be either maternal or fetal. The Aberdeen data are more compatible with the fetal genotype hypothesis whereas Chesley's observations fit better the maternal genotype hypothesis. It is of course conceivable that both mother and fetus could be involved in some type of genotype interaction.] ◀

Preeclampsia: State of Mother-Fetus Immune Imbalance. The cause of preeclampsia is not completely known, but both hereditary and acquired factors seem to be involved. Sporadic observations have been made of a reduced lymphocyte response to blast transformation, suggesting low immune responsiveness in preeclamptic women. S. A. Birkeland and K. Kristofferson[3-18] (Odense Univ.) monitored immune responsiveness in 5 women with preeclampsia and 22 normal women; respective average ages were 26.2 and 29.6 years. Four preeclamptic women and 16 normal women were completing their first pregnancies.

One preeclamptic woman had antibody to the father's leukocytes. The preeclamptic women had lower B lymphocyte counts at time of diagnosis and after delivery. The T cell counts were lower than in the normal group toward the end of pregnancy. Children born to preeclamptic women had increased B cell counts. Responses to phytohemagglutinin stimulation were significantly lower in preeclamptic women at diagnosis and after delivery. Preeclampsia developed in 1 woman who was initially considered to have a normal pregnancy; her phytohemagglutinin response fell to very low values between the fourth and sixth months of gestation when preeclampsia became apparent. The response to *Escherichia coli* also fell markedly, and the response to tuberculin purified protein derivative was below normal throughout.

Preeclampsia is associated with low T and B lymphocyte counts and low phytohemagglutinin responses. Fathers of infants born of preeclamptic women also have low B lymphocyte counts. It appears that maternal and paternal immune hyporesponsiveness, and child immune hyperresponsiveness, contribute to the development of preeclampsia and to the similarity between preeclampsia and the graft-

(3–18) Lancet 2:720–723, Oct. 6, 1979.

vs.-host reaction. Future studies will include measurement of T suppressor cells.

▶ [These differences in lymphocyte subtype populations between patients with preeclampsia, their husbands, and their children, on the one hand, and normal controls, on the other hand, are interesting, but, because of the small study population, the findings must be considered to be preliminary. How does preeclampsia associated with hydatidiform mole fit into the scheme?] ◀

Effect of Prostaglandin A₁ on Renal Hemodynamics in Pregnancy Toxemia.

Effect of Prostaglandin A$_1$ on Renal Hemodynamics in Pregnancy Toxemia. The A prostaglandins have been isolated from the renal medulla and implicated as possible mediators of a specific renal antihypertensive function. They are believed to be involved in the control of renal blood flow and in the fine adjustment of intrarenal blood distribution. Hypertensive patients have depressed plasma prostaglandin A (PGA) levels, and infusion of PGA induces a hypotensive response in such patients. M. Toppozada, A. Ghoneim, Y. A. Habib, L. El-Ziadi, and H. El-Damarawy[3-19] (Univ. of Alexandria) infused PGA$_1$ in 35 pregnant women in the third trimester. Ten normal women received 1 μg/kg per minute for 2 hours. Twenty patients with signs of pregnancy toxemia received similar infusions, whereas 5 others received 0.5 μg/kg per minute for 2 hours.

The high-dose PGA$_1$ infusion produced a hypotensive response in toxemia patients, but it did not alter blood pressures significantly in controls. The low-dose infusion resulted in an insignificant reduction in blood pressure in toxemic patients. The infusion was a weak uterine stimulant in all subjects. A significant increase in glomerular filtration rate was seen on PGA$_1$ infusion in both toxemic and control subjects. In toxemic patients the preexisting deficit resolved. Renal plasma flow increased markedly in all groups. No significant changes in plasma or urine sodium, potassium, or chloride, plasma osmolality, or blood urea values were observed. No appreciable diuresis occurred with the 2-hour infusion.

Prostaglandin A$_1$ appears to offer advantages as a therapeutic measure in toxemia of pregnancy. It has beneficial effects on renal and cardiovascular hemodynamics and may be of value for induction of labor. Its clinical use should at present be restricted to well-equipped institutions with facilities for continuous fetal and maternal monitoring. The optimum dosage and duration of PGA$_1$ therapy remain to be finally established.

▶ [Pregnancy normally involves the elaboration of something that protects the gravida against the hypertensive effects of increased renin activity. That "something" may be missing in toxemia patients, and if this line of reasoning is correct, the pathogenesis of toxemia involves a missing component rather than a toxin. One of the prime candidates for the role of "something" is prostaglandins of the A series. They are vasodilator substances that appear to be produced in the placenta, and depressed peripheral levels have been found in hypertensive patients. This interesting study indicates that PGA infusions lower blood pressure in toxemic (but not in normal) patients and improve renal function. With the higher dose, an oxytocic action was observed. These observations are exciting but we must realize that this is far from being a clinically applicable approach at present. More research is needed. After all, the history of preeclampsia therapy is loaded with treatments that enjoyed brief popularity before being discarded for one reason or another.] ◀

(3–19) Am. J. Obstet. Gynecol. 135:581–585, Nov. 1, 1979.

Hemodynamic Observations in Severe Preeclampsia With Flow-Directed Pulmonary Artery Catheter. Thomas J. Benedetti, David B. Cotton, John C. Read, and Frank C. Miller[3-20] (Univ. of Southern California) evaluated cardiopulmonary hemodynamics in ten patients with severe preeclampsia who were managed in a standardized manner during and after labor. All were in early labor when first studied. Patients were receiving an infusion of magnesium sulfate at a rate of 1.5 gm/hour and crystalloid solution at a rate of 75–100 ml/hour. Only a narcotic analgesic and a pudendal anesthetic were used for vaginal delivery. Four patients had a cesarean section.

The findings are summarized in the table. An elevated cardiac output was seen secondary to increases in both heart rate and stroke volume. Systemic vascular resistance was slightly elevated compared with normotensive patients in early labor. Pulmonary artery pressures did not differ significantly in the two groups. No consistent changes were noted between early labor and the early puerperium. In three cases, central venous pressures did not reflect pulmonary artery wedge pressures.

Pregnancy with severe preeclampsia appears not to affect pulmonary artery pressures. An elevation in left ventricular stroke work index was found in the present cases of severe preeclampsia, which suggests a hyperdynamic state. The pulmonary artery catheter may provide useful information in patients with hemorrhage or oliguria and in those who require a regional or general anesthetic.

▶ [These results indicate that cardiac output appears to be increased in patients with preeclampsia, in comparison with previously reported findings in normal subjects. The increase reflected elevations in both pulse rate and stroke volume. Because all preeclamptic women were receiving magnesium sulfate, it is not certain whether the difference is due to the disease or to treatment, though the former seems more likely. One important observation is the lack of a consistent relationship between central venous pressure and pulmonary artery wedge pressure; other studies in a variety of disease states have concluded that the Swan-Ganz catheter is preferable to the central venous pressure catheter when this type of hemodynamic monitoring is indicated.

Other enthusiastic reports of the Swan-Ganz catheter in management of acute cardiopulmonary problems in pregnancy were published by Berkowitz and Rafferty (Obstet. Gynecol. 55:507, 1980; and Am. J. Obstet. Gynecol. 137:127, 1980).] ◀

Hydrostatic Mechanism in Roll-Over Test. An increase in the diastolic blood pressure of ≥20 mm Hg that occurs on movement from the left lateral recumbent to the supine position (the roll-over test) reportedly predicts the development of hypertension during the third

HEMODYNAMICS IN SEVERE PREECLAMPSIA VS. NORMOTENSIVE LABOR			
	CO (L/min)	*HR*	*SV (ml)*
Severe pre-eclampsia—early labor	7.4	91	83
(Mean and SE)	(0.32)	(4.7)	(5.1)
Normotensive —early labor	5.5	83	69
(Mean and SE)	(0.54)	(5.4)	(7.3)

(3–20) Am. J. Obstet. Gynecol. 136:465–470, Feb. 15, 1980.

trimester of pregnancy. Previous studies have not considered the potential hydrostatic effect of the location of the arm in which the blood pressure is measured with respect to the level of the heart. B. Sobel, D. Laurent, S. Ganguly, L. Favro, and C. Lucas[3-21] (Wayne State Univ.) investigate the role of this hydrostatic mechanism in the blood pressure rise observed in the roll-over test.

METHOD.—Figure 3–2 demonstrates positioning of the patient and placement of the pressure cuff for these studies. First, 9 men and 8 nonpregnant women, aged 19–40 years, were tested. Blood pressure was measured in the right arm (superior side); when the diastolic pressure was constant, the subject assumed the supine position and the blood pressure was again measured. After a short interval, the procedure was repeated, using the left (inferior) arm.

The study was also performed in 10 normotensive primigravidas, aged 14–27 years, who were between 24 and 33 weeks of pregnancy. Blood pressure was recorded simultaneously in both arms. Blood pressure measurements were also taken during the roll-over test in 6 patients undergoing cardiac catheterization.

The results indicate that diastolic blood pressure appears to in-

Fig 3–2.—In roll-over test, blood pressure is recorded in right (superior) arm (A), and in left (inferior) arm in left lateral recumbent position (B) and then after the supine position is assumed. (Courtesy of Sobel, B., et al.: Obstet. Gynecol. 55:285–290, March 1980.)

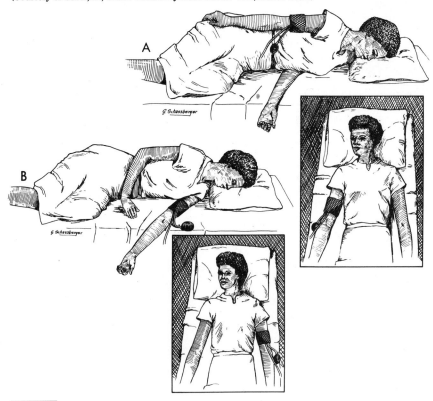

(3–21) Obstet. Gynecol. 55:285–290, March 1980.

DIASTOLIC BLOOD PRESSURE CHANGES IN PREGNANT WOMEN*

Position of subject	Right arm (superior)	Left arm (inferior)
Left lateral	53.6 ± 5	71.3 ± 7
Supine	70.2 ± 7	68.0 ± 7
Roll-over response	16.6 ± 4	−3.2 ± 2

*Values in mm Hg ± SD.
Mean distance between the two points where blood pressure was obtained was 22.1 ± 0.76 cm. Mean calculated hydrostatic pressure was 17.40 and was not significantly different from roll-over response obtained in right vs. left arm (16.6 mm Hg to −3.2 mm Hg = 19.8 mm Hg).

crease in both men and nonpregnant women when the right arm is used during the roll-over test. However, the opposite blood pressure response is seen when the left arm is used. This paradoxical response can be explained in terms of the hydrostatic effect of the arm position during the test. When blood pressure is taken in the right arm with the subject in the left lateral recumbent position, the arm is above the level of the heart, but when the left arm is used, that arm is below the level of the heart. When the subject rolls from the left lateral to the supine position, the blood pressure measured in the right arm would increase even if no physiologic change in blood pressure occurred at heart level. The diastolic pressure is consistently higher in the left (inferior) arm when the subject is in the left lateral position.

No change in central blood pressure was observed during the roll-over test in the catheterized patients.

The difference between the right and left arm blood pressures is also seen in pregnant patients (table). However, a significant difference is seen between pregnant and nonpregnant patients in the mean blood pressure readings when either arm is used. The actual increase in blood pressure is greater for both arms in pregnant patients, suggesting that a real increase in central blood pressure occurs in pregnant patients during the roll-over test.

▶ [These results are relevant not only to the roll-over test, but also to any other determination of blood pressure in a patient's arm. Hydrostatic factors may help explain some of the divergent values frequently recorded on a patient's chart.

Kassar et al. have also commented on the effects of hydrostatic pressure changes on the roll-over test (Obstet. Gynecol. 55:411, 1980).] ◀

Fetal Growth and Placental Function Assessed by Urinary Estriol Excretion Before Onset of Preeclampsia. Several reports suggest that placental function may be abnormal before preeclampsia becomes clinically apparent. Peter A. Long, David A. Abell, and Norman A. Beischer[3-22] (Univ. of Melbourne) evaluated fetoplacental function in 919 patients with preeclampsia by measuring urinary estriol excretion before (744 patients) and after (366 patients) onset of clinical signs of the disease.

(3–22) Am. J. Obstet. Gynecol. 135:344–347, Oct. 1, 1979.

TABLE 1.—FETAL OUTCOME ACCORDING TO ESTRIOL EXCRETION BEFORE AND AFTER ONSET OF PREECLAMPSIA

	Before onset of pre-eclampsia		After onset of pre-eclampsia	
Time of onset of pre-eclampsia	Small-for-dates infants (%)	Perinatal death rate (%)	Small-for-dates infants (%)	Perinatal death rate (%)
Less than 37 weeks' gestation:				
Normal estriol excretion	6.5*	3.3***	8.0***	0.8***
Low estriol excretion	22.6	12.9	35.2	14.8
More than 37 weeks' gestation:				
Normal estriol excretion	5.2**	—	9.3	—
Low estriol excretion	14.1	1.6	8.3	8.3
Total series:				
Normal estriol excretion	5.4***	0.5***	8.7***	0.4***
Low estriol excretion	16.8	5.3	29.5	13.4

*P <0.05.
**P < 0.01.
***P < 0.001.
These probabilities show significance of difference between groups of patients with normal and subnormal estriol excretion.

Low estriol excretion had a highly significant association with fetal growth retardation and perinatal death both before and after the onset of clinical signs of preeclampsia (Table 1). When assessed in terms of the incidence of low estriol excretion, fetal growth retardation, and perinatal wastage, preeclampsia of early onset (before 37 weeks) was considered a malignant disease in comparison with preeclampsia of late onset (after 37 weeks). Although the incidence of fetal growth retardation in the 919 patients with preeclampsia was only slightly higher than that of the hospital population, distribution of fetal growth retardation was sharply polarized between preeclampsia of early and late onset, there being a large and significant increase in its incidence in patients with early-onset disease.

When compared with the total obstetric population, patients destined to have early-onset preeclampsia had a high incidence (25.4%) of subnormal estriol excretion (Table 2). In this group there was further deterioration of placental function after the onset of clinical disease, with the incidence of subnormal estriol excretion increasing to 41.3%. Thus, fetal growth and prognosis are already determined, presumably due to impaired placental function, before the onset of clini-

TABLE 2.—INCIDENCE OF LOW ESTRIOL EXCRETION BEFORE AND AFTER ONSET OF PREECLAMPSIA

		Before onset of pre-eclampsia		After onset of pre-eclampsia	
Time of onset of pre-eclampsia	No. of patients	No. of patients screened	Low estriol excretion (%)	No. of patients screened	Low estriol excretion (%)
Less than 37 weeks' gestation	249	122	25.4***	213	41.3***
More than 37 weeks' gestation	670	622	10.3*	153	15.7 N.S.
Total series	919	744	12.8	366	30.6

*P < 0.05.
***P < 0.001.
N.S., not significant.
Probabilities represent significance of difference compared with hospital incidence of low estriol excretion (13.7% in 5,000 patients).

cal signs of preeclampsia when the disease occurs before 37 weeks' gestation.

Fetal Growth Retardation and Preeclampsia. P. A. Long, D. A. Abell, and N. A. Beischer[3-23] (Univ. of Melbourne) examined 2,434 consecutive singleton pregnancies with preeclampsia seen over a 7-year period to test their previous findings in 1977 that suggested fetal growth retardation frequently preceded signs of the disease in patients with early-onset preeclampsia and that hypoglycemia was directly related to the cause of perinatal death. Patients were grouped according to whether preeclampsia was diagnosed before (early onset) or after (late onset) the beginning of the 37th week of gestation.

The prevalence of fetal growth retardation was 8.7% compared with 8.6% in the total hospital population. The prevalence was increased in early-onset preeclampsia (18.2%) and reduced in late-onset preeclampsia (5.6%). In patients in whom early-onset preeclampsia with fetal growth retardation developed, the prevalence of subnormal estriol excretion was significantly increased (79.5%), compared to the late-onset group (25.0%), as was the prevalence of hypoglycemia (33.3%) compared to all patients with preeclampsia (13.8%). Placental abruption was more common in patients with early-onset preeclampsia and fetal growth retardation. In patients with early-onset preeclampsia, the perinatal mortality was 28.7% in those who had fetal growth retardation, compared to 6.4% in those who showed no fetal growth retardation.

Clinical signs of preeclampsia were observed for not more than a week before delivery in almost half of the patients in this study with both early-onset disease and fetal growth retardation. The brief duration of signs in so many and the high frequency of subnormal estriol excretion before the detection of early-onset preeclampsia suggests that fetal growth retardation in severe preeclampsia frequently precedes manifest disease. Significantly increased hypoglycemia in these patients corroborated the evidence from urinary estriol assays that confirmed this finding.

The strong association of hypoglycemia with perinatal mortality also implicated hypoglycemia in the cause of perinatal mortality. The study supported previous reports that placental insufficiency commonly precedes placental abruption.

▶ [Late-onset preeclampsia did not predispose to intrauterine growth retardation, as did early-onset preeclampsia. Those patients with early-onset disease had an increased likelihood of low estriol excretion and placental abruption as well. The central difference between the two groups probably relates to a greater prevalence of underlying vascular or renal disease in those patients with early-onset preeclampsia.] ◀

Management of Severe Toxemia in Patients at Less Than 36 Weeks' Gestation. The treatment of severe toxemia remains controversial, particularly in patients seen before 36 weeks' gestation. T. R. Martin and W. R. C. Tupper[3-24] (Dalhousie Univ.) evaluated a conservative approach to severe toxemia occurring before 36 weeks' gesta-

(3–23) Br. J. Obstet. Gynaecol. 87:13–18, January 1980.
(3–24) Obstet. Gynecol. 54:602–605, November 1979.

tion in 55 patients seen in 1973 to 1978, 39 primigravidas and 16 multiparas. These patients had persistent proteinuria and repeated blood pressures of 160/110 mm Hg or above.

Patients were placed at bed rest and given phenobarbital in doses of 60–120 mg 4 times daily, and magnesium sulfate if there was hyperreflexia or if the blood pressure approached 170/110 mm Hg. Magnesium was given either intramuscularly in a dose of 5 gm every 6 hours for four doses or intravenously in a dose of 2–4 gm, followed by an infusion of 1 gm/hour for about 24 hours. Antihypertensive agents were used for later exacerbations if the blood pressure approached 180/120 mm Hg.

Twelve patients received antihypertensive drugs, alone or with a diuretic. Three of 9 infants at 23 to 30 weeks' gestation died; 1 had multiple and lethal anomalies. Ten patients went into labor spontaneously, and 45 pregnancies were terminated, most often for fetal lung maturity or worsening maternal disease. Cesarean section delivery was performed in 53% of the cases. Over half of the 53 live neonates, including one set of twins, were severely growth-retarded. Two had severe respiratory distress syndrome, and 1 died of the disease. The perinatal mortality was 8.9%, and the corrected rate was 7.1%. Eleven of 47 patients followed for a mean of 25 months after delivery were hypertensive. Four had had hypertensive-renal disease before pregnancy, whereas 11 acquired essential hypertension after delivery.

Immediate antihypertensive drug therapy is not favored in this setting. Further study of the value of glucocorticoid therapy is needed.

▶ [The approach to the patient with severe toxemia at less than 36 weeks' gestation outlined by the authors is more conservative (perhaps a better term would be "more expectant") than is our own. In the absence of rapid in-hospital improvement in these patients, we generally effect delivery. The unfavorable nature of the uterine environment in this condition is underscored by the 57% rate of intrauterine growth retardation.] ◀

Relationship Between Maternal Hypertensive Disease of Pregnancy and Incidence of Idiopathic Respiratory Distress Syndrome. Jing Ja Yoon, Schuyler Kohl, and Rita G. Harper[3-25] (New York) analyzed the relationship between maternal hypertensive disease of pregnancy (HDOP) and idiopathic respiratory distress syndrome (IRDS) in a series of 2,105 premature infants weighing 1,000–2,199 gm at birth between 1968 and 1975. Gestational ages were 28 to 36 weeks. Twins were excluded. Hypertensive disease of pregnancy developed in 250 mothers. Mothers with mild preeclampsia were managed by bed rest and phenobarbital. Those with severe preeclampsia and eclampsia were treated with anticonvulsants, chiefly magnesium sulfate given parenterally, and antihypertensive drugs, chiefly hydralazine, and delivery.

Idiopathic respiratory distress syndrome was diagnosed in 28.2% of infants, including 15.2% of infants of mothers with HDOP and 29.9% of other infants, a significant difference. A significant difference was found for infants of gestational ages 32 weeks or less and 33 weeks

(3–25) Pediatrics 65:735–739, April 1980.

or more. The low rate of IRDS in the HDOP group persisted after infants with known predisposing and protecting factors were eliminated from consideration. The rate of IRDS was inversely related to the severity of maternal toxemia. Total mortality and mortality with IRDS did not differ significantly in the HDOP and non-HDOP groups. Among infants who did not develop IRDS, mortality in the HDOP group was significantly higher than that in the non-HDOP group, particularly for infants of lower gestational ages.

A decreased incidence of IRDS was found in infants of HDOP mothers in this study. The mechanism responsible for this is unclear, but chronic stress may accelerate fetal lung maturation. The data suggest that when stress is significant enough to accelerate fetal lung maturation, premature infants have no IRDS but have a higher mortality rate.

▶ [This study confirms a general impression that pregnancy-induced hypertension exerts some protective effect against respiratory distress, presumably mediated through glucocorticoid release with chronic stress. Though the frequency of respiratory distress syndrome was less in hypertensive than in nonhypertensive pregnancies, the overall mortality rates were not different. Thus, premature infants born to hypertensive women were *less* likely to die of respiratory distress syndrome but apparently were *more* likely to die of other causes.] ◀

Diagnosis of Multiple Pregnancy. Perinatal mortality is increased in twin pregnancies, and there are hazards to the second twin. In some series almost a third of twin pregnancies were not diagnosed until the second stage of labor. G. J. Jarvis[3-26] (Sheffield, England) reviewed the experience in the diagnosis of multiple pregnancy at a hospital where diagnostic ultrasound is in regular, but not routine, use. Ninety-four sets of twins were born in 1975–78, an incidence of 1 set per 115 pregnancies. Nine twin pregnancies were not diagnosed before the start of labor. Seventy-five were clinically suspected, and 10 were diagnosed unexpectedly in the antenatal period, 9 by ultrasonic examination. The initial clinical suspicion of multiple pregnancy arose from finding a large-for-dates uterus in 66 women, polyhydramnosis in 5, and multiple fetal parts on palpation in 4. Ultrasonic studies were done in 3 patients because of uncertain dates. The mean time between the initial suspicion of twin pregnancy and its confirmation was 1.6 weeks. Eighty twin pregnancies ultimately were diagnosed by ultrasonography.

Ultrasonic examination has substantially reduced the incidence of undiagnosed twin pregnancies. Some 20% of patients having ultrasonography done in the presence of a twin pregnancy, however, were reported on at least one occasion to have a singleton pregnancy. Ultrasonography must be done at least twice before multiple pregnancy can confidently be excluded.

▶ [This is a good news-bad news situation. The good news is that 90% of the twin pregnancies were diagnosed prior to labor. This is a higher figure than that usually reported, due in part to the 11% diagnosed unexpectedly, usually by ultrasound performed for some other reason. The bad news is that 14 of the 80 patients with diagnosed twins had at least one previous ultrasound in which only a single fetus was noted. Therefore, if we clinically suspect twins, we should not dismiss our suspicion

(3–26) Br. Med. J. 2:593–594, Sept. 8, 1979.

simply because a previous ultrasound report on the chart notes a singleton pregnancy. A second examination is indicated.] ◄

Sonar Cephalometry in Twins: Table of Biparietal Diameters for Normal Twin Fetuses and Comparison with Singletons. Sonography has become the preferred method for detecting twin pregnancies. Once two separate biparietal diameters (BPDs) are recognized, prediction of gestational age is based on BPD tables derived from singleton pregnancies; however, the accuracy of predicting the gestational age of twin pregnancies with the use of such data is unknown. Kenneth J. Leveno, Rigoberto Santos-Ramos, Johann H. Duenhoelter, Joan S. Reisch, and Peggy J. Whalley[3-27] (Univ. of Texas Southwestern Med. School) examined the relationship between mean BPDs of twin singleton fetuses at 16 to 40 weeks' gestation. Study was made of 123 otherwise uncomplicated twin pregnancies yielding normal infants, in all of which the BPDs were within 4 mm of one another. The mean number of sonar studies per pregnancy was 2.8. Initial sonar cephalometry was done before 28 weeks' gestation in 61% of cases.

The mean gestational age at delivery was 37 weeks. Nearly 80% of infants were at or below the 50th percentile, and 25% were below the 10th percentile for body weight. Mean BPDs of twin fetuses were con-

PREDICTED BPDs* OF TWIN FETUSES BETWEEN
16 AND 40 WEEKS' GESTATION

Weeks' gestation	Mean BPD (mm)
16	32.9
17	36.7
18	40.5
19	44.1
20	47.6
21	51.0
22	54.2
23	57.4
24	60.4
25	63.3
26	66.1
27	68.7
28	71.3
29	73.7
30	76.0
31	78.2
32	80.3
33	82.2
34	84.1
35	85.8
36	87.4
37	88.8
38	90.2
39	91.4
40	92.5

*Measurements on bistable scope with the use of outer-to-outer edge.

(3–27) Am. J. Obstet. Gynecol. 135:727–730, Nov. 15, 1979.

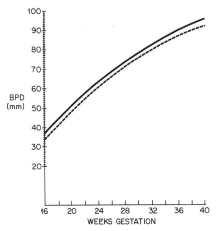

Fig 3–3.—Smoothed mean twin *(dashed line)* and singleton *(solid line)* biparietal diameters between 16 and 40 weeks' gestation. Smoothing was done by the use of polynomial regression equations. The equation for twins is: Predicted BPD = $-45.097 + 5.827$ weeks $- 0.0597$ (weeks)^2. The equation for singletons is: Predicted BPD = $-39.424 + 5.694$ weeks $- 0.0578$ (weeks)^2. (Courtesy of Leveno, K. J., et al.: Am. J. Obstet. Gynecol. 135:727–730, Nov. 15, 1979.)

sistently smaller than those of singletons, the difference averaging 3.3 mm at 16 to 30 weeks' gestation and increasing to 3.8 mm as pregnancy advanced. Predicted BPD values are given in the table. The correlation coefficient for the polynomial regression equation predicting mean twin BPDs was 0.968. Predicted mean twin and singleton BPDs are compared in Figure 3–3.

This table of BPDs for normal twin pregnancies permits a more accurate assessment of twin gestational age and fetal growth.

▶ [This report provides new and valuable information about BPD growth in twins. Its most important finding is that the heads of twins are consistently smaller than those of singleton infants throughout at least the last two thirds of intrauterine life. Thus, the general concept from birth weight data that twins grow at the normal rate until the middle of the third trimester and then slow does not seem to apply to growth of the BPD. The data in the table will provide a useful reference.

In contrast to these findings, Crane et al. (Obstet. Gynecol. 55:678, 1980) reported that like-size twins have biparietal growth that is similar to that of singletons appropriate for gestational age in their population at all stages of gestation. The BPD growth curve of twins is considered in more detail in the following article.] ◀

Zygosity and Intrauterine Growth of Twins. Recent findings indicate that the biparietal diameter (BPD) growth curve of second twins runs consistently below that of first twins. Monozygotic twins are generally lighter at birth and have greater intrapair weight differences than dizygotic twins. Lars Grennert, Per-Håkan Persson, Gerhard Gennser, and Bo Gullberg[3-28] (Univ. of Lund) examined the association between zygosity and intrauterine BPD growth in a group of twins undergoing longitudinal monitoring of the BPD. A total of 678 sonar measurements of fetal BPD were used to assess the growth of 182 twins from 18 to 40 weeks' gestation. Pregnancies lasting less

(3–28)   Obstet. Gynecol. 55:684–687, June 1980.

than 28 weeks were excluded. Most deliveries were induced before week 40.

The growth curve for the dizygotic first twin was consistently above that of the monozygotic first twin. The same relationship was observed between dizygotic and monozygotic second twins. In intrapair comparisons, first twins from both monozygotic and dizygotic pairs had the larger BPD values. The differences were apparent at 18 to 25 weeks' gestation. Dizygotic twins were insignificantly heavier than monozygotic twins at birth. Intrapair differences in weight were greater in dizygotic pairs. Total placental weight was greater for dizygotic twin pairs. Five of 45 monozygotic twin pairs had a clinical diagnosis of transfusion syndrome.

This is the first study to demonstrate an association between zygosity and intrauterine growth of the BPD in twins. The lower growth profile of the head diameter in monozygotic twins should be regarded as more significant than the previously observed birth weight differences. Discrepancy in head growth between monozygotic and dizygotic twins appears to be determined at an early stage. It is unclear whether monozygotic twinning by its pathogenesis might be associated with reduced growth potential. Bulmer showed in lower vertebrates that factors such as lack of oxygen can lead to monozygotic twinning through retardation of early development.

▶ [In this study, the mean BPD of dizygotic twins was greater than that of monozygotic twins and the mean BPD of the "first" twin was greater than that of the "second" twin regardless of zygosity. Although dizygotic twins were somewhat heavier than monozygotic twins, this difference did not reach statistical significance. In contrast to earlier reports, monozygotic twins showed smaller intrapair weight differences than did dizygotic twins in the present study.] ◀

Double-Blind Trial of Ritodrine and Placebo in Twin Pregnancy. Premature delivery occurs in over 30% of twin pregnancies in most reported series, and is largely responsible for the high perinatal mortality associated with twinning. The value of prophylactic bed rest in the last trimester appears doubtful, and cervical cerclage has proved ineffective in reducing premature deliveries. M. C. O'Connor, H. Murphy, and I. J. Dalrymple[3-29] carried out a double-blind trial of ritodrine therapy in 49 patients with twin pregnancies, confirmed by ultrasound at 20 to 34 weeks' gestation. Twenty-five patients received 40 mg ritodrine by mouth daily, whereas 24 received a placebo. Treatment was stopped at 37 weeks' gestation, and patients who had not already delivered had labor induced at 38 to 40 weeks.

Ritodrine therapy was begun at a mean of 28.4 weeks' gestation. Spontaneous premature deliveries were comparably frequent in the ritodrine-treated and placebo groups, and there was no significant difference in mean gestational age at delivery. The induction rate was 43% in the ritodrine group and 52% in the placebo group. Birth weights were similar in the two groups. Ritodrine therapy did not significantly reduce the number of infants with birth weights below the 10th or 5th percentile. No reduction in the rate of low Apgar

(3–29) Br. J. Obstet. Gynaecol. 86:706–709, September 1979.

scores was observed. Muscle tremor occurred in nearly all patients, and over half had palpitations from ritodrine therapy. One patient had sinus tachycardia.

Oral ritodrine did not prevent premature delivery or improve intra-uterine growth in twin pregnancies in this study. A double-blind trial of fenoterol in adequate dosage is needed, but further evaluation of the prophylactic use of ritodrine in twin pregnancies probably is un-justified.

▶ [In this controlled double-blind study of ritodrine prophylaxis in twin pregnancy, spontaneous labor before 37 weeks' gestation occurred in 5 of 25 (20%) treated patients compared with 9 of 23 (39%) controls. The difference was not statistically signif-icant, though it might become so with a larger series. Nevertheless, from these obser-vations it does seem unlikely that β-adrenergic agents will prove to be the answer to the major problem with multiple gestation.] ◀

Comparison of Uteroplacental Blood Flow in Normal and in Intrauterine Growth-Retarded Pregnancy: Measurements With Indium-113m and a Computer-Linked Gamma Camera. N. O. Lunell, B. Sarby, R. Lewander, and L. Nylund[3-30] (Huddinge Univ. Hosp., Huddinge, Sweden) used a computer-linked gamma camera technique for the time-activity analysis of ^{113m}In, as a noninvasive means of comparing uteroplacental blood flow in relative terms in normal and intrauterine growth retardation (IUGR) pregnancies, de-fined as a fetal weight below the tenth percentile for sex and gesta-tional age.

Eleven normal and eight IUGR pregnancies were evaluated in the last trimester. Each subject received 1 mCi ^{113m}In-chloride by intra-venous injection. Placental blood flow was expressed as an index or ratio between the maximum of the time-activity curve and the rise time of the curve.

The mean placental blood flow in the IUGR pregnancies was only one fourth of corresponding mean values in the normal group. The difference between the two groups was highly significant. Rise times were longer in the IUGR cases, and the flow-volume ratios were lower. Activity maxima also were lower in the IUGR cases.

It is often difficult to diagnose IUGR prenatally, especially if the gestational age is uncertain. An acute reduction in uteroplacental blood flow resulting in placental insufficiency might not produce IUGR and might be overlooked clinically. The present method might help detect such states. The radiation dose to the fetus is only 10 mrad.

▶ [This study found that placental blood flow was decreased in patients with growth-retarded fetuses. We do not know the maternal conditions associated with growth re-tardation in these patients, but the results are not surprising. The determinations were generally done late in pregnancy and cause vs. effect is unclear. Blood flow was in-ferred in this tracer study by the rate of uptake and maximal uptake at the placental site. The technique, assumptions, and mathematics are complex, but, if the authors truly are describing placental blood flow, they have an important tool. So often in ob-stetrics, we speculate as to the effects of various diseases and treatments on placental blood flow. Perhaps we will gain real information in this most important area.] ◀

Platelet Life Span in Pregnancies Resulting in Small-for-Ges-tational-Age Infants. Henk C. S. Wallenburg and Piet H. van Kes-

(3–30) Gynecol. Obstet. Invest. 10:106–118, 1979.

sel[3-31] (Erasmus Univ., Rotterdam, Netherlands) measured platelet number and life span during the last trimester of pregnancy in 22 women in whom insufficient fetal growth was confirmed by ultrasound examinations and who were delivered of infants small for gestational age and in 21 randomly selected women delivered of infants having normal birth weights. Platelet life span was determined by a nonradioisotopic method involving the use of acetylsalicylic acid. Except for insufficient fetal growth in the first group, all pregnancies were uncomplicated.

As shown in Figure 3–4, mean platelet life span was 7.2 days in the women delivered of small infants and 9.2 days in those delivered of normal infants. Mean platelet concentration was $235 \times 10^9/L$ in women delivered of small infants and $208 \times 10^9/L$ in women delivered of normal infants. There was no significant correlation between platelet number and life span. Platelet life span was restudied at 2 months

Fig 3–4.—Platelet life span in pregnancies resulting in infants who are small for gestational age *(A)* and in infants with normal birth weights *(B)*. Bar represents the mean ± SD. (Courtesy of Wallenburg, H. C. S., and van Kessel, P. H.: Am. J. Obstet. Gynecol. 134:739–742, Aug. 1, 1979.)

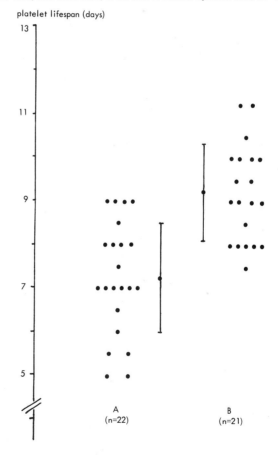

(3–31)   Am. J. Obstet. Gynecol. 134:739–742, Aug. 1, 1979.

post partum in 2 patients delivered of small infants; their platelet life spans of 6.5 and 7 days had returned to normal values of 9 and 10 days, respectively.

The reduced platelet life span and increased platelet concentration in pregnant women with insufficient fetal growth indicate a compensated thrombocytolytic state with increased platelet turnover. This could be explained by increased platelet consumption in the uteroplacental arterial bed.

▶ [An interesting observation is described here. "Normal" patients delivering babies small for gestational age had shortened platelet life spans. The authors speculate that this may be due to platelet aggregation in the uteroplacental vessels that would interfere with maternal-placental exchange. Although this is an intriguing speculation, at this point that is all it is.] ◀

Coitus and Associated Amniotic Fluid Infections. Amniotic fluid infections in the presence of intact fetal membranes appear to be the most common cause of fetal and neonatal death in the United States. The bacteria responsible usually reach the amniotic fluid through the cervical os, and coitus may contribute to the genesis of these infections. Richard L. Naeye[3-32] (Pennsylvania State Univ.) investigated this possibility by analyzing data from 26,886 pregnancies in the Collaborative Perinatal Project. Amniotic fluid infection was

FREQUENCY AND OUTCOME OF AMNIOTIC FLUID INFECTIONS			
CHARACTERISTIC	COITUS*	NO COITUS	P VALUE
Gestational age 20–24 wk			
Cases/1000 births	688 (33)†	354 (23)†	<0.05
Deaths/100 cases	60.6 (20)†	47.8 (11)†	>0.1
Perinatal mortality rate	416.7†	169.2†	<0.05
Gestational age 25–28 wk			
Cases/1000 births	374 (40)†	286 (52)†	>0.1
Deaths/100 cases	52.5 (21)†	32.7 (17)†	>0.1
Perinatal mortality rate	196.3†	93.4†	<0.05
Gestational age 29–32 wk			
Cases/1000 births	251 (58)†	207 (114)†	>0.1
Deaths/100 cases	20.7 (12)†	7.9 (9)†	<0.05
Perinatal mortality rate	51.9†	16.3†	<0.02
Gestational age 33–36 wk			
Cases/1000 births	158 (106)	153 (308)†	>0.1
Deaths/100 cases	4.7 (5)	1.9 (6)	>0.1
Perinatal mortality rate	7.4	3.0‡	>0.1
Gestational age 37–38 wk			
Cases/1000 births	116 (81)	118 (410)	>0.1
Deaths/100 cases	3.7 (3)	1.7 (7)	>0.1
Perinatal mortality rate	4.3	2.0	>0.1
Gestational age >38 wk			
Cases/1000 births	137 (299)	106 (1803)	<0.001
Deaths/100 cases	2.3 (7)	0.9 (16)	<0.05
Perinatal mortality rate§	3.2	0.9	<0.01

*Coitus once a wk or more during mo. before delivery. Figures in parentheses denote no. of cases.

†$P < 0.001$ as compared with value in gestational age category more than 38 wk.

‡$P < 0.01$ as compared with value in gestational age category more than 38 wk.

§Number of fetal and neonatal deaths per 1,000 births.

(3–32) N. Engl. J. Med. 301:1198–1200, Nov. 29, 1979.

diagnosed when there was acute inflammation in the subchorionic plate of the placenta.

Mothers who reported having coitus once a week or more often in the month before delivery had more frequent amniotic fluid infections before 33 weeks' gestation than others (table). Infections were also more frequent if coitus was reported after 38 weeks' gestation. At all gestational ages, perinatal mortality due to the infections was two to three times greater when coitus had taken place. The frequency with which local infections in the extraplacental membranes spread to the amniotic fluid decreased with advancing gestational age. At 38 weeks, the rates of spread were 76% with coitus and 51% without it. More blacks than whites had coitus during pregnancy and this, with socioeconomic status, explained most of the increased frequency of infection-related deaths observed in blacks. Many more mothers were found to be having coitus if data collected in the antepartum clinic were used from any given gestational period.

Coitus during pregnancy may increase the frequency and severity of amniotic fluid infections and thereby increase fetal and neonatal mortality. It may be that fastidious perineal cleaning by the coital partners or the use of condoms can reduce the frequency and improve the outcome of these infections, but further clinical studies are needed to elucidate the reasons for the association of coitus with amniotic fluid infections.

▶ [This article suggesting that coitus in late pregnancy increases both the frequency and the severity of amniotic fluid infections will likely cause reverberations around the world. While it is certainly provocative, several things argue for caution in interpretation. Two general features of the Collaborative Perinatal Project must be kept in mind: (1) the study was conducted 15–20 years ago and applicability of its findings to the contemporary situation is problematic and (2) the data gathering in this multi-institutional study was undoubtedly done by individuals with little interest in the study itself or how the results might be used. There must be some inherent skepticism about patient responses to such an emotion-laden topic as sex. The article states that the incidence of infections increased only slightly when the frequency of intercourse was reported to be twice or more weekly as opposed to once weekly, and this lack of a "dose-response" relationship seems curious. Finally, as indicated in the table, the fatality rate (i.e., deaths per 1,000 cases) was higher with coitus in each gestational age interval but statistically significantly so in only the 29- to 32-week and >38-week periods.

In another report from the same data base, Naeye (Lancet 1:192, 1980) examined patients with premature rupture of the membranes and found again that coital frequency seemed to increase the severity (i.e., more infection-related deaths) but not the incidence of amniotic fluid infections.] ◀

Bacterial Colonization of Amniotic Fluid From Intact Fetal Membranes. With rare exceptions, intact membranes have been considered to be a barrier to infection of the amniotic fluid. Joseph M. Miller, Jr., Marcos J. Pupkin, and Gale B. Hill[3-33] (Duke Univ.) collected amniotic fluid from 45 patients by amniocentesis or needle amniotomy before or during labor, or by needle aspiration at cesarean section. Fluid was cultured and examined directly by use of a Gram stain. All the patients had intact membranes. In 23 of 31 patients in labor the gestational age was under 35 weeks. Most specimens were delivered within 2 hours.

(3–33) Am. J. Obstet. Gynecol. 136:796–804, Mar. 15, 1980.

Only 1 of the 14 patients not in labor had bacteria isolated from broth culture. Thirteen amniotic fluid cultures from 31 patients in labor were positive on primary cultures from 31 patients in labor were positive on primary plating mediums, and 5 others grew in broth only. Of the 13 patients with more than 10^2 colony-forming units (CFU)/ml, 8 had clinical chorioamnionitis; 3 of the 5 patients without fever or symptoms had premature labor. Six positive cultures yielded only aerobes and 5, only anaerobes. Bacteria and leukocytes on the Gram stain of unspun amniotic fluid were significantly associated with cultures yielding more than 10^2 CFU/ml. Both bacteria on the stain and more than 10^2 CFU/ml on culture were significantly associated with clinical chorioamnionitis. Neither of the 2 mothers with postpartum endometritis was febrile before delivery. One of them had a positive amniotic fluid culture.

A wider spectrum of bacteria colonizing amniotic fluid from intact membranes was found in this study than has previously been appreciated. A direct Gram stain in addition to culture of the amniotic fluid can provide valuable diagnostic information. Not all patients with clinical chorioamnionitis have significant bacterial growth in the amniotic fluid. The infection could be limited to the membranes or placenta, or other microorganisms could be involved.

▶ [This study documents that bacterial invasion of the amniotic sac can occur with intact membranes, especially with labor. Moreover, the number of different bacterial species found is greater than that generally appreciated. Of particular importance is the high incidence (half of positive cultures) of anaerobic organisms.] ◀

Psychosocial Stress in Pregnancy and Its Relation to Onset of Premature Labor. Richard W. Newton (Manchester, England), Pat A. C. Webster, P. S. Binu, Neal Maskrey, and A. B. Phillips[3-34] (Hull, England) attempted to define the extent to which psychosocial stress determines the onset of premature labor. Stress was measured by a modified form of the Life Events Inventory developed by Cochrane and Robertson. The inventory was validated in a study of 160 women and the validated inventory was presented to 132 consecutive women entering labor over a 4-month period at two institutions. Eighty-three were at term, whereas 30 were at 33 to 36 weeks' gestation, and 19 were under 33 weeks' gestation. The three groups were comparable in age, gravidity, and parity.

Only 43% of mothers whose pregnancies went to term experienced any major life events, compared with 67% of those who went into preterm labor at 33 to 36 weeks and 84% of those whose labor was earlier. Numbers of major life events per pregnancy are given in Table 1 and numbers of events in relation to social class in Table 2. Psychosocial stress was significantly higher with more premature labors, although the difference between the two preterm groups was not significant. Descending socioeconomic class was associated with increase in the number of major life events recorded per pregnancy in the term and preterm groups.

Pregnancies resulting in premature labor are far more likely to

(3–34) Br. Med. J. 2:411–413, Aug. 18, 1979.

TABLE 1.—MEAN NUMBER OF MAJOR LIFE EVENTS PER PREGNANCY IN
THREE STUDY GROUPS

	≥37 weeks (n = 83)	33–36 weeks (n = 30)	<33 weeks (n = 19)
Mean No of life events per pregnancy	0·63	1·33	1·95
Mean No of life events in last week per pregnancy	0·04	0·27	0·42

TABLE 2.—MEAN NUMBER OF MAJOR LIFE EVENTS PER PREGNANCY
ACCORDING TO SOCIAL CLASS IN GROUPS WITH GESTATION UNDER OR OVER
37 WEEKS

	Social class				
	I	II	III	IV	V
≥37 weeks		0·43	0·44	0·75	0·84
<37 weeks	1·0	1·2	1·35	2·00	2·13

have been stressful. This is particularly striking because fewer major life events would be expected in a shortened pregnancy. The provision of more specially trained social workers at antenatal clinics might be indicated. Should these findings be ignored, the authors believe that the prevalence of premature labor cannot be further reduced, and perinatal mortality and morbidity resulting from psychosocial stress may soon reach an irreducible minimum.

▶ [Since premature labor is the foremost obstetric problem, this report showing a relationship between premature labor and "major life events" independent of social class is intriguing. Much more needs to be learned, however. Many of the listed "life events" are quite subjective and hard to interpret. For example, do arguments between husband and wife *cause* premature labor or does the stress of the abnormally early parturition with its attendant anxiety create strains in the marital relationship?] ◀

Antepartum Aminophylline Treatment for Prevention of Respiratory Distress Syndrome in Premature Infants. Corticosteroids enhance the maturation of fetal lungs but may produce side effects. Studies with pregnant rabbits suggest that aminophylline administration produces earlier maturation of fetal lungs. E. Hadjigeorgiou, S. Kitsiou, A. Psaroudakis, C. Segos, D. Nicolopoulos, and D. Kaskarelis[3-35] conducted a clinical trial of aminophylline treatment in 142 women (148 neonates) at risk of premature delivery who were admitted to Alexandra Maternity Hospital, Athens. None had conditions known to affect fetal pulmonary maturation, membranes which had ruptured more than 48 hours before admission, or small-for-dates babies.

All women received isoxsuprine in an initial dose of 0.25 to 0.5 mg/minute intravenously for 40 to 60 minutes and subsequently in a dose of 5 to 20 mg intramuscularly every 3 to 6 hours for 24 hours. Oral administration of the same dosage followed. Delay of delivery was attempted only for 48 hours. The 67 women randomly assigned to also receive aminophylline were given 250 mg intramuscularly on admission and every 12 hours thereafter for 3 days. If, as rarely happened, delivery was delayed for more than 7 days after aminophylline

(3–35) Am. J. Obstet. Gynecol. 135:257–260, Sept. 15, 1979.

CORRELATION BETWEEN DURATION OF GESTATION AND FREQUENCY OF IDIOPATHIC RESPIRATORY
DISTRESS SYNDROME*

Gestation (wk.)	Aminophylline group		Control group		Statistical analysis
	No. of neonates	IRDS	No. of neonates	IRDS	
28-30	25	3 (13%)	17	9 (53%)	S(p < 0.01)
30-32	16	1 (6.2%)	21	6 (28.6%)	NS
32-34	29	2 (6.9%)	40	8 (20%)	NS
Total	70	7 (10%)	78	23 (29.5%)	S(p < 0.01)

*IRDS, idiopathic respiratory distress syndrome; NS, not significant.

was discontinued, a similar 3-day regimen of aminophylline administration was repeated every week until the 34th week of pregnancy was approached.

The frequency of idiopathic respiratory distress in infants of 28 to 34 weeks' gestation was 10% in the aminophylline group, compared with 29.5% in the control group (table). A significant decrease in frequency of respiratory distress after aminophylline treatment was noted in infants whose mothers had their membranes ruptured for more than 24 hours and when the time between the first injection and delivery was longer than 24 hours. The perinatal mortality rate was 7.1% in the aminophylline group and 17.9% in the controls. No complications or side effects of aminophylline administration were noted in the mothers or the infants.

► [This preliminary study suggests that aminophylline administered to mothers at risk for premature delivery decreases the frequency of the respiratory distress syndrome in their premature offspring. Statistical significance was reached for the group that delivered from 28 to 30 weeks' gestation. As with antenatal glucocorticoid treatment, more needs to be learned about efficacy and safety, but the results reported here are intriguing.] ◄

4. Antepartum Fetal Surveillance

Simple Technique for Visualization of Vagina During Ultrasound Scanning. The indications for ultrasound scanning in obstetrics and gynecology are rapidly expanding; the study is done almost routinely during pregnancy to evaluate intrauterine development of the fetus. Improved visualization of the pelvic organs may contribute greatly to proper diagnosis. Y. Beyth and M. Ron[4-1] (Hadassah Univ. Hosp.) describe a simple method of clearly visualizing the vagina during ultrasound scanning. If it is performed with the bladder full and well outlined, mistakes in localizing the uterus and ovaries will be avoided. A 10-ml syringe is filled with sterile water, sealed, cleaned with aqueous chlorhexidine solution, and introduced into the vagina before scanning (Fig 4−1).

This procedure simplifies localization of the pelvic organs and permits a more precise interpretation of the scan findings, particularly when gray-scale equipment is not available. The method may aid in differentiating intrauterine and tubal pregnancies, solid ovarian tumors, and uterine fibroids. Its use is contraindicated in women with cervical incompetence associated with a dilated cervix. It should not be used in patients with amniotic fluid leakage. Use of the cylinder is not necessary when vaginal bleeding is present. The procedure is safe

Fig 4−1.—Longitudinal midline section of ultrasound scanning performed at 11 weeks' gestation. The vagina is well outlined and clearly visualized. *U*, uterus; *B*, bladder; *V*, vagina. (Courtesy of Beyth, Y., and Ron, M.: Isr. J. Med. Sci. 16:118−120, February 1980.)

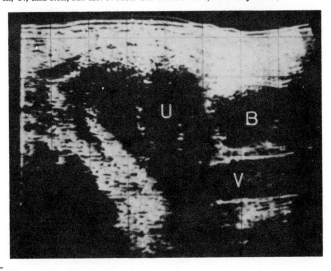

(4−1) Isr. J. Med. Sci. 16:118−120, February 1980.

and easy to carry out. There is no patient discomfort, and the slight distortion of pelvic anatomy that results does not interfere with improved interpretation of the scan findings.

▶ [This article describes a neat little trick for use as an adjunct in ultrasound scanning—vaginal insertion of a plastic syringe container filled with water. It is probably not necessary with gray-scale techniques, but it might prove helpful in other situations.] ◀

Prediction of Intrauterine Growth Retardation via Ultrasonically Measured Head-Abdominal Circumference Ratios. Biparietal measurements can be used to detect intrauterine growth retardation (IUGR), but two major shortcomings exist: false positive results and the need to obtain two ultrasound recordings at least 2 to 3 weeks apart. James P. Crane and Mazie M. Kopta[4-2] (Washington Univ., St. Louis) assessed the proposal made by Campbell and Thoms (1977) that the head-abdominal circumference (H-A) ratio could be used to detect IUGR related to uteroplacental insufficiency because uteroplacental insufficiency typically results in asymmetric growth retardation, with the liver (thus, abdominal circumference) affected to a greater extent than the brain (thus, head circumference). This would make the H-A ratio unusually high in an asymmetrically growth-retarded fetus.

Ultrasound measurements were made of fetal head and abdomen diameters, from which circumferences were calculated, of 47 patients. Of these, 28 were referred for initial ultrasound examination during the third trimester because of clinically suspected IUGR. The other 19 had baseline scans during the second trimester and were evaluated with the H-A ratio because of subsequent flattening of biparietal diameter growth on serial scans during the third trimester.

Of the 28 patients (Fig 4–2), 21 had one or more H-A ratios that

Fig 4–2.—Head-abdominal ratio in 28 fetuses with clinically suspected intrauterine growth retardation and an initial biparietal diameter < -2 SD for gestational age. Solid circles indicate head-abdominal values obtained from 21 fetuses average for gestational age. Open circles indicate values for 7 fetuses small for gestational age. (Courtesy of Crane, J. P., and Kopta, M. M.: Obstet. Gynecol. 54:597–601, November 1979.)

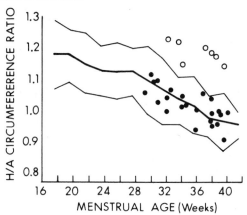

(4–2) Obstet. Gynecol. 54:597–601, November 1979.

were normal for gestational age, and all 21 infants were classified at birth as appropriate for gestational age. The other 7 fetuses had H-A ratios that were abnormally high, and IUGR related to uteroplacental insufficiency was predicted; at birth, all 7 infants were classified as small for gestational age.

Of the 19 patients with suspected IUGR based on suboptimal increases of biparietal diameter, 16 had one or more normal H-A ratio measurements despite the fact that little or no increment in biparietal diameter was noted on serial examinations during the third trimester; at birth, all 16 infants were classified as adequate for gestational age. The remaining 3 fetuses had elevated H-A ratios, and all 3 were classified as small for gestational age at birth.

The H-A ratio is a sensitive index of IUGR related to uteroplacental insufficiency. Use of this method minimizes the possibility of false diagnosis in women referred for initial evaluation late in pregnancy and in patients who show abnormal slowing of third-trimester biparietal growth for reasons other than uteroplacental insufficiency.

▶ [The H-A circumference ratio effectively identified asymmetrically growth-retarded fetuses in this study. More numbers are needed to know whether the separation between fetuses appropiate for gestational age and small for gestational age is as good as it seems. The technique (using "area" rather than "circumference") has been successfully used by others. Read on.] ◀

Ultrasound Assessment of Fetal Growth. Thankam R. Varma, H. Taylor, and C. Bridges[4-3] (St. George's Hosp. and Med. School, London) obtained consecutive ultrasonic measurements of the fetal head area, thorax area, abdomen area, head-thorax area ratio, and head-abdomen area ratio from 100 patients with normal pregnancies and 186 with suspected intrauterine fetal growth retardation. All measurements were made from B-scan echograms obtained using a diasonograph with a 2.5-MHz transducer. Biparietal diameter was measured by the combined A- and B-scan method. Thirty-five patients in the study group were delivered of light for dates infants. Twenty-six of these infants had birth weights at or below the fifth percentile, whereas 9 had weights between the fifth and tenth percentiles.

With one measurement of the head area 10 days before delivery, 74.3% of light for dates infants were identified. With measurement at 33 weeks' gestation, only 57% were identified. A single thoracic area measurement at 33 weeks and at 10 days before delivery led to identification of 71.4% and 82.9% of light for dates infants, respectively. About 80% of the diagnoses also were made from abdominal area measurements. A single measurement of the head-thorax area identified 77% of cases at 33 weeks and 83% within 10 days before delivery. The head-abdomen area ratio was the best means of identifying fetal growth retardation. One measurement identified 82.9% of light for dates infants at 33 weeks and 85.7% within 10 days of delivery. The respective false negative rates were 17.1% and 14.3%. The false positive rates were low.

A single measurement of fetal abdomen area and the head-abdomen area ratio appears to be the most reliable and efficient means of

(4–3) Br. J. Obstet. Gynaecol. 86:623–632, August 1979.

identifying intrauterine fetal growth retardation. Ideally, fetal maturity would be assessed early in all at-risk pregnancies, with measurement of the fetal abdomen at 32 to 33 weeks' gestation and a repeat measurement at 36 to 38 weeks. The head-abdomen area ratio provides a method for identifying the type of growth retardation that is important in further management of the pregnancy.

▶ [In this study, the head-abdomen area ratio was found to be the most reliable diagnostic index of fetal growth retardation tested, correctly identifying 83–86% of cases, with a false negative rate of 14–17% and a false positive rate of 8–9%. The fetal liver is generally considered to be affected first and most severely with fetal malnutrition, whereas the brain is generally spared. Thus, the head-abdomen area ratio is a larger value with the growth-retarded fetus than in the normally growing fetus.] ◀

Assay of a Placental Protein to Determine Fetal Risk. Lin et al. in 1973 isolated pregnancy-associated plasma protein A (PAPP-A) from pregnant women. It is produced in the placenta and its concentration increases with growth of the placenta as pregnancy advances. Graeme Hughes, Paul Bischof, George Wilson and Arnold Klopper[4-4] (Univ. of Aberdeen) estimated plasma concentrations and total amounts of PAPP-A in 272 patients at 34 weeks' pregnancy with the use of a simple immunoelectrophoretic technique to determine whether the screening of large numbers of patients is feasible. Ninety-six patients had clinical obstetric abnormalities, some of them at the time of evaluation at 34 weeks' pregnancy.

The mean plasma concentration and mean total amount of PAPP-A were closely related and were significantly elevated in 28 patients who subsequently had preeclampsia, 12 who went into premature labor and 10 who suffered from antepartum hemorrhage. The mean values were also increased in all patients delivering growth-retarded infants, but no difference remained when the results for such patients who also had other complications were excluded.

The PAPP-A assay is easily performed and may be a useful means of screening pregnant women to detect those at risk of acquiring preeclamptic toxemia. More needs to be learned about the function of this protein before the full potential of the assay can be realized. The assay is of no value in diagnosing fetal growth retardation, since the protein is of placental origin. Untoward immune responses have often been implicated in preeclampsia and there is increasing evidence that PAPP-A participates in the immunologic interaction between trophoblast and maternal tissues. If PAPP-A is a locally active, nontoxic biologic immunosuppressive agent, it may find applications in such areas as transplant surgery.

▶ [This preliminary report suggests that PAPP-A levels are higher in maternal plasma in patients destined to develop preeclampsia, antepartum hemorrhage, or premature labor than in controls. Considerable overlap exists. As we have previously been disappointed in the predictive value of other placental proteins (eg, human placental lactogen), we will sit on the sidelines for now.] ◀

Intrauterine Supraventricular Tachycardia. Jane W. Newburger and John F. Keane[4-5] (Harvard Med. School) report 6 cases of intrauterine supraventricular tachycardia (SVT) and review 31 previ-

---

(4–4) Br. Med. J. 1:671–673, Mar. 8, 1980.
(4–5) J. Pediatr. 95 (Pt. 1):780–786, November 1979.

ously reported cases. Two undocumented cases were included in the authors' series. No structural heart disease was apparent in 81% of the total group. Seven infants (19%) in the combined series had an identifiable possible cause of SVT other than preexcitation. Four had structural cardiac abnormalities, 1 had possible myocarditis and 1 had congenital cytomegalovirus infection. Twenty-three infants had signs of congestive heart failure within the first hours after delivery. Myocardial function was poor in 4 infants who were catheterized in the first days of life.

Thirteen infants (35%) converted to normal sinus rhythm during or shortly after delivery, spontaneously or on vagal stimulation. One infant with repetitive SVT in utero was asymptomatic postnatally. Twenty-three patients received antiarrhythmic agents, 4 in utero. Maternal digitalization was ineffective in 3, but 1 fetus converted during maternal propranolol therapy. Digitalis was successful when given postnatally in all but 3 of 17 patients. The others received quinidine or propranolol. Digoxin toxicity was reported in 5 infants. Sixteen infants had recurrent arrhythmia within the first month of life and 9 had a recurrence after age 1 month. All 3 infants who died had structural abnormalities; 2 of them had persistent arrhythmia.

The prognosis of infants with intrauterine SVT in this series depended on the underlying cardiac status. Maternal digitalization is reasonable when intrauterine SVT is recognized. Digoxin is safe and effective for infants with SVT at birth who exhibit mild to moderate congestive heart failure. Severely compromised infants require electric cardioversion. Digoxin is continued in all cases for 1 year. Rarely, quinidine or propranolol may have to be added.

▶ [Fetal supraventricular tachycardia is rare. Only 31 cases have been reported previously and the present report adds 6 additional cases. In the total series, 81% were unassociated with structural abnormalities of the heart and those infants generally did well, whereas the outcome was less favorable in the 19% with cardiac diseases. Congestive failure was evident at or shortly after birth in 62% and generally responded quite well to digitalis neonatally. The few attempts to digitalize the fetus, however, did not seem particularly successful, presumably because therapeutic blood levels were not reached in mother or fetus. Digitalis apparently crosses the placenta quite freely.

We recently encountered a similar case in our service. Ultrasound findings suggested that congestive heart failure was developing in the fetus. Maternal digitalization and propranolol administration were ineffective in slowing the fetal heart rate, and even direct fetal injection of digitalis was unsuccessful. After delivery by cesarean section at 34 weeks, the infant required intensive treatment for cardiac failure but survived and has subsequently done well.

Lingman et al. (Br. J. Obstet. Gynaecol. 87:340, 1980) reported a case of fetal supraventricular tachycardia that was successfully converted by (or coincident with) maternal digoxin administration.] ◀

Physicians' Subjectivity in Evaluating Oxytocin Challenge Tests. Much of the care of high-risk pregnant patients has been based on the oxytocin challenge test (OCT). Theodore M. Peck[4-6] (Washington Univ.) sought to determine whether readings of OCTs are as objective as the listed criteria used in determining the test results. Five physicians specializing in maternal-fetal medicine evaluated 50 OCTs, 33 of them originally read as positive, 16 as negative, and 1 as

(4–6)   Obstet. Gynecol. 56:13–16, July 1980.

icious. All interpreters were American-trained, board-certified
tricians and gynecologists.

agreement among the physicians was considerable. Two agreed
...ie average only 52% of the time on any 1 OCT. Disagreement
was great when the physicians evaluated fetal heart rate reactivity
patterns, if present. Reasonable correlation with neonatal outcome
was observed when 3 or more physicians agreed on the OCT result,
fetal heart rate reactivity, or both. The presence or absence of fetal
heart accelerations with fetal motion correlated well with the neonatal outcome, regardless of the OCT reading. Among infants with accelerations, no difference was found in the outcome that accorded
with whether the OCT was positive or negative.

The reading of OCTs, even by highly trained obstetricians, is subjective. The "window" concept should be used, according to which any
ten-minute space containing three consecutive contractions of appropriate length without late deceleration makes the test negative. Only
technically acceptable tracings should be evaluated. Fetal movements
should be marked by an observer or by the patient. Most false positive results can be avoided by using nonstress tests as the basic
screening measure.

▶ [This study confirms what is probably predictable—that antepartum heart rate monitoring interpretation is highly subjective. Even among "experts," the degree of variation between observers was great. Variation within observers at different times was not
tested but had it been, we suspect it also would have been appreciable. Of the fetal
heart rate indices, accelerations with fetal movements seemed more reliable than late
decelerations, supporting the use of the nonstress test over the contraction stress test
as a primary screening mechanism.] ◀

Role of Trial of Labor With Positive Contraction Stress Test.
Noting that most patients with a positive contraction stress test
(CST) who underwent a trial of closely monitored labor were safely
delivered vaginally, John M. Bissonnette, Katherine Johnson, and
Christine Toomey[4-7] (Univ. of Oregon Health Sciences Center) attempted to learn which CST parameters could predict fetal status
during a subsequent labor. Data on 812 patients who underwent antepartum fetal heart rate (FHR) testing during a 28-month period
were retrospectively reviewed; 28 patients were found to have had a
positive CST. Their records were then analyzed for duration of the
test, number of contractions, number of contractions associated with
late deceleration, baseline FHR, number of accelerations, duration of
latency period, defined as the time from onset of contraction to onset
of late deceleration (Fig 4–3), and amplitude of deceleration.

Of the 28 patients, 11 had a cesarean section without a trial of
labor, and 15 underwent a closely monitored trial. There were 2 antepartum fetal deaths. Eleven of the 15 patients (73%) were delivered
vaginally, all of vigorous infants.

Analysis of the CST records of the 11 patients with no trial of labor,
the 9 with no late decelerations during labor, and the 8 with fetal
death in utero or persistent late deceleration in labor suggested that
two parameters separated patients who tolerated labor without per-

(4–7) Am. J. Obstet. Gynecol. 135:292–296, Oct. 1, 1979.

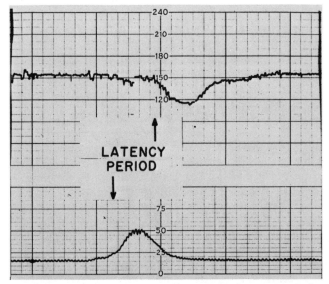

Fig 4–3.—Record of contraction stress test shows method of measuring the latency period. (Courtesy of Bissonnette, J. M., et al.: Am. J. Obstet. Gynecol. 135:292–296, Oct. 1, 1979.)

sistent late decelerations from those with late deceleration or a fetal death in utero: the presence or absence of acceleration during the CST and the duration of the latency period (table). Seventy percent of patients with FHR accelerations labored without late decelerations, whereas only 29% of patients without accelerations failed to go on to either fetal death or late decelerations in labor. Duration of the latency period was a more accurate predictor of fetal status during a subsequent labor: labor without late decelerations was achieved by 82% of patients with a latency period of 45 seconds or longer but by none of the patients with a latency period of less than 45 seconds.

A positive CST is an excellent indicator of fetuses at risk, but it does not indicate the mode of delivery that should be undertaken. It

PATTERN OF CONTRACTION STRESS TEST AS A PREDICTOR OF
FETAL STATUS DURING A TRIAL OF LABOR*

Pattern	No. of cases	No. with late deceleration or fetal death in utero	No. without late decelerations
FHR accelerations			
Present	10	3	7
Absent	7	5	2
Latency period:			
≥45 sec	11	2	9
<45 sec	6	6	0

*Trend shown with presence or absence of fetal heart rate acceleration is not significant ($\chi^2 = 2.84$, $P > 0.05$), but the difference seen with a latency period ≥45 seconds compared to that of <45 seconds does achieve significance ($\chi^2 = 10.43$, $P < 0.01$).

is reasonable to allow a trial of closely monitored labor in patients with a positive CST. Absence of accelerations (nonreactive CST) and a latency period of less than 45 seconds predict persistent late deceleration during labor or fetal death in utero.

▶ [This report adds to our knowledge of the contraction stress test. The presence of fetal heart rate accelerations during the test or of a latent period before the late decelerations of 45 seconds or more indicated that most fetuses would tolerate labor without developing late decelerations. How to manage the patient with a positive contraction stress test depends on many factors (the length of gestation, estriol levels, fetal presentation, state of the cervix, etc). Attention to the presence or absence of fetal heart rate accelerations and the length of the latent period should help refine our clinical judgment in these cases.] ◀

Fetal Movements in Human Pregnancies in the Third Trimester. Maternal awareness of decreased or absent fetal movements (FM) has traditionally been considered to be a sign of impending fetal difficulty. Frank A. Manning, Lawrence D. Platt, and Louise Sipos[4-8] (Univ. of Southern California) examined the relation between the frequency of FM in a 20-minute period, as determined with a real-time B-scan method, and pregnancy outcome in 50 women in the third trimester of pregnancy. The transducer was placed on the maternal abdomen to obtain a longitudinal scan of the fetus in either the coronal or the sagittal plane. Fetal movements were defined as flexion or extension of the limbs, trunk, or both.

A total of 195 observations of FM were made. All subjects delivered within a week of examination. Fetal movements did not vary significantly with gestational age. The frequency of FM was not abnormal in pregnancies complicated by diabetes, hypertension, or placenta previa, but it was significantly reduced in cases of Rh isoimmunization with a severely affected fetus. The frequency of FM was greater where fetal breathing movements were present and with a reactive nonstress test. Among 46 cases in which FM were present on the last observation before delivery, 2 fetuses died in utero and 3 infants had low 5-minute Apgar scores. Fetal movements were absent before delivery in 4 instances. Three of these fetuses died in utero, and the other had a positive contraction stress test and was normal at delivery after labor was induced. In 3 of these cases, FM were absent only on the last observation before delivery. The frequency of FM varied widely in the 42 patients in whom serial observations were made.

The findings confirm a relation between FM and fetal well-being. The presence of at least one fetal movement in a 20-minute recording period is a reassuring sign of a normal fetus, but if FM are absent, further biophysical variables should be evaluated.

Subjective Recording of Fetal Movement. Sadovsky and Yaffe, and Pearson and Weaver, showed that changes in counts of fetal movements recorded by mothers can help predict fetal death and fetal asphyxia. C. Wood, M. Gilbert, A. O'Connor, and W. A. W. Walters[4-9] (Melbourne) reviewed findings among 137 patients, including 113 with obstetric complications, who recorded fetal movements by a subjective method for three 20-minute periods each day. An automatic

(4–8) Obstet. Gynecol. 54:699–702, December 1979.
(4–9) Br. J. Obstet. Gynaecol. 86:836–842, November 1979.

timing device and counter were used. Counts for the last 46 days of pregnancy were calculated.

Fetal movement counts decreased over the 46 days preceding delivery. The percentile distribution of movements was not influenced by age, parity, ethnic origin, or a number of antepartum complications. Infant sex, malformations, amniotic fluid volume, umbilical cord length, infant length, and neonatal morbidity also failed to influence fetal movement counts. Apgar scores did not correlate significantly with the counts. Low counts were associated with maternal cigarette smoking and prolongation of pregnancy, and high counts were associated with maternal ingestion of sedatives or tranquilizers, an abnormal fetal heart rate in labor, and a true knot in the umbilical cord. The absence of fetal movement in four consecutive counting sessions was not associated with a poor fetal outcome.

Further studies are needed to assess the usefulness of fetal movement counting by pregnant women.

▶ [This article and the preceding one deal with the assessment of fetal movements (FM) in 20-minute periods (by ultrasound in California, by patient report in Australia) and perinatal outcome. In both series, abnormal pregnancy conditions were not generally associated with differences in FM counts. No effect of length of gestation on FM count was found in the preceding article, although the Australian workers suggest a decline in late pregnancy. As far as outcome is concerned, four patients in the California study had no FM on the last determination before delivery and three stillbirths occurred. Three other patients, however, had FM absent on one occasion, with a subsequent return of activity and normal outcome. In the Australian study, FM were absent on from two to four consecutive occasions in from 7% to 14% of patients. No stillbirths occurred. We doubt that the counting of FM by ultrasound will play much of a role in the determination of fetal well-being. The role of subjective recording of FM in 20-minute segments is problematic as well. This is not to say that we should not inquire about fetal activity in our antepartum patients or that we should ignore a patient's concern about decreased activity. The question involves the value of FM determinations in specific 20-minute "windows." Can't the poor fetus rest?] ◀

▶ ↓A more optimistic report follows. Read on. ◀

Fetal Movements as an Indicator of Fetal Well-Being. Many unexpected perinatal deaths continue to occur in infants without serious congenital malformations. The problem of delivering these infants in time has not been solved. Steen Neldam[4-10] (Univ. of Copenhagen) evaluated the usefulness of fetal movements (FM) as an indicator of intrauterine fetal well-being in a prospective trial of 2,250 pregnant women seen over a 4-month period during 1978. Half were allocated to the study group, and half were used as controls. Study subjects counted FM 2 hours after meals while lying down, once a week to 32 weeks' gestation, and then three times a week. A count of less than three per hour was considered to be an alarm signal and an indication for ultrasound study and cardiotocography. If a motionless fetus did not respond to manual stimulation, and intrauterine asphyxia was suggested by cardiotocography in a mother not taking a sedative, the fetus was delivered as soon as possible by cesarean section. Controls were not given any specific instructions about counting FM.

Eight intrauterine deaths occurred in fetuses weighing more than

(4–10)   Lancet 1:1222–1224, June 7, 1980.

1,500 gm without major congenital malformations. All were in the control group. All the women had felt fewer FM, and some no FM, 2 to 5 days before contacting the hospital. Nine study mothers reported a decrease in FM. Three outpatients were delivered by acute cesarean section, and 1 had labor induced with oxytocin. Two inpatients with preeclampsia had acute cesarean section, and 1 had oxytocin induction. Seven infants had no perinatal problems. Two had respiratory distress syndrome, but they survived. The cause of decreased FM counts was unclear in three normal pregnancies.

All pregnant women should be taught how to count FM, particularly those with high-risk pregnancies, in whom FM counting is a reliable test of fetal well-being. Fetal movements are also useful in timing delivery when the ultrasound, cardiotocographic, or hormonal findings are abnormal.

▶ [This controlled, prospective study with random patient assignment to the "treatment" and "control" groups strongly endorses the value of maternal monitoring of FM. Apparently, those in the FM group spent 6 hours per week after the 32d week of gestation lying down and counting movements. A count of fewer than 3 FM per hour was regarded as an alarm signal. Patients in the control group had noticed fewer or no FM, but decided to "wait and see."

Unless further studies cast doubt on the validity of these results, it would seem prudent for all of us to discuss fetal activity with our patients. Patients who note markedly decreased or absent FM should be encouraged to contact us and not to "wait and see." This history from a patient should serve as an indicator of risk sufficient for fetal heart rate to be tested. Apparently, fewer than 1% of the patients in the "FM group" in this study reported decreased movements. We are surprised that this figure is not higher.] ◀

The Lung Profile—*I. Normal pregnancy.*—Marie V. Kulovich, Mikko B. Hallman, and Louis Gluck[4-11] (La Jolla, Calif.) obtained lung profiles by two-dimensional thin-layer chromatography in 200 amniotic fluid specimens from 158 women with apparently normal pregnancies. Specimens from 57 other women who had been delivered after low lecithin-sphingomyelin (L/S) ratios (under 2.0) also were analyzed. The L/S ratio was determined along with percentages of disaturated (acetone-precipitated) lecithin, phosphatidyl inositol (PI), and phosphatidyl glycerol (PG).

The coefficient of correlation between mean L/S ratios and weeks of gestation for subjects free of high-risk conditions was 0.986. The percentage of acetone-precipitated disaturated lecithin correlated with gestational age with a coefficient of 0.948. The correlation coefficient for percentage of PG in total phospholipid was 0.943. The percentage of PI increased until about 35 to 36 weeks' gestation and then declined. The lung profile form is shown in Figure 4–4. Of 57 pregnancies with low L/S ratios, 69% were diagnosed correctly by L/S ratio alone where the newborn infants had respiratory distress syndrome. The lung profile extended the ability to diagnose unsuspected maturity in infants with low L/S ratios, detected by the presence of PG, to 93%.

In certain infants of early gestational age, lung maturity characterized by the accelerated appearance of PG may occur at L/S ratios be-

(4–11) Am. J. Obstet. Gynecol. 135:57–63, Sept. 1, 1979.

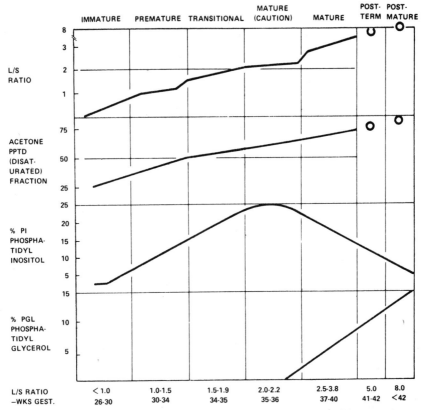

Fig 4–4.—Form used to report lung profile. The four determinations are plotted on the ordinate and weeks of gestation on the abscissa (as well as L/S ratio as an "internal standard"). When these are plotted, they fall with a high frequency into a given grid that then identifies the stage of development of the lung as shown in the upper part of the form. The designation "mature (caution)" refers to patients other than those with diabetes who can be delivered *if necessary* at this time; if the patient has diabetes she can be delivered with safety when values fall in the "mature" grid. (Courtesy of Kulovich, M. V., et al.: Am. J. Obstet. Gynecol. 135:57–63, Sept. 1, 1979; copyright 1977 by the Regents of the University of California.)

low 2.0. The lung profile increases the predictability of fetal lung maturity to close to 100% and also may signal an abnormal pregnancy. The physician can in this way obtain reliable information on the status of the maturing lung, when to expect maturity, and when, if necessary, to do a repeat study of fetal lung maturity on amniotic fluid.

II. Complicated pregnancy. Questions exist about the reliability of applying the criterion for fetal lung maturity in normal pregnancy, an L/S ratio of 2.0 or above, to diabetic pregnancies. Kulovich and Gluck[4-12] analyzed 220 amniotic fluid samples from 187 women with diabetes, 104 samples from 92 women with rupture of membranes (ROM) for more than 24 hours, and 116 samples from 89 women with hypertension. All specimens were obtained transabdominally on medical indication for monitoring fetal lung maturity. The mean time for

(4–12) Am. J. Obstet. Gynecol. 135:64–70, Sept. 1, 1979.

sampling in ROM was 61 hours. Most hypertensive patients had terminal preeclampsia with mild to moderate hypertension and mild proteinuria.

No significant differences in L/S ratios according to gestation were seen among different classes of diabetics, and no class differed significantly from the curve for normal pregnancy. Seven of 43 class A (pregnancy-induced diabetes) patients had delayed maturation of the L/S ratio. Similar findings were obtained for percentage of disaturated lecithin measured after acetone precipitation. A prolonged high percentage of PI was seen in class A diabetics, in which the level did not decline until 37 or 38 weeks of gestation, compared to about 35 weeks in normal subjects and other classes of diabetics. The appearance of PG was clearly delayed in class A diabetics, in whom the mean time of its appearance was 37 to 39 weeks of gestation. In patients with class F and R diabetes, PG appeared as early as 29 or 30 weeks. The findings in hypertensive patients with mild problems were normal, but accelerated maturation was noted in the prolonged ROM group, with higher mean and earlier mature L/S ratios and an earlier than normal mean appearance of PG.

It is concluded that diabetic pregnancies of any class can safely be delivered free of respiratory distress syndrome after PG appears in the amniotic fluid.

▶ [Much of our current knowledge of fetal pulmonary maturation has come from the extensive studies of Doctor Gluck, and this two-part article from his laboratory can be considered a "state of the art" report on fetal lung maturity assessment. In addition to the familiar L/S ratio, Gluck's "lung profile" includes the percentages of disaturated acetone-precipitated lecithin, phosphatidylinositol (PI), and phosphatidylglycerol (PG). As we have observed several times in previous editions of the YEAR BOOK, conventional amniotic fluid tests of fetal maturation are usually quite accurate in predicting maturity but considerably less so in predicting immaturity; specifically, a substantial percentage of instances with L/S <2 are not associated with respiratory distress syndrome. This issue is addressed in the first article, on normal pregnancy, and the data indicate that the multifaceted approach of the lung profile yields a false negative rate of only 7%. In the second article, abnormal gestations are considered. The results suggest that the propensity to respiratory distress syndrome exhibited in maternal diabetes (along with falsely mature L/S) derives from delay in the appearance of PG. Further, an accelerated maturation with premature rupture of membranes (itself a controversial issue) and chronic hypertension results from the early appearance of PG.] ◀

Developmental Study of a Lamellar Body Fraction Isolated From Human Amniotic Fluid. Surfactant apparently is secreted into amniotic fluid as intact lamellar bodies. Surfactant material has been recovered in a pellet fraction of amniotic fluid after differential centrifugation, and measurement of this fraction may provide a specific index of fetal pulmonary maturity. M. Oulton, T. R. Martin, G. T. Faulkner, D. Stinson, and J. P. Johnson[4-13] (Dalhousie Univ.) investigated the properties of a pellet fraction obtained by centrifuging amniotic fluid specimens, taken at various stages of gestation, at 10,000 g for 20 minutes. A developmental profile was defined, which appears to describe the maturational process of the fetal lung surfactant system.

At 14 to 18 weeks' gestation the pellet fraction consisted of mem-

(4–13 Pediatr. Res. 14:722–728, May 1980.

CORRELATION OF AMNIOTIC FLUID ANALYSIS AND RESPIRATORY STATUS OF NEWBORN WITH INDIVIDUAL STAGES OF DEVELOPMENT OF FETAL LUNG SURFACTANT SYSTEM*

10,000 × g pellet analysis	Phospholipid concentration (μg/ml)	Composition†			Gestation (wk)	Respiratory status‡	Developmental stage
Electron microscopy		% PC	% PI	% PG			
I Nonlamellated vesicles	<5	<SPH	<10	0	14–18	No infants delivered	Presurfactant
II No electron microscopy performed	<25	>SPH	<10	0	30	100% RDS	Onset of surfactant synthesis
III Lamellar bodies	>25	>75	>10	0	34–36	75% RDS 84.6% RDS and TRD	Early lamellar body
IV Lamellar bodies	>50	>75	>10	>0<1	36–37	0% RDS in NDM 50% RDS in ODM	Biochemical maturation of lamellar bodies
V Lamellar bodies	>>50	>75	<10	>1	36–37	0% RDS 1.7% TRD	

*Values shown for phospholipid concentration and composition represent summary of data obtained from 6 to 117 specimens at each stage. Electron microscopic examination was performed on 1 to 5 individual specimens for each stage indicated. Gestations represent approximate time at which each stage was first observed. Stage of fetal lung surfactant system was assigned on basis of these analyses.
†PC, lecithin; PI, phosphatidylinositol; PG, phosphatidylglycerol; SPH, sphingomyelin.
‡TRD, transient respiratory distress; NDM, nondiabetics; ODM, overt diabetics.

brane-bound vesicles without internal lamellae. The major phospholipid was sphingomyelin. After 30 to 32 weeks' gestation the phospholipid concentration of the pellet fraction increased continuously. Lecithin and phosphatidylinositol increased at 30 to 35 weeks' gestation. From 36 weeks on, the fraction contained structures resembling lamellar inclusion bodies. Early formed lamellar bodies lacked phosphatidylglycerol and had a high content of phosphatidylinositol. A phosphatidylglycerol value above 1% of total phospholipids appeared to represent the stage of maturity at which there was no risk of respiratory distress syndrome. Data on the various stages are summarized in the table.

The development of respiratory distress syndrome appears to be highly dependent on the stage at which biochemical maturation of the fetal lung surfactant system is interrupted. Detailed phospholipid analysis of the isolated surfactant fraction of amniotic fluid can provide an index of the precise stage of fetal lung maturity.

▶ [This article describes results of electron microscopic and phospholipid analysis of a pellet obtained by high-speed centrifugation of amniotic fluid. The authors believe the pellet fractions contain surfactant. The analytic results at various stages of gestation permit one to trace the sequence of biochemical development of the lung. Prior to 20 weeks, there is no surfactant and the main phospholipid is sphingomyelin. Beginning in the early third trimester, phospholipids (lecithin and phosphatidylinositol [PI]) increase; once phosphatidylglycerol (PG) appears at about 36 weeks, maturity is certain. There are, however, some major problems in correlating the results of this study with clinical experience. For example, in stage III in which lecithin represents >75% of phospholipids and PI >10% with no PG present, corresponding to 34 to 36 weeks' gestation, the occurrence of respiratory distress syndrome is said to be 75%, which is far greater than it really is at this gestational age.] ◀

Saturated Phosphatidylcholine in Amniotic Fluid and Prediction of Respiratory Distress Syndrome. Mason et al. (1976) developed a rapid method for isolating saturated phosphatidylcholine (SPC), the major component of pulmonary surfactant. John Torday, Linda Carson, and Edward E. Lawson[4-14] (Harvard Med. School) compared the predictive values of the lecithin-sphingomyelin (L/S) ratio and the concentration of SPC in 322 amniotic fluid samples obtained

Fig 4–5.—Amount of SPC *(solid bars)* and non-SPC *(open bars)* in amniotic fluid *(A),* contaminant (either blood or meconium) *(B);* amniotic fluid and contaminant *(C);* and amniotic fluid, contaminant, and osmium tetraoxide *(D).* (Courtesy of Torday, J., et al.: N. Engl. J. Med. 301:1013–1018, Nov. 8, 1979.)

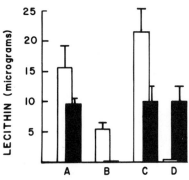

PREDICTION OF RESPIRATORY DISTRESS SYNDROME IN ALL AMNIOTIC
FLUID SPECIMENS STUDIED

TEST	RESPIRATORY-DISTRESS SYNDROME	NO RESPIRATORY-DISTRESS SYNDROME	TOTAL
L/S ratio			
Positive (≤2/1)	25 true positive	20 false positive	45
Negative (>2/1)	13 false negative	264 true negative	277
SPC (μg/dl)			
Positive (≤500)	35 true positive	7 false positive	42
Negative (>500)	3 false negative	277 true negative	280

within 72 hours before birth, 75% of which were contaminated or obtained during complicated pregnancies.

Positive results predictive of respiratory distress syndrome were taken as an L/S ratio of 2:1 or below and an SPC below 500 μg/dl. Respiratory distress syndrome was correctly predicted in 25 of 45 cases (55.5%) with L/S ratios of 2:1 or less, and in 35 of 42 cases (82%) with criterion SPC levels. The false negative rate for the L/S ratio was 4.7% and that for the SPC was 1.1%. Blood or meconium did not alter the SPC concentration of amniotic fluid in vitro (Fig 4–5), but the L/S values were altered by these contaminants.

The two methods were comparably predictive in uncontaminated cases and in women with uncomplicated pregnancies, but in the total study population the SPC method provided marked predictive improvement (table). Sensitivity was increased from 66% to 92%, and the predictive value of a positive test from 55.5% to 83%. Specificity was also improved, from 93% to 97.5%. The predictive value of a negative test rose from 95% to 99%.

The assay of SPC in amniotic fluid is a practical means of more reliably predicting respiratory distress syndrome than use of either the L/S ratio or the foam stability test.

▶ [The use of osmium tetroxide permits a better separation of saturated lecithin (SPC) from unsaturated lecithin than does cold acetone precipitation, according to this report. Since the former is considered to be the major component of pulmonary surfactant, the Harvard University workers think they are measuring what counts. Blood or meconium contamination is not a problem. The authors found fewer false premature ("false positive" in their nomenclature) tests with SPC than with the L/S ratio. Because a concentration and not a ratio is measured, abnormalities of amniotic fluid volume could cause problems, but the authors did not encounter them in diabetic patients with polyhydramnios. The test is not a "quickie"; however, if others confirm its accuracy, the SPC test will probably have a place in the evaluation of fetal lung maturity.] ◀

Amniotic Fluid Optical Density and Neonatal Respiratory Outcome. A simple, rapid, economical, and accurate test to assess fetal pulmonary maturity on a 24-hour basis seven days a week, is urgently needed. A positive correlation between amniotic fluid optical density readings and lecithin-sphingomyelin (L/S) ratios has previously been reported. Curtis L. Cetrulo, Anthony J. Sbarra, Ratnam J. Selvaraj, Kenneth A. Kappy, Marguerite J. Herschel, Robert J.

Knuppel, Charles J. Ingardia, Joseph L. Kennedy, and George W. Mitchell[4-15] (Boston) report the development of a 15-minute amniotic fluid optical density test that correlates well with fetal pulmonary maturity.

Amniotic fluids were obtained from 300 patients. Specimens containing gross meconium, blood, or bilirubin were excluded, as were specimens which had been frozen and thawed. After centrifugation of 3–5 ml fluid, optical density readings at 650 nm were made on the supernatant.

Betamethasone was usually given when the optical density was 0.15, gestational age was <34 weeks, and delivery appeared imminent. Betamethasone was also given in a few instances when gestational age was >34 weeks.

Respiratory distress syndrome did not develop in any infant whose mother's amniotic fluid optical density was ≥0.15. Gestational ages at the time of amniocentesis in these cases were 33–42 weeks. In 14 of 169 patients in whom the optical density reading was <0.15, respiratory distress syndrome did develop, proving fatal in 2 infants. The gestational ages in the group having optical densities <0.15 were 24–40 weeks, most being under 35 weeks.

If the amniotic fluid optical density at 650 nm is <0.15, respiratory distress syndrome may develop. In this study the true incidence of respiratory distress syndrome is unknown, because most of the mothers received steroid treatment. As a result, this syndrome developed in only 8.3% of the infants, most of them surviving.

These results indicate that optical density measurements of amniotic fluids are of value in assessing fetal lung maturity and in making management decisions. With optical density readings >0.15, pulmonary maturity may be assumed and steroid treatment is not required. However, with optical density readings <0.15 and presumably immature L/S ratios, inhibition of labor and steroid management may be considered. With this plan, 91.7% of the infants in this series did not experience respiratory distress. The mothers of 6 of the 14 infants in whom the syndrome did develop had not received adequate steroid treatment.

▶ [This is the latest in the continuing controversy about the value of amniotic fluid optical density at 650 nm in fetal maturity estimation, written by the same group that made the original observation. From the data presented, it appears that optical density at 650 nm is a good predictor of maturity but a much less reliable index of immaturity. So what else is new? Read on.] ◀

Assessment of Fetal Lung Maturity: Comparison of Lecithin-Sphingomyelin Ratio and Tests of Optical Density at 400 and 650 Nm. Simpler tests of fetal lung maturity have been developed because of the problem of obtaining accurate laboratory measurements of the lecithin-sphingomyelin (L/S) ratio at small obstetric units. W. N. Spellacy, W. C. Buhi, A. C. Cruz, S. R. Gelman, K. R. Kellner, and S. A. Birk[4-16] (Univ. of Florida) compared optical density (OD) test readings at both 400 and 650 nm with the classic amniotic

(4–15) Obstet. Gynecol. 55:262–265, February 1980.
(4–16) Am. J. Obstet. Gynecol. 134:528–531, July 1, 1979.

fluid L/S ratio test. Seventy-eight amniotic fluid samples were taken by transabdominal amniocentesis from women being considered for delivery for medical reasons and if there was a question of fetal maturity. No fetal or maternal complications resulted. Optical density readings were made with a recording spectrophotometer.

The OD at 650 nm (OD_{650}) gave an excellent prediction of the L/S ratio. The coefficient of correlation for the L/S ratio and OD_{400} was 0.55, and for the OD_{650}, 0.49; both were significant. The false negative and false positive rates for the 650-nm reading at 0.15 were 14.1% and 3.8%, respectively. When an OD reading at 400 nm of 0.28 or above was used as an index of fetal maturity, the false positive rate was 22.1% and the false negative rate, 5.2%. When an OD_{400} reading of 0.35 or above was used, the false positive rate was 9.1% and the false negative rate was 14.3%. Optical density readings fell for two days when amniotic fluid specimens were refrigerated, probably because of flocculation of the fluid proteins. This effect could bring "mature" fluids to "immature" readings at both wavelengths.

The OD_{650} test on fresh amniotic fluid is a rapid, inexpensive means of determining fetal lung maturity. All samples with values below 0.15 must also be tested for their L/S ratio, because some infants with such values may be mature. It may be that tests more complicated than the L/S ratio, such as measurements of phosphatidylglycerol and phosphatidylinositol, are necessary for backup.

▶ [Measurement of amniotic fluid OD_{650} has been proposed as a simple alternative to the L/S ratio. Several studies have given conflicting results. This one represents a generally favorable review, particularly with respect to the correlation between an L/S >2 and OD_{650} >0.15. Particularly important is the portion of the study demonstrating a progressive decline in OD_{650} with refrigerated storage, which may explain the high false negative rates in other studies.] ◀

Amniotic Fluid Palmitic Acid-Stearic Acid Ratios, Lecithin-Sphingomyelin Ratios and Palmitic Acid Concentrations in Assessment of Fetal Lung Maturity in Diabetic Pregnancies. Both the L/S ratio and the palmitic acid concentration have proved unreliable in assessing fetal lung maturity in diabetes. A. G. Andrews, J. B. Brown, P. E. Jeffery, and I. Horacek[4-17] (Royal Women's Hosp., Victoria, Australia) obtained evidence that measurement of the palmitic acid-stearic acid (P/S) ratio in the acetone-insoluble fraction is a more reliable indicator of fetal lung maturity.

All three measurements were made on amnoitic fluid from 66 diabetic women. Twenty patients delivered live infants within 48 hours of the last estimate. Six were gestational diabetics, and 14 were insulin-dependent diabetics. Studies also were done in 127 nondiabetic patients. Amniotic fluid was obtained by transabdominal amniocentesis, at amniotomy, or at cesarean section.

The L/S ratio and palmitic acid concentration were considerably higher in diabetics at 35 to 40 weeks' gestation, whereas the P/S ratio was similar throughout gestation in both diabetics and nondiabetics. The P/S ratio correctly predicted fetal lung maturity in 19 of 20 patients (95%). In the exceptional case, the L/S ratio and palmitic acid

(4–17) Br. J. Obstet. Gynaecol. 86:959–964, December 1979.

concentration were also incorrect. The palmitic acid concentration prediction was incorrect in 8 patients (40%) and the L/S ratio prediction in 10 patients (50%).

These findings confirm the unreliability of the L/S ratio in diabetic pregnancies. The palmitic acid concentration does not seem to be any more reliable in predicting respiratory distress syndrome in diabetic pregnancies, but the P/S ratio was correct in 95% of the present cases. The P/S ratio appears to be superior to the others in predicting fetal lung maturity in the presence of maternal diabetes. The P/S ratio should be determined within 48 hours of birth, with the use of the acetone precipitation method.

▶ [An appreciable false positive rate of the L/S ratio (ie, despite mature values) with maternal diabetes has been found by many, but not all (see Gabbe et al.: Am. J. Obstet. Gynecol. 128:757, 1977) investigators. This study confirms a lack of reliability of L/S and palmitic acid level as well, whereas the palmitic acid–stearic acid ratio seemed to correlate much better with fetal pulmonary status. It should be noted that fatty acid measurements require gas chromatography, which may be beyond the capability of some laboratories. The other major approach to the diabetic "problem" in amniotic fluid maturity studies, phosphatidyl glycerol, is the subject of a number of articles in this and previous editions of the YEAR BOOK.] ◀

Evaluation of the FELMA Microviscosimeter in Predicting Fetal Lung Maturity. The FELMA is a commercially available device that measures surfactant in amniotic fluid by making use of the principle that a lipid-soluble dye excited by polarized light fluoresces light that is also polarized. Steven H. Golde, John F. Vogt, Steven G. Gabbe, and Luis A. Cabal[4-18] (Univ. of Southern California) compared its ability to predict fetal lung maturity with that of the standard Lecithin-sphingomyelin (L/S) ratio.

A total of 236 amniotic fluid samples were tested with the FELMA; an L/S ratio was determined for 154 of them. When FELMA scores were plotted against L/S ratios, a wide scattering of scores was found in the direction of maturity, with a significant correlation between FELMA scores and L/S ratios. Any FELMA scores below 0.320 were taken to indicate mature fetal lungs.

When 102 infants born within 48 hours of sampling were studied (Table 1) it was found that no neonate with hyaline membrane disease had a FELMA score below 0.320, and all infants deemed mature by the FELMA scores were free of the disease. Comparison of FELMA scores with L/S ratios in the 64 infants delivered within 48 hours of sampling (Table 2) showed that no neonate with a mature FELMA

TABLE 1.—NEONATAL RESPIRATORY OUTCOME BY 102 FLUORESCENCE POLARIZATION SCORES

FP score	HMD present	HMD absent
< 0.320	0	83
≥ 0.320	5	14

$\chi^2 = 22.97, P < 0.001.$
HMD, hyaline membrane disease.

(4–18) Obstet. Gynecol. 54:639–643, November 1979.

TABLE 2.—NEONATAL OUTCOME IN 64 PATIENTS DELIVERED WITHIN 48 HOURS OF TESTING*

	HMD present		HMD absent	
Score	L/S ≥ 2.00	L/S < 2.00	L/S ≥ 2.00	L/S < 2.00
FP < 0.320	0	0	45	4
FP ≥ 0.320	2	3	7	3

$\chi^2 = 22.5$; if 3, $P < 0.001$.
*HMD, hyaline membrane disease; FP, fluorescence polarization; L/S, lecithin-sphingomyelin ratio.

score had hyaline membrane disease. Of 5 neonates with the disease, 2 had mature L/S ratios. The L/S ratio technique had a false positive error rate of 3.7% and a false negative rate of 70.0%, whereas the FELMA score had rates of 0% and 64.3%, respectively.

The FELMA score and the L/S ratio had similar correlations with neonatal outcome regarding immature fetuses as well as those that were mature by gestational age, outcome, and L/S ratio. The FELMA score was slightly, but insignificantly, better than the L/S ratio in predicting hyaline membrane disease. The FELMA technique, while as predictive as the L/S ratio, was technically easier to perform and required only 30 minutes (incubation time of dye with the fluid sample) until the score was known.

▶ [These findings are generally consistent with those of Elrad et al. (1979 YEAR BOOK, p. 123). The two studies differ somewhat in laboratory methodology and in what is considered a mature FP value, but both suggest the microviscosimeter to be of value in assessing fetal lung maturity. Falsely immature readings were more common in this study than in the earlier one. We are certain to see other evaluations of this amniotic fluid maturity test.] ◀

Antenatal Prediction of Graduated Risk of Hyaline Membrane Disease by Amniotic Fluid Foam Test for Surfactant. The foam or shake test is a rapid and simple method of determining the presence of pulmonary surfactant in amniotic fluid. High concentrations of surfactant, positive tests, are associated with absence of hyaline membrane disease (HMD); low concentrations, negative tests, are associated with a high incidence of HMD. False positive results are rare, but false negative results are not uncommon. Mureen A. Schlueter, Roderic H. Phibbs, Robert K. Creasy, John A. Clements, and Wil-

TABLE 1.—COMPOSITION OF TUBE DILUTIONS FOR THE FOAM TEST

	Tube No.		
	1	2	3
Dilution (cc)	1:1	1:1.3	1:2
Amniotic fluid	1.0	0.75	0.5
Saline (0.9% NaCl)	—	0.25	0.5
Alcohol (95% ethanol)	1.0	1.0	1.0

liam H. Tooley[4-19] (Univ. of California, San Francisco) report that this test can give a graded estimate of risk of development of HMD as well.

METHOD.—Saline and alcohol are added to test tubes containing amniotic fluid to give three dilutions (Table 1). The tubes are capped, shaken vigorously by hand for 15 seconds, placed in a rack, and left undisturbed for 15 minutes. The air-liquid interface of each tube is then examined for the presence of stable bubbles. Contents of a tube are recorded as being positive when there are enough bubbles present to form a complete ring around the tube, intermediate when small bubbles are present but not in sufficient numbers to form a complete ring around the tube, and negative when there are no bubbles (Fig 4–6).

Of 410 infants born within 24 hours after a foam test, 205 had positive tests in all three dilutions, and HMD developed in only one. For the other 205 infants the reaction was intermediate or negative in one or more dilutions; HMD developed in 64 of these infants.

Because the test has three possible reactions in each of 3 dilutions, the results were ranked according to 8 degrees of reaction as a titer of amniotic fluid surfactant. A progressive increase in incidence of HMD was found with decreasing reaction, with the infants falling into five groups (Table 2). Infants in groups I and II were heavier and more mature than those in groups III to V. However, among infants of equivalent gestational age or birth weight, the incidence of HMD

Fig 4–6.—Schematic representation of eight possible results of the foam test and their interpretation. (Courtesy of Schlueter, M. A., et al.: Am. J. Obstet. Gynecol. 134:761–767, Aug. 1, 1979.)

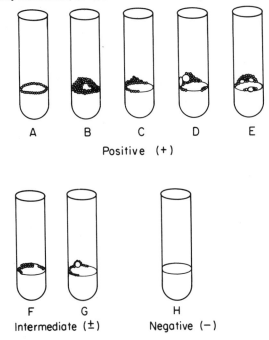

TABLE 2.—RISK FOR DEVELOPING HYALINE MEMBRANE DISEASE
IF DELIVERY IS WITHIN 24 HOURS OF AMNIOTIC FLUID FOAM TEST

	Amniotic fluid dilution			*Outcome*	
Risk group	*1:1*	*1:1.3*	*1:2*	*HMD/total*	*% HMD*
I	+	+	+	1/205	<1
II	+	+	±	10/97	10
	+	±	±		
III	+	±	−	11/44	25
	±	±	±		
IV	±	±	−	9/22	41
V	±	−	−	33/42	79
	−	−	−		

TABLE 3.—INDEPENDENT ASSOCIATIONS OF FOAM TEST AND GESTATIONAL AGE WITH THE RISK
OF HYALINE MEMBRANE DISEASE

	GA (wk)					
	≤29	*30-32*	*33-35*	*36-38*	*39-41*	*≥42*
Risk group	*HMD/total*	*HMD/total*	*HMD/total*	*HMD/total*	*HMD/total*	*HMD/total*
I	0/1	0/1	0/12	1/55 (2%)	0/102	0/34
II	0/2	3/11 (27%)	3/14 (21%)	3/40 (8%)	1/27 (4%)	0/3
III	6/6 (100%)	3/8 (38%)	1/12 (8%)	1/10 (10%)	0/8	
IV	2/2 (100%)	2/3 (67%)	2/5 (40%)	3/9 (33%)	0/3	
V	6/6 (100%)	10/10 (100%)	7/9 (78%)	10/16 (62%)	0/1	

still correlated significantly with the foam test results. Within each risk group the incidence of HMD was equal among infants delivered by vagina and by cesarean section and was slightly greater among boys than girls. At a given level of foam test reaction, the risk of HMD decreased as length of gestation increased, but at a given gestational age, the risk of HMD decreased as surfactant titer increased (Table 3). There were no false negative tests among the less mature infants, and all infants born before 33 weeks' gestation in group V had HMD.

The foam test can be used to accurately predict a graded risk of development of HMD in an infant delivered within 24 hours after the test. The eight levels of foam test reaction appear to span most of the range of surfactant concentration from the immature to the fully matured lung, thus giving a semiquantitative measure of surfactant concentration.

▶ [This is an important follow-up report on the shake test. As with other amniotic fluid maturity tests, a "mature" result is a better predictor of no respiratory distress syndrome (RDS) than is an "immature" result a predictor of RDS. The decreased risk of RDS with advancing gestational age for a given shake test result is clearly illustrated in Table 3. The results of an amniotic fluid maturity test should not be interpreted in isolation. Other factors (the most important of which is gestational age) must also be considered. It is of interest that, although others have described the shake test as a simple bedside maneuver that can be done by anyone, these authors, the developers of the test, suggest that it be done by an experienced technician to ensure reliability.] ◄

5. Labor and Operative Obstetrics

Simultaneous Determination of Seven Unconjugated Steroids in Maternal Venous and Umbilical Arterial and Venous Serum in Elective and Emergency Cesarean Section at Term. Evidence has been obtained for active involvement of the fetal adrenal cortex in initiation of the spontaneous onset of human labor. Wolfgang G. Sippell, Helmut G. Dörr, Henning Becker, Frank Bidlingmaier, Harald Mickan, and Kurt Holzmann[5-1] (Univ. of Munich) assessed specific glucocorticoid and mineralocorticoid functions in the mother and fetoplacental unit in relation to labor. Serum hormone levels were determined by specific radioimmunoassays in 16 normal nulliparous

Fig 5–1.—Comparison of mean umbilical cord arteriovenous differences of seven unconjugated steroids in the elective cesarean section group I *(open columns)* and in the indicated cesarean section group II *(black columns)*. Figures denote percentage of change of mean arteriovenous difference between the groups. (Courtesy of Sippell, W. G., et al.: Am. J. Obstet. Gynecol. 135:530–542, Oct. 15, 1979.)

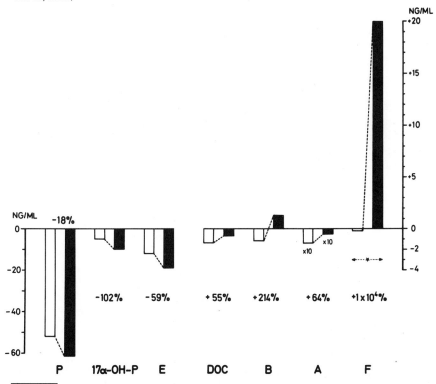

(5–1) Am. J. Obstet. Gynecol. 135:530–542, Oct. 15, 1979.

pregnant women, 8 at term but not in labor (group I) and 8 in spontaneous labor (group II). All were undergoing cesarean section with general anesthesia, group I patients for breech presentation and group II patients after a mean duration of spontaneous labor of 11.5 hours. Maternal age, gestational age, and neonatal and placental weights were comparable in the two groups.

The mean maternal serum levels of all the steroids measured were greater in group II than in group I. The increases were most marked for cortisol (F) and deoxycorticosterone (DOC). The other steroids determined included unconjugated aldosterone (A), corticosterone (B), progesterone (P), 17-hydroxyprogesterone (17-OHP), and cortisone (E). Arteriovenous differences in umbilical steroid levels showed the placental origin of P, 17-OHP, and E, with greater (more negative) mean arteriovenous differences noted after labor. The negative arteriovenous differences of DOC, B, A, and F seen in group I decreased after labor and became positive in the cases of B and F (Fig 5–1).

These findings demonstrate stimulation of both the glucocorticoid- and mineralocorticoid-producing pathways of the maternal adrenals by spontaneous labor. It appears that, in association with spontaneous labor, the fetus actively produces not only the glucocorticoids B and F, but also, to a lesser extent, the mineralocorticoids DOC and A.

High-Risk Prematurity: Progestin Treatment and Steroid Studies. A previous double-blind study showed reductions in prematurity and perinatal mortality in patients at risk for preterm delivery who received 17α-hydroxyprogesterone caproate (17α-OHP-C). John W. C. Johnson, Peter A. Lee, Annelies S. Zachary, Shirley Calhoun, and Claude J. Migeon[5-2] (Johns Hopkins Univ.) attempted to substantiate the risk-benefit ratio of 17α-OHP-C treatment in 70 patients with at least two previous preterm deliveries, two spontaneous miscarriages, or one miscarriage and one preterm delivery immediately preceding the current pregnancy. Patients received 250 mg of 17α-OHP-C weekly, intramuscularly, from gestational week 16 to week 36 or to the onset of spontaneous labor.

Twenty-one of 27 additional high-risk patients took 17α-OHP-C, and 16 delivered after 36 weeks' gestation. Two of the 6 unmedicated patients delivered preterm. When the results in these 27 patients are added to those of the original 43 patients, the overall rate of prematurity was 12.8% in treated patients and 40.9% in untreated patients. The respective perinatal mortality rates were 5% and 25%. No congenital anomalies were observed. Plasma progesterone values in treated patients delivering after 36 weeks were significantly higher than in patients delivering before 36 weeks. Levels of plasma 17α-OHP also were significantly higher in successfully treated patients. No significant differences in plasma estradiol or cortisol were observed.

These findings support the progesterone block theory as an important mechanism in preterm delivery in high-risk cases. It appears that 17α-OHP-C may act to prevent prematurity by increasing

(5–2) Obstet. Gynecol. 54:412–418, October 1979.

plasma progesterone levels. Although birth defects were not noted in the present series, extreme caution remains necessary with use of this medication. Much larger studies will be required to determine the true risk-benefit ratio of such treatment.

▶ [This represents the latest report by Johnson and associates of the prophylaxis of premature labor with 17α-OHP-C, and the clinical outcome seems to confirm earlier studies demonstrating efficacy of the therapy. The steroid levels appear at first glance to indicate that the mechanism involves increasing either progesterone or 17α-OHP levels in maternal blood, which presumably blocks the onset of labor prior to term. However, careful examination of the data confuses us because the patients who delivered prematurely and who had significantly lower mean levels of P and 17α-OHP were 5 subjects who were fully treated, 3 who received treatment for 3 weeks or less, and 2 who refused therapy. While this heterogenous group had lower steroid levels than either of the other groups (ie, normal controls and treated subjects who carried to term), the question remains as to whether the difference is in the treatment or in the patients.] ◀

Inhibition of Premature Labor With Indomethacin. Prostaglandins appear to be important in mediating uterine contractions in labor and in spontaneous abortion and may be involved in triggering premature labor. Inhibition of prostaglandin synthesis has been suggested as a possible means of inhibiting premature labor.

Jennifer R. Niebyl, David A. Blake, Robert D. White, Karen M. Kumor, Norman H. Dubin, J. Courtland Robinson, and Patricia G. Egner[5-3] (Johns Hopkins Univ.) during 1976 to 1978 administered indomethacin to inhibit premature labor in a prospective double-blind, placebo-controlled study of women in premature labor at 24 to 35 weeks of gestation who had intact fetal membranes. Criteria for premature labor were at least 2 cm of cervical dilatation, 75% effacement or change in the cervix, and painful or regular contractions less than 5 minutes apart. Patients were randomly assigned to receive 50 mg indomethacin (Indocin) followed by 25 mg every 4 hours for 24 hours or a placebo.

The 15 indomethacin-treated and 15 placebo patients did not differ significantly with respect to age, parity, gestational age, cervical effacement, and plasma estradiol and progesterone levels. Indomethacin was significantly more effective than placebo in inhibiting premature labor during the 24 hours of therapy. Only 1 indomethacin patient was a treatment failure, compared to 9 placebo patients. Three indomethacin patients received a second course of indomethacin and were delivered within 24 hours after the last dose. Three placebo patients received isoxsuprine and 1 received intravenous alcohol, but all delivered within the next 3 days. Two indomethacin patients were considered treatment failures within 72 hours in association with unrecognized chorioamnionitis with intact membranes. Plasma levels of PGFM (15-oxo-13,14-dihydroprostaglandin F_{2a}) decreased markedly in indomethacin-treated patients.

Infants in the two treatment groups did not differ significantly with respect to birth weight, neonatal morbidity, and complications. There was no evidence of premature closure of the ductus arteriosus or increased bleeding in infants exposed to indomethacin in utero.

(5–3) Am. J. Obstet. Gynecol. 136:1014–1019, Apr. 15, 1980.

Prostaglandin inhibitors, which are easily administered and well tolerated by the mother, are an attractive alternative to other drugs used to inhibit premature labor. Fetal toxicity remains a possibility, and indomethacin should still be considered an experimental treatment.

▶ [Theoretically, prostaglandin inhibitors are the most appealing agents, in terms of efficacy, in treating premature labor. In this small series, indomethacin was significantly more effective than placebo in preventing delivery during the 24 hour period of treatment and for 24 hours thereafter, which correlated with substantial suppression of plasma prostaglandin metabolite levels. We agree with the authors that prostaglandin inhibitors are the most "experimental" of agents for treatment of premature labor. For a suggestion of their possible adverse effects, read on.] ◀

Oligohydramnion, Meconium, and Perinatal Death Concurrent With Indomethacin Treatment in Human Pregnancy. Indomethacin arrests premature labor and concurrently produces undesirable sequelae in the fetus and newborn. Joseph Itskovitz, Haim Abramovici, and Joseph M. Brandes[5-4] (Rambam Med. Center, Haifa) describe 3 patients in whom indomethacin was used alone with resultant fetal death associated with oligohydramnion and meconium.

CASE 1.—Woman at 34 weeks' gestation and in premature labor was treated with 100 mg indomethacin rectally and 25 mg orally after baseline external monitoring. Two additional 100 mg doses were given 2 and 4 hours later. The contractions subsided and the patient was given an oral maintenance dose of the drug. On the fourth day, contractions began again and the cervix dilated to 5 cm. When the membranes ruptured, only a few drops of thick meconium-stained fluid appeared. Delivery was rapid and a 2,400 gm male was born. Apgar scores were 6 at 1 minute and 8 at 5 minutes, and the infant was meconium stained. At 15 minutes he had mild cyanosis and slight retraction. Despite ventilation and other measures, his condition deteriorated and he died within 3 hours after delivery. The newborn did not urinate and immediate postmortem catheterization produced no urine. Autopsy revealed a normal heart with a ductus arteriosus of 2 mm, marked congestion of the lung capillaries, and submucous hemorrhage in the esophagus and stomach.

CASE 2.—Woman at 33 weeks' gestation began taking oral indomethacin on an ambulatory basis for 6 days. On the seventh day the patient did not feel any fetal movement and no fetal heart tones were detected. After removal of a cervical suture and induction of labor, a 1,900 gm stillborn female was delivered. The fetal skin and membranes were meconium stained, and there was severe oligohydramnios.

CASE 3.—Woman, having premature contractions at 32 weeks' gestation, was treated with indomethacin after external monitoring. On the fourth day, fetal heart tones were no longer heard. On the fifth day, induction of labor was begun. When the membranes ruptured, only a few milliliters of thick meconium were found. The membranes and skin were meconium stained. The placenta showed multiple infarctions. Autopsy revealed slight maceration and a small cervical myelocele.

If indomethacin is given during the third trimester, careful monitoring should be undertaken for signs of placental insufficiency. If delivery occurs despite indomethacin therapy, one should be prepared to handle the newborn's cardiopulmonary disturbances. There are

(5–4) J. Reprod. Med. 24:137–140, March 1980.

theoretical reasons to believe that indomethacin may jeopardize the fetus, but further controlled studies are needed.

▶ [This collection of 3 perinatal deaths in cases treated with indomethacin is sobering, although, to be sure, there is no indication of the total population from which they were derived. Of special concern is the fact that the 3 patients were between 32 and 34 weeks' gestation of the time of treatment. In our judgment, pharmacologic efforts to inhibit suspected premature labor are seldom, if ever, indicated after 32 weeks. Neonatal survival in good neonatal intensive care units is quite acceptable after this time—in our own case, 96% of infants born alive at 32 to 34 weeks' gestational age now leave the hospital alive—so there is not a great deal to be gained by inhibiting labor after 32 weeks.] ◀

Ritodrine Hydrochloride: Betamimetic Agent for Use in Preterm Labor: II. Evidence of Efficacy. Irwin R. Merkatz, John B. Peter, and Tom P. Barden[5-5] reviewed the findings of a series of randomized, prospective, multicenter, double-blind comparisons of ritodrine hydrochloride with ethanol or placebo in the treatment of idiopathic preterm labor. Clinical studies were carried out at 11 university centers. A total of 366 gravid women entered the studies between 1972 and 1977; 223 received ritodrine parenterally and 77, ethanol intravenously. Successful parenteral ritodrine therapy was followed by oral maintenance therapy. Efficacy was analyzed in a total of 313 singleton pregnancies with intact amniotic membranes. Mean fetal age at entry in the ritodrine group was 30.9 weeks.

Among patients with onset of labor before 33 weeks' gestation, neonatal mortality was significantly lower in the ritodrine-treated group. A sizable reduction in the incidence of respiratory distress syndrome was also apparent in this group. More ritodrine-treated patients achieved gestations of 36 weeks or longer, and a significantly greater mean gestational age was obtained. The mean times gained in utero were 40.9 days in the ritodrine group and 24.4 days in controls, a highly significant difference. Ritodrine therapy was associated with an increase in infants weighing over 2,500 gm at birth. The findings are summarized in the table.

These results and its generally acceptable side effects have contributed to ritodrine's becoming the first drug approved for the treatment of preterm labor in the United States. It is expected that release of ritodrine for widespread use will increase interest in the management

RITODRINE SUMMARY: ANALYSIS OF ALL CASES			
Efficacy criterion	Ritodrine	Control	Significance
Neonatal death	5%	13%	$P < .05$
Neonatal RDS*	11%	20%	$P < .05$
Attaining ≥ 36 weeks' gestation	52%	38%	$P < .05$
Weeks' gestation at delivery	35.5	34.5	$P < .05$
Mean days gained	32.6	21.3	$P < .001$
Birth weight ≥ 2500 g	58%	43%	$P < .05$

*RDS: respiratory distress syndrome.

(5–5) Obstet. Gynecol. 56:7–12, July 1980.

of preterm labor. Research into newer and more specific tocolytic agents must be encouraged.

▶ [At this writing, it is anticipated that ritodrine will shortly be released for clinical use and thus will become the first "Food and Drug Administration-approved" drug for treatment of preterm labor. This article summarizes the efficacy of ritodrine in the extensive clinical testing conducted in the United States. The drug clearly improves outcome with statistically significant benefits in terms of survival, incidence of respiratory distress syndrome, and continuation of pregnancy to 36 weeks and/or 2,500 gm. However, it is no cure-all, for, after all, the improvements are relatively modest (eg, mean continuation of pregnancy of 40.9 days vs. 24.4 days with controls). Of particular importance is the fact that when the data are analyzed with respect to gestational age at the start of treatment, statistically significant improvement in the incidence of respiratory distress syndrome, achievement of 36 weeks' gestation or birth weight of 2,500 gm occurred only in the group treated before 33 weeks. As we have commented earlier, in our judgment, pharmacologic treatment of preterm labor is primarily indicated prior to 32 completed weeks' gestation; after 34 weeks it is probably never indicated.] ◀

Oral Ritodrine Maintenance in Treatment of Preterm Labor. Preterm parturition is the leading cause of neonatal morbidity and mortality. β-Adrenergic stimulants have been shown to reduce preterm and term uterine contractions, and clinical trials of ritodrine hydrochloride have suggested that it is safe and effective in delaying preterm births. Robert K. Creasy, Mitchell S. Golbus, Russell K. Laros, Jr., Julian T. Parer, and James M. Roberts[5-6] (Univ. of California, San Francisco) evaluated ritodrine therapy in 70 patients with preterm labor and intact membranes at 20 to 36 weeks' gestation. Estimated fetal weight was below 2,500 gm. Three or four regular contractions were documented in a 20-minute period, and there was documented progress in cervical effacement, dilation, or both. Patients with more than 3 to 4 cm of cervical dilatation were excluded. Ritodrine was given intramuscularly in doses of 5 to 10 mg every 2 to 4 hours. If tocolysis succeeded, oral therapy was begun with 10 to 20 mg of ritodrine every 3 or 4 hours or with placebo.

Ten patients delivered within 24 hours. Thirty-five of 69 patients were delivered after 36 weeks' gestation. The oral ritodrine and placebo groups were comparable in mean duration of pregnancy and number of days gained after the start of treatment. Among patients on oral therapy, significantly more recurrent preterm labors requiring repeated parenteral therapy occurred in the placebo than in the ritodrine group. The neonatal findings were similar in the two groups. Side effects of treatment were common but not clinically serious. Medication was discontinued because of undesirable side effects in 3 patients.

This study is the first to show that a maintenance program of continued oral β-adrenergic therapy, after successful inhibition of preterm labor, reduces the incidence of relapse. It has not been proved that the rate of preterm births is decreased, but this approach can diminish the need for repeated hospitalization, improving overall quality of life for the rest of the pregnancy.

▶ [The results of this well-designed study are somewhat difficult to interpret. Although

(5–6) Am. J. Obstet. Gynecol. 137:212–216, May 15, 1980.

oral ritodrine therapy was associated with fewer relapses of threatened premature labor than occurred in the placebo group, there was no difference between groups in the length of gestation at delivery or in the number of days gained after initial treatment. Whether long-term oral β-adrenergic treatment should be given to patients whose threatened premature labor has been successfully suppressed with parenteral therapy remains unknown.] ◄

Effect of Ritodrine on Labor After Premature Rupture of Membranes. β-Adrenergic receptor-stimulating drugs inhibit labor in patients with intact fetal membranes. In a double-blind study, Karen Kvist Christensen, Ingemar Ingemarsson, Ture Leideman, Hore Solum, and Niels Svenningsen[5-7] investigated the effect of ritodrine in prolonging pregnancy in 30 patients with premature rupture of the membranes.

Criteria for inclusion in the study were 28–32 weeks of gestation, a single fetus, cervical dilation of 4 cm or less, and absence of signs of uterine infection. Of the 30 patients, 14 received ritodrine and 16 were given placebo.

The fetal heart rate was monitored for 30 minutes before the ritodrine or placebo infusion was started. The infusion continued for 24 hours. Two hours before the infusion was stopped, oral treatment with ritodrine or placebo was started; this was continued to the end of 35 weeks' gestation. If uterine activity recurred during oral treatment, a new sequence of infusions was begun. Labor was induced at 36 weeks' gestation or when signs of infection appeared.

Of the 14 patients treated with ritodrine, none delivered within 24 hours, whereas 6 of the 16 control patients delivered within this time. This difference is significant. However, after 24 hours there was no difference between the two groups with respect to length of pregnancy. The 1 ritodrine-treated patient who reached 36 weeks' gestation had oxytocin induction of labor.

In 23 patients uterine activity recurred after the initial infusion. In 11 of these the cervix dilated to >4 cm shortly thereafter, so that they did not receive a second infusion. A second infusion was given to 6 patients in each group, but was uniformly unsuccessful in preventing premature delivery.

No serious side effects of treatment were noted in either group. There was no difference between the two groups with respect to obstetric operations and complications.

One patient from each group with suspected intrauterine infection had labor induced. Infections developed in 2 other patients after delivery and were easily controlled.

There was no significant difference between the two groups in mean birth weight or Apgar score of the infants. One infant whose mother received ritodrine was born at 29 weeks' gestation after almost 2 days of premature rupture of the membranes; he subsequently died. The rate of idiopathic respiratory distress syndrome was low.

The potential benefit for the preterm infant, and the low risk of

(5–7) Obstet. Gynecol. 55:187–190, February 1980.

infection to the mother and child, seem to justify prolongation of pregnancy for at least 24 hours. The value of attempts to inhibit labor beyond 24 hours after premature rupture of the membranes needs further investigation.

▶ [Rupture of the membranes has been considered a relative contraindication to pharmacologic inhibition of premature labor, less because of any particular risk than because of lack of efficacy. These results, though the numbers are small, seem confirmatory. The only significant difference was in delivery within 24 hours. Thus, it may be possible to forestall delivery immediately with ritodrine, but it is questionable whether birth can be delayed any significant length of time when the membranes are ruptured. If one is considering glucocorticoid administration, then a delay of 24 hours or so might be desirable. However, many authorities question whether glucocorticoid treatment with premature rupture longer than 24 or 48 hours confers any benefit.] ◀

Role of Glucocorticoids, Unstressful Labor, and Atraumatic Delivery in Prevention of Respiratory Distress Syndrome. J. Gerald Quirk, Jr., Richard K. Raker, Roy H. Petrie, and Athanasia M. Williams[5-8] (Columbia-Presbyterian Med. Center) report a 37-month review of the effects of glucocorticoids and uncompromised labor with atraumatic delivery on the incidence of respiratory distress syndrome (RDS) in 85 infants delivered by 79 mothers. Patients in premature labor with intact membranes received magnesium sulfate. Glucocorticoids were given according to the protocol of Liggins and Howie (1972). Glucocorticoids were given for at least 12 hours. All infants weighed 2,000 gm or less at birth. Control patients were matched with the glucocorticoid group for gestational age, race, and mode of delivery.

No significant difference in the incidence or severity of RDS was found between steroid-treated and control groups. Nine neonatal deaths and 1 stillbirth occurred in the study group. Three neonatal deaths were in infants with RDS who died of intraventricular hemorrhage while on mechanical ventilation; all were under 28 weeks' gestation. Ten neonatal deaths and 1 stillbirth occurred in the control group. Four neonatal deaths were in infants with RDS; 3 of these infants had intraventricular hemorrhage as the terminal event. In a total of 170 infants, only 1 who weighed more than 1,250 gm died with a diagnosis of RDS, and she died of group B streptococcal sepsis. The rate of RDS was 16.5% in the study group and 14.1% in the control group. Survival rates for infants with RDS in the two groups were 79% and 67%, respectively.

A nonstressful labor and atraumatic delivery appear to be as effective as glucocorticoids in reducing the incidence of RDS. There may be a role for glucocorticoid therapy in institutions where the incidence of RDS is relatively high. Careful attention to the management of the labor and delivery of low birth weight infants, however, so reduces the rate of RDS that the pulmonary maturational effects of glucocorticoid therapy are not clinically apparent.

▶ [The central point here is that the incidence of RDS was low and survival rates high whether or not glucocorticoids were administered. The study is not prospective, but a reasonable control group was chosen. Intensive fetal monitoring, avoidance of traumatic delivery, and effective neonatal resuscitation were the key factors, according to

(5–8) Am. J. Obstet. Gynecol. 134:768–771, Aug. 1, 1979.

the authors. The cesarean section rate (37%) was high. Whether or not cesarean section per se predisposes to RDS remains unresolved. The overall outcome results reported here are excellent. More study is needed to know which of the various management steps are the truly important ones.] ◄

Maternal Glucocorticoid in Unplanned Premature Labor: Controlled Study on Effects of Betamethasone Phosphate on Phospholipids of the Gastric Aspirate and on Adrenal Cortical Function of the Newborn Infant. Liggins and Howie showed in 1972 that maternal betamethasone therapy prevents respiratory distress syndrome in premature infants born before the end of week 32 of pregnancy, but glucocorticoid therapy has potential side effects. Kari Teramo, Mikko Hallman, and Kari O. Raivio[5-9] (Univ. of Helsinki) examined the effects of betamethasone on surfactant composition and neonatal adrenal function in a double-blind, placebo-controlled study of 74 patients at risk for premature delivery. Gestational ages ranged from 28 to 35 weeks. Nylidrine or ritodrine was infused to suppress uterine activity, and either 12 mg of betamethasone or placebo was injected intramuscularly. β-Adrenergic drug infusion was continued for at least 12 hours, and the drug was then given intramuscularly and then by mouth. Phospholipid studies were done on 23 newborn infants.

The overall incidence of respiratory distress syndrome was low, and no difference was found between the betamethasone and placebo groups. Phospholipid patterns in gastric aspirates were similar in the two groups of newborn infants. Adrenocortical responsiveness, determined by ACTH testing at age 24 hours, did not differ between the study and placebo groups.

The low incidence of respiratory distress syndrome in this study (3 cases in each group) is ascribed in part to a high rate of prolonged fetal membrane rupture. The findings do not exclude the possibility that antenatal maternal betamethasone administration could prevent respiratory distress syndrome in other defined high-risk infants, such as those born before 32 weeks' gestation. The safety and efficacy of glucocorticoid prophylaxis require further controlled studies before its widespread application is warranted.

► [These results, although consistent with those of the preceding report, are somewhat in conflict with several previous studies in that the incidence of respiratory distress syndrome was similarly low in both betamethasone-treated and control infants. Several features of the study could be responsible. (1) Pregnancies up to 35 weeks' duration were included. (2) The incidence of premature membrane rupture, which is thought by some to accelerate pulmonary maturity, was appreciable. (3) β-Adrenergic drugs, which appear to stimulate surfactant synthesis themselves (see Kanjanpone et al.: Pediatr. Res. 14:278, 1980), were given to all mothers.] ◄

Maternal Pulmonary Edema Resulting From Betamimetic and Glucocorticoid Therapy. Although few reports in the American literature have detailed adverse maternal cardiovascular effects of betamimetic drug therapy, the European literature contains several reports of serious maternal morbidity and mortality related to the simultaneous use of betamimetic agents and corticosteroids. Mark M. Jacobs, Alfred B. Knight, and Fernando Arias[5-10] (Washington

(5–9) Pediatr. Res. 14(Pt. 1):326–329, April 1980.
(5–10) Obstet. Gynecol. 56:56–59, July 1980.

RELATIVE CONTRAINDICATIONS TO USE OF BETAMIMETIC
AND CORTICOSTEROID DRUGS IN PATIENTS WITH
PREMATURE LABOR

Hyperthyroidism

Unstable diabetes mellitus

Asthma already treated by betamimetics

Uncontrolled hypertension

Severe preeclampsia

Moderate to severe cardiac disease, especially aortic stenosis, idiopathic hypertrophic subaortic stenosis, pulmonic stenosis, and mitral stenosis

---

Univ.) report 4 cases of pulmonary edema in women with no primary heart disease who were receiving terbutaline, alone or with glucocorticoids, for treatment of premature labor. Fluid overload triggered the decompensation in these cases. All 4 patients recovered after delivery. Cardiac embarrassment and pulmonary edema were life threatening in 2 patients and moderately severe in the other 2. All had evidence of hemodilution and potassium values below 3 mEq/L.

The vulnerability of pregnant patients given betamimetic drugs and glucocorticoids to sudden cardiac embarrassment and pulmonary edema depends on the development of a compensated high cardiac output state during pregnancy. Terbutaline and other betamimetic drugs cause peripheral vasodilatation and redistribution of blood flow to several organs and increase cardiac output. They may also cause sodium and water retention and may be directly cardiotoxic. These drugs can produce paradoxical postcapillary pulmonary venoconstriction. Anemia and hypokalemia, besides liberal use of crystalloid solutions, predispose to cardiac embarrassment when these drugs are administered. Contraindications to their use are listed in the table. Fluid intake should be maintained at 1.5 to 2 L daily, and total sodium intake at 4 to 6 gm daily. Serum potassium and glucose concentrations should be determined frequently. Patients treated with these drugs should be managed at centers that have facilities for intensive maternal and neonatal care.

▶ [This report of 4 cases calls attention to a recently reported complication of tocolytic therapy, particularly with β-agonists and especially when combined with glucocorticoids and large amounts of intravenous fluids. It reminds us of the observation of Harold Kaminetzky a number of years ago (Obstet. Gynecol. 21:512, 1963): "There are no really 'safe' biologically active drugs. There are only 'safe' physicians." The cautious obstetrician will prescribe these agents only on strict indications where risk-benefit considerations favor their usage. Furthermore, patients should be carefully monitored and fluid administration limited to 1.5 or 2 L per 24 hours. Finally, we cannot resist pointing out that the 4 patients described here were at 27, 32, 34, and 35 weeks' gestation when treated; the indication in the last 2 cases is highly questionable.] ◀

Effects of Betamethasone on Plasma Levels of Estriol, Cortisol, and HCS in Late Pregnancy. Corticosteroids have been used for some time to prevent respiratory distress syndrome. They suppress maternal blood concentrations of estriol and cortisol, whereas the concentration of human chorionic somatomammotropin (hCS) is unaltered. Jan Martin Maltau, Kjell Torgeir Stokke, and Narve

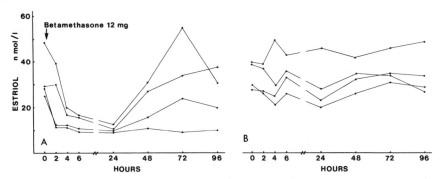

Fig 5-2.—Concentration of unconjugated estriol in maternal plasma. Four patients in each group. *A,* after betamethasone, 12 mg, given intramuscularly; *B,* control group. (Courtesy of Maltau, J. M., et al.: Acta Obstet. Gynecol. Scand. 58:235–238, 1979.)

Moe[5-11] (Rikshosp., Oslo) examined the time course of hormonal changes in maternal plasma after a single corticosteroid dose in 4 patients in the last trimester of pregnancy. One of the corticosteroid-treated patients received therapy to inhibit uterine contractions. Patients received 12 mg of betamethasone intramuscularly. Four patients who did not receive betamethasone served as controls.

Moderate suppression of plasma unconjugated estriol was evident 2 hours after betamethasone administration (Fig 5-2), and a 46% decrease was found at 4 hours. Between 6 and 24 hours the concentration was 33% of baseline. A precipitous increase occurred in 3 patients on the second or third day. A decrease in plasma cortisol concentration occurred after 2 hours, with the lowest value, about 30% of baseline, present after 24 to 48 hours; a gradual rise ensued. The concentration of hCS in maternal plasma was unaffected by the single dose of betamethasone.

A single dose of betamethasone led to a rapid, marked fall in maternal plasma estriol concentration in this study, probably reflecting placental transfer of the corticosteroid and subsequent suppression of fetal production of estriol precursors. The maternal plasma estriol determination will be misleading as a measure of fetal well-being for several days if betamethasone has been given the mother. Human chorionic somatomammotropin, however, is produced by the placenta and is uninfluenced by betamethasone administration to the mother.

▶ [This study illustrates the rapid appearance in the fetus of the effects of maternal betamethasone administration. Maternal plasma estriol levels fell by 50% at 4 hours. The degree of estriol suppression at 24 hours is marked, reminding us to be careful in our interpretation of estriol results in a patient receiving corticosteroids, including acute short-term therapy as described here.] ◀

A Study of the Benefits and Acceptability of Ambulation in Spontaneous Labor. R. M. Williams, Margaret H. Thom, and J. W. W. Studd[5-12] (Dulwich Hosp., London) studied the feasibility of ambulation on 300 consecutive patients and recorded the effects on prog-

(5–11)   Acta Obstet. Gynecol. Scand. 58:235–238, 1979.
(5–12)   Br. J. Obstet. Gynaecol. 87:122–126, February 1980.

ress and outcome of labor as well as patient and nursing acceptability.

Only patients with no at-risk factors were admitted to the study and were divided into two groups according to odd or even hospital numbers on admission. Odd-numbered patients were allocated to the control group, who were nursed in the conventional recumbent fashion with routine labor observations made every 15 minutes and the fetal heart checked by electronic monitor (Sonicaid). Even-numbered patients comprised the study group and were informed about the possible benefits of ambulation and encouraged to walk around during the first stage of labor. Routine labor observations were made at 15-minute intervals with the patient sitting in a chair.

Patients who refused ambulation or requested to return to bed were allowed to do so. Those who had abnormalities of fetal heart rate or showed fresh meconium staining of the amniotic fluid were returned to bed for continuous fetal monitoring. Patients who requested or were advised to have epidural anesthesia also returned to bed, but those requiring oxytocin carried their intravenous infusions with them.

Only 103 patients met the criteria for entry into the study; 48 were ambulant and 55 acted as controls. The ambulant patients returned to bed before the second stage, but all found ambulation during the early first stage acceptable. The nursing staff found ambulation satisfactory, and there were no difficulties with the monitoring procedures used. No difference in the length of first or second stage of labor, incidence of fetal distress, or mode of delivery was observed in the two groups.

The study indicated no reason related to fetal well-being to justify advising that ambulation should be recommended in the management of labor. However, it is not harmful and many patients enjoy the opportunity for mobility. Therefore, facilities for ambulation should be available and ambulation should not be discouraged.

▶ [No harm from ambulation in labor was noted in this study, but no real benefit occurred either. An article in the 1979 YEAR BOOK (p. 132) came to similar conclusions. A subsequent report (1980 YEAR BOOK, p. 144) suggested shorter labors and healthier babies with ambulation. The study designs seem similar. In our view, therefore, the question remains open.] ◀

Prospective Study of Different Methods and Routes of Administration of Prostaglandin E₂ to Improve the Unripe Cervix.
Cervical ripening is associated with loosening of the collagen fiber arrangement in the cervix, probably a result of chemical changes in the ground substance. An absolute loss of collagen may also be involved. There is evidence of direct involvement of E prostaglandins in the ripening process. P. J. Toplis and C. D. Sims[5-13] (London) evaluated various methods of prostaglandin therapy in 60 patients with Bishop scores of 3 or below in whom induction of labor was planned. Patients received a vaginal pessary containing 3 mg of prostaglandin E₂ in a fatty acid base (group A); vaginal paste containing the same dosage (group B); or an extra-amniotic paste with 500 µg of prosta-

(5–13) Prostaglandins 18:127–136, July 1979.

glandin E_2 (group C). Prostaglandin was administered the evening before planned induction.

The groups were similar in maternal age, Bishop scores, and length of gestation, but primigravidas predominated in groups A and B. The number of patients in established labor before formal induction was similar in the various groups. The number requiring oxytocic stimulation was greatest in group A. Failed inductions and cesarean sections were most frequent in groups A and B; all such patients were primigravidas. No uterine hypertonus was noted and there were no differences in mean 5-minute Apgar scores. One fourth of group C patients were febrile during labor, but there were no proved genitourinary or neonatal infections. No patient vomited or had diarrhea. Two patients in group A and 1 in group B had vaginal irritation and discomfort during and after labor; all had been treated antenatally for genital moniliasis.

Considering cost, ease of preparation and storage, and patient and staff convenience, prostaglandin E_2 in pessary form is a superior form of prostaglandin administration to improve the unripe cervix. The use of 3 mg in pessaries is now routine for cervical ripening and induction of labor at the authors' institution. Over 500 inductions have been carried out with no major problems. A wide range of indications, Bishop scores, and gestational ages is represented.

▶ [We have been told by several British investigators that the application of prostaglandin E to the cervix "ripens" the cervix and virtually eliminates the problem of the patient with an unfavorable cervix with the need for induction. This study indicates that there is little difference in applying the agent extra-amniotically, as a paste in the vagina, or as a vaginal pessary. The authors state that the vaginal pessary technique is the easiest and most convenient and has been adopted as the standard approach to cervical ripening for induction. One disadvantage is fever during labor, which occurred in 13% of all subjects and in 25% of those who received the agent extra-amniotically; this is not serious per se but must cause some concern that it indicates infection.

It is unclear to us whether this effect of prostaglandin E on cervical ripening reflects an action on the cervix directly or occurs indirectly via inducing contractions. The former is suggested by the rather remarkable increases in Bishop scores, from a mean of about 2 to 1 of 4 or 5. On the other hand, 25% of the subjects went into labor "spontaneously" after prostaglandin treatment but before induction. In this regard, Liggins (Prostaglandins 18:167, 1979) has shown a 65–85% success rate in inducing labor with prostaglandin E_2 vaginal suppositories. Hutchon and colleagues (Int. J. Gynaecol. Obstet. 17:604, 1980) found that 50% of patients given prostaglandin E_2 gel went into labor, compared with 8.6% of controls.] ◀

Comparison of Prostaglandin E_2 and Intravenous Oxytocin for Induction of Labor. Ulf Ulmsten, Lars Wingerup, and Karl-Erik Andersson[5-14] (Univ. of Lund) studied 100 nulliparas at term who were randomly given oxytocin intravenously or prostaglandin E_2 (PGE_2) gel intracervically. The PGE_2 was prepared by mixing hydroxypropyl methylcellulose with an ethanol solution of PGE_2 as previously described (1978). Each of 50 women received 4 ml gel containing 0.5 mg PGE_2. Each of the other 50 women received oxytocin intravenously with the aid of an electronic infusion pump: 2 mU/minute, increased by 2 mU every half hour up to 24 mU/minute.

In patients with a favorable cervical state (Bishop score of >5),

(5–14) Obstet. Gynecol. 54:581–584, November 1979.

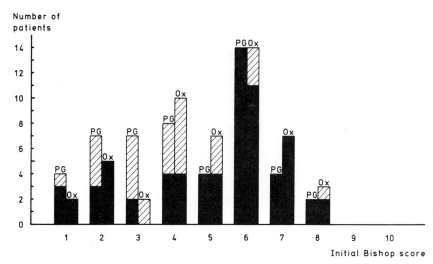

Fig 5–3.—Results of induction in 100 nulliparas randomly given 0.5 mg of PGE_2 gel intracervically or intravenous oxytocin. *Solid bars,* delivered after primary induction; *hatched bars,* undelivered after primary induction; *PG,* patients given PGE_2 gel; *Ox,* patients given oxytocin. (Courtesy of Ulmsten, U., et al.: Obstet. Gynecol. 54:561–584, November 1979.)

both methods seemed equally efficacious in inducing labor (Fig 5–3). However, when the cervical state was unfavorable (Bishop score ≤5), 53% of the patients were delivered within 24 hours with PGE_2 gel compared with 31% when oxytocin was given. In patients with a highly unfavorable cervical state (Bishop score <3), 8 of 18 subjects given PGE_2 delivered within 24 hours compared to 0 of 9 given oxytocin, a significant difference (P < 0.02).

In patients not induced into labor, PGE_2 gel caused a considerable ripening of the cervix, with a mean change in the Bishop score from 2.9 to 6.3. In patients undelivered after oxytocin stimulation, no change in the Bishop score occurred. This effect of locally applied PGE_2 gel on cervical ripening was highly significant (P < 0.001). No adverse maternal or perinatal effects were noted with either mode of treatment.

Results of this study indicate that, in patients with an unfavorable cervix, locally applied PGE_2 gel seems more efficient than intravenous oxytocin for induction of labor. More important is that, unlike oxytocin, intracervically applied PGE_2 gel causes marked ripening of the cervix. Also, PGE_2 has no antidiuretic properties, which may be an asset if labor is to be induced in patients with preeclampsia or cardiac disease.

▶ [These results with 0.5 mg of *intracervical* PGE_2 are quite impressive. The low dose used obviated the gastrointestinal side effects usually associated with prostaglandins. Delivery rates and improvement in Bishop scores in those patients with unfavorable cervices initially were much better in the prostaglandin E_2 group than in the oxytocin group. The authors of this article are convinced that there is a local cervical effect, as many patients with marked cervical ripening after treatment were unaware of uterine contractions.] ◀

OUTCOME ON MORNING AFTER TREATMENT OF CERVIX

—	Placebo	Relaxin
No. of patients	30	30
Delivered at 15 h	0	7
Established in labour	0	3
Average change in cervical score	0·86	3·38
Average change where labour did not supervene	0·86	2·08
No. with no change	18	5

Ripening of Human Cervix and Induction of Labor with Purified Porcine Relaxin. In many species, relaxin plays a major role in cervical ripening before parturition. However, its part in human parturition has yet to be established. In women, serum levels of relaxin do not rise at the end of pregnancy, but cervical tissue levels do. Purified porcine relaxin is now available, and Alastair H. MacLennan, Roslyn C. Green, Gillian D. Bryant-Greenwood, Frederick C. Greenwood, and Robert F. Seamark[5-15] investigated its effect on cervical ripening and parturition in a randomized double-blind study of 60 patients. Treatment and control groups were closely matched, except that the mean initial cervical score of the relaxin group was 1.6 points higher than the placebo group, using a modified Bishop score. Patients received the relaxin or placebo as an intravaginal gel.

A comparison of the placebo and relaxin groups is illustrated in the table. Within 15 hours, 10 of the 30 patients given relaxin went into labor, but none of the control group did; this difference is highly significant. There was also a significant improvement in the cervical score of the relaxin group, even in those patients who did not go into labor. The improvement was seen regardless of initial cervical score, parity, or gestation.

Significantly fewer women who received relaxin required oxytocin to enhance labor, as compared to controls. The treatment group also had shorter labors. No significant difference was seen between the two groups in mode of delivery, degree of analgesia, or Apgar scores.

No side effects of relaxin were noted in the women, nor were there neonatal complications.

This trial suggests that endogenous relaxin may be important in ripening the human cervix and in initiation of parturition.

▶ [Much interest recently has been directed at means of ripening the cervix prior to the induction of labor. These efforts are well placed. The present study concerns porcine relaxin (the polypeptide hormone found in animals and in the corpora lutea of pregnant women). The authors of this report think the striking effects illustrated in the table are due to a direct effect of relaxin on the cervix rather than to an effect mediated through uterine contractions. A weakness of this study is that despite random assignment, the relaxin group had much more favorable cervices to begin with than did the placebo group. Whether relaxin really relaxes the cervix remains to be seen.] ◀

(5–15) Lancet 1:220–223, Feb. 2, 1980.

Sinusoidal Fetal Heart Rate: Clinical Significance. The sinusoidal fetal heart rate is usually considered indicative of severe fetal jeopardy. Bruce K. Young, Miriam Katz, and Stephen J. Wilson[5-16] (New York Univ.) reviewed the sinusoidal fetal heart rate in 16 neonates with respect to perinatal outcome, fetal scalp and umbilical arterial pH, and characteristics of the fetal heart rate (FHR) pattern. Sinusoidal heart rate was defined as an FHR pattern of regular variability, resembling a sine wave, having a relatively fixed periodicity of 3–5 cpm and an amplitude of 5–40 beats/minute from the basal FHR, and lasting at least 10 minutes.

The incidence of sinusoidal heart rate was <0.3% of monitored patients. There were 10 high-risk pregnancies. A sinusoidal heart rate occurred only in the first stage of labor in 11 patients and only in the second stage in 2; it occurred during both stages, during the antepartum and intrapartum periods, and only during unstressed monitoring in 1 patient each.

There were no perinatal deaths in this series. Two fetuses were delivered by normal spontaneous vaginal delivery, 8 by low forceps, and 6 by primary cesarean section.

Apgar scores were 6 or less at 1 minute in 5 neonates. Only 1 had an Apgar score under 6 at 5 minutes; this was partially attributed to meconium aspiration.

In 11 fetuses the sinusoidal heart rate was monitored by fetal scalp blood sampling. In this group 5 fetuses were preacidotic or acidotic, having pH levels less than 7.25; 4 had pH values of 7.20 or less. Three of the 11 fetuses had repeated pH values of 7.20 or less, and Apgar scores of 6 or less at 1 minute. Conversely, 7 had normal scalp pH levels and Apgar scores of 7 or more. When scalp pH is compared with the amplitude of the sinusoidal heart rate there is a highly significant correlation: low pH is correlated with increased amplitude. In the 8 fetuses also monitored by umbilical artery pH levels, a similar, highly significant inverse relationship was demonstrated between pH and sinusoidal heart rate amplitude. Acidosis appears to be associated with an amplitude of at least 15 beats/minute.

The pathophysiology of sinusoidal heart rate is not understood. These data suggest that acidosis may follow the development of sinusoidal heart rate, but is not intrinsic to it. The sinusoidal heart rate may begin without acidosis being present and may persist in normal or preacidotic conditions.

In the non-Rh-isoimmunized pregnancy, the sinusoidal heart rate does not necessarily imply impending fetal demise or necessitate emergency delivery. Management decisions should be based on biochemical monitoring, with labor and vaginal delivery indicated unless the fetus becomes acidotic.

▶ [When the sinusoidal heart rate was first recognized, it was thought to have a very ominous prognosis in that most fetuses exhibiting the pattern died. Subsequently, it has become clear that the sinusoidal pattern indicates a potentially serious, but not hopeless, situation. In this careful clinical analysis, the frequency of low scalp pH or low Apgar score was about 1 in 2 or 3; there were no perinatal deaths, due in all likeli-

(5–16) Am. J. Obstet. Gynecol. 136:587–593, Mar. 1, 1980.

hood to prompt and appropriate management. Clearly, scalp pH measurement is indicated immediately upon recognition of a sinusoidal pattern.] ◄

Influence of Occiput Posterior Position on Fetal Heart Rate Pattern. In fetal heart rate monitoring, decelerations of various types are important indicators of fetal condition during delivery. Eva Ingemarsson, Ingemar Ingemarsson, Thore Solum, and Magnus Westgren[5-17] (Univ. Hosp., Lund, Sweden) investigated the possible influence of the occiput posterior position on the fetal heart rate.

The 138 infants born in the occiput posterior position were matched with infants born in the occiput anterior position. Age, parity, duration of labor, and monitoring rate were similar in the two groups. Epidural nerve block was used in approximately 20% of the patients in each group.

Early and late decelerations occurred in 25% and 3% of the patients, respectively, in both groups. Variable decelerations occurred much more frequently in the occiput posterior position group (59%) compared to controls (33%).

Variable decelerations of 30 to 60 beats occurred with the same frequency in both groups, but decelerations of more than 60 beats were significantly more frequent in the occiput posterior position group.

There was no significant difference between the groups in incidence of cord complications at birth. Similarly, the incidence of low Apgar scores was comparable.

This study indicates that not all variable decelerations are caused by cord compression; the occiput posterior position of the fetal head is at least partly responsible for some of these events. However, these periodic fetal heart rate patterns do not always reflect an increased risk of fetal distress.

► [This is a very interesting clinical observation. Variable decelerations, especially those lacking an initial acceleration, were much more common in fetuses delivered in the occiput posterior position. The incidence of apparent cord complications did not differ between the two groups. Although it would be nice to know when in labor the decelerations occurred, we are presumably looking at a vagal response to a pressure phenomenon that is dependent on fetal position. Hopefully, others will analyze their monitor tracing data in an attempt to confirm or refute this finding.] ◄

Pediatric Follow-up of Randomized Controlled Trial of Intrapartum Fetal Monitoring Techniques. Sharon Langendoerfer, Albert D. Haverkamp, James Murphy, Kenneth D. Nowick, Miriam Orleans, Frank Pacosa, and William van Doorninck[5-18] (Univ. of Colorado) evaluated methods of fetal surveillance in a prospective, randomized, controlled trial in offspring of high-risk mothers in labor after at least 34 weeks' gestation. A total of 690 such women were assigned randomly to monitoring by auscultation alone, electronic monitoring alone, or electronic monitoring with the option to obtain the fetal scalp pH. Brazelton examinations were performed at ages 48 to 72 hours, and the infants were reevaluated at age 9 months with the Bayley Scales of Infant Development and the Milani-Comparetti

(5–17) Obstet. Gynecol. 55:301–304, March 1980.
(5–18) J. Pediatr. 97:103–107, July 1980.

Development Test. The different monitoring groups were comparable with respect to clinical and sociodemographic characteristics.

The three groups of offspring did not differ significantly in neonatal mortality or morbidity, Apgar scores, cord blood gas values, or Brazelton examination results at ages 2 to 3 days. Reevaluation at age 9 months showed no significant differences in growth or development among infants in the different monitoring groups. Cesarean section delivery was significantly more frequent in the electronically monitored group than in the auscultated group.

This study demonstrated no benefit from electronic fetal monitoring, as compared with auscultation alone, for high-risk but relatively mature fetuses. Auscultatory monitoring allows more flexibility in hospital rules to accommodate the wishes of parents regarding labor and delivery. Careful auscultation provides a medically acceptable alternative when electronic monitoring is undesirable for other reasons. The wide variety of circumstances in maternity services calls for variety of policies regarding fetal surveillance.

▶ [This follow-up report of the Denver electronic monitoring study considers infant development at 9 months of age. The monitored groups fared no better than the auscultated group. Again, it must be emphasized that the auscultated group received excellent, intensive nursing care (cf. 1980 YEAR BOOK, pp. 150–151).] ◀

Intrapartum Fetal Heart Rate: Correlation with Scalp pH in Preterm Fetus. The relationship of fetal heart rate (FHR) patterns and fetal scalp blood pH is well documented in the term fetus. Monitoring of the FHR has been increasingly used in the intrapartum management of the preterm fetus. Bernardino Zanini, Richard H. Paul, and James R. Huey[5-19] (Univ. of Southern California) reviewed the records of 62 patients who had FHR monitoring and scalp blood pH determinations during 1966 to 1975. All were at 36 weeks' gestation or less, had birth weights under 2,500 gm, and were appropriate for gestational age. The FHR data in the 20 minutes preceding the pH determination were analyzed for the level and variability of the baseline FHR. The presence or absence of short- and long-term variability was noted. Periodic accelerations or decelerations were independently tabulated for each uterine contraction.

In 13 cases (31%), fetal tachycardia occurred. Bradycardia occurred in one case. The pH distributions in the tachycardic group and in that with normal FHRs were similar. The absence of both short-term variability and long-term variability of FHRs was associated with a significantly lower mean pH regardless of periodic FHR patterns. Of the 62 fetuses, 37 (60%) demonstrated accelerations in the periodic FHR patterns. The mean pH of the group with accelerations was significantly higher than that of those without. There was a positive linear correlation between pH and the percentage of uterine contractions with accelerations. When accelerations were associated with absent short-term variability, the mean pH was significantly lower.

There was no correlation between the occurrence of early decelerations and pH values. There was no significant difference in the mean

(5–19) Am. J. Obstet. Gynecol. 136:43–47, Jan. 1, 1980.

pH of the groups with or without variable deceleration patterns, although the pH was significantly lower when variable decelerations occurred with more than 75% of the uterine contractions. The group with late deceleration of FHRs had a significantly lower pH level compared with those without such patterns. There was a negative linear correlation between pH and the percentage of uterine contractions with late decelerations. All pH values under 7.20 occurred in patients with late decelerations. Only 8 fetuses (42%) with late decelerations had normal pH values.

The general trends in FHR and pH observed in the mature fetus are also valid in the preterm fetus, although the preterm fetus may abruptly demonstrate FHR patterns that progress in their degree of severity more rapidly than the mature fetus.

▶ [Virtually all authorities agree that fetal blood sampling is an essential part of fetal monitoring. Normative data for fetal pH values were derived from term fetuses and their applicability to the premature fetus, whereas there is no reason to doubt it, has not been proved. Because premature labor is one of the clear indications for fetal monitoring, this question is of some consequence. As demonstrated by this study, the correlation between FHR and scalp pH seems to apply to the premature fetus in much the same way as in the term fetus.] ◀

Normal Values for Fetal Scalp Tissue pH during Labor. T. Weber and Suzanne Hahn-Pedersen[5-20] (Univ. of Copenhagen) measured normal values for fetal scalp tissue pH during labor by using a glass electrode and compared them to normal values for fetal scalp blood. A total of 132 recordings were obtained and 84 (64%) were of good quality.

Of the 84 patients with recordings of good quality, 64 had infants with an Apgar score of 9 or 10 at 1 and 5 minutes after delivery. The 64 recordings showed pH values (mean ± 2 SEM) of 7.38 ± 0.12 at 6 hours before delivery and 7.28 ± 0.12 at time of delivery. Between the 5th and 55th minutes of the second stage of labor, the pH (mean ± 2 SEM) fell from 7.30 ± 0.14 to 7.20 ± 0.13 (Fig 5–4).

The authors have previously found a very close correlation between fetal tissue and scalp blood pH values. Their pH values resemble most closely the highest values observed for fetal scalp blood.

Other authors have emphasized the variation of fetal scalp blood pH values between one clinic and another. This variation was thought to be due to variations in management of labor and in the techniques used for fetal blood sampling.

Because the tissue pH is measured by an implanted electrode, some of the technical reasons for variations in pH in different clinics will be removed, leaving only the difference in management of labor.

Continuous measurement of fetal tissue pH is relatively new, but the similarity between normal values in labor for tissue pH and fetal scalp blood pH suggests that tissue pH measurements will ultimately play a role in fetal monitoring. Advantages of tissue pH measurements are that they are continuous, less traumatic to the fetal scalp, and less time-consuming than measurement of pH in fetal scalp blood

(5–20) Br. J. Obstet. Gynaecol. 86:728–731, September 1979.

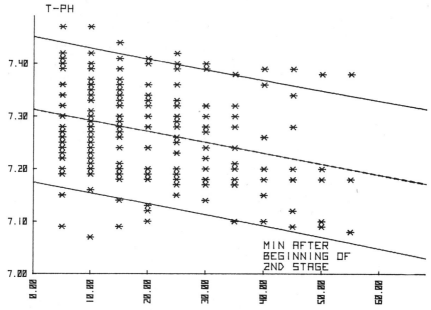

Fig 5–4.—Normal values of fetal scalp tissue pH in second stage of labor (64 patients). *Dotted line,* mean. *Upper* and *lower lines,* 95% confidence limits. (Courtesy of Weber, T., and Hahn-Pedersen, S.: Br. J. Obstet. Gynaecol. 86:728–731, September 1979.

samples. The disadvantage is the high (36%) rate of unsuccessful recordings, but this will probably be overcome by improvements in the design of tissue pH electrodes.

▶ [The technique of continuous fetal tissue pH measurement is now in the clinical trial stage. This article describes normal values, which seem to correlate quite closely with what is known from intermittent fetal blood determinations. At complete dilation, the mean was 7.32 and the normal range 7.17–745; pH fell progressively during the second stage to an average value of 7.25 at 1 hour. Technical problems exist—only 64% of the recordings were of "good" quality—but this is clearly the most promising approach to intrapartum fetal assessment on the horizon.] ◀

Acid-Base Characteristics of Fetuses With Intrauterine Growth Retardation During Labor and Delivery. Intrauterine growth retardation (IUGR) accounts for a large proportion of perinatal morbidity and perinatal mortality. Chin-Chu Lin, Atef H. Moawad, Philip J. Rosenow, and Philip River[5-21] (Univ. of Chicago) investigated the acid-base status of IUGR fetuses at birth and related it to fetal heart rate (FHR) decelerations. Study was made of 37 IUGR fetuses and 108 normally grown fetuses during 1977 and 1978.

Both maternal and fetal blood lactate concentrations increased with the progress of labor; the fetal values were higher. In the absence of intrapartum FHR decelerations, IUGR fetuses were not significantly different from control fetuses with respect to umbilical arterial lactate, pH, or blood gas values. Late deceleration was observed in 30% of the IUGR group and 7% of controls. In the presence of FHR

(5–21) Am. J. Obstet. Gynecol. 137:553–559, July 1, 1980.

decelerations, IUGR fetuses exhibited significantly higher lactate concentrations than controls. Apgar scores did not differ significantly in the groups with and without FHR decelerations. There was no difference in section rates between the IUGR and the control groups. The groups did not differ significantly in any maternal high-risk factors. Gestational age did not appear to be important in the occurrence of fetal metabolic acidosis.

Growth-retarded fetuses tolerate labor less well than normally grown fetuses. In the absence of FHR decelerations, it appears to be safe to allow IUGR fetuses to go through labor and vaginal delivery. Earlier intervention is preferable in the presence of late FHR decelerations because of the increased risk of metabolic acidosis.

▶ [In this study, no difference in acid-base status was found in growth-retarded and normal fetuses as long as the FHR pattern was normal. In the presence of late decelerations, however, IUGR infants exhibited a greater degree of lactic acidemia, presumably reflecting lesser reserve against hypoxia, than did normal infants. Suspected fetal growth retardation is probably the clearest indication for FHR monitoring in labor, and these data underscore the need for prompt investigation (ie, fetal blood sampling) in the presence of any FHR abnormality, particularly when the fetus is growth retarded.] ◀

Controlled Intravenous Bicarbonate and Fetal-Maternal Acid-Base Balance: I. Primipara. The fetus is in a state of relative acidosis during labor and delivery, and marked acidosis has deleterious effects on oxygenation and glycolysis, contributing to fetal hypoxia. Eliahu Caspi, Raphael Ron-El, and David Modai[5-22] (Tel Aviv Univ.) examined the effects of controlled material sodium bicarbonate administration on maternal and fetal acid-base balance during labor in primiparas with uncomplicated singleton pregnancies who entered labor spontaneously at term, with no signs of fetal distress. Ten sodium bicarbonate-treated patients were compared with 12 controls. Sodium bicarbonate was given in a dosage of 2 mEq/kg, starting at cervical dilation of 6 cm and continuing until full dilation occurred. The total amount infused ranged from 102 to 176 mEq.

Highly significant changes in pH, base excess, and plasma bicarbonate were noted in both mothers and fetuses, appearing in the latter after a time lag of about 2 hours. No adverse effects were seen in the mothers or fetuses. The maternal pH after sodium bicarbonate infusion was 7.51 at cervical dilation of 8 cm, compared with 7.42 in the control group. Fetal pH also was significantly higher in the treated group. No significant differences in P_{CO_2} were noted. Apgar scores at 1 minute were comparable in the treated and control groups.

Controlled sodium bicarbonate infusion led to a significant reduction in relative fetal acidosis in this study. The results warrant further studies of the potential of this method for use in high-risk deliveries and during intrapartum fetal distress.

▶ [This interesting study demonstrates that the fetal pH can be elevated by maternal sodium bicarbonate administration. Bicarbonate transfer across the placenta is thought to be a slow process, which probably explains the 2-hour lag from the start of the infusion to an observed fetal effect. Whether this demonstration of acid-base gymnastics has any clinical relevance is unknown. We must be careful not to conclude

(5–22) Obstet. Gynecol. 54:615–623, November 1979.

from these data that a distressed fetus would be helped if bicarbonate were given to the mother. Much more study is needed.] ◄

Fetal Breathing in Labor. Fetal breathing movements occur normally in late pregnancy. Peter Boylan and Peter J. Lewis[5-23] (London) investigated fetal breathing movements during labor in 42 patients who subsequently delivered healthy infants. Fetal breathing activity was recorded with a real-time B mode ultrasonic scanner. A sagittal section through the fetal chest wall and upper abdomen was recorded on videotape. Fetal breathing was considered to be continuous if more than one breath was observed every 6 seconds. Twenty-two patients were studied twice in an open trial, ante partum after the 38th week of pregnancy and again during labor, for periods of 25 to 50 minutes. All patients received a 50-gm glucose drink 30 minutes before the antepartum study. A double-blind study was done in 12 women given 0.2 gm of glucose per kg intravenously or Hartmann solution. Eight patients were studied in conjunction with artificial rupture of the membranes.

All pregnancy outcomes were normal. Breathing movements were seen in each case prenatally; the mean fetal breathing index, or time that continuous breathing occurred, was 36%. The mean fetal body movement index was 6.6%. The mean maternal blood glucose concentration rose from 62.9 to 92.9 mg/dl 1 hour after glucose ingestion. In only 3 of the 22 cases was fetal breathing observed during labor, and the mean index was below 1%. No significant change in fetal breathing was observed after glucose injection in the double-blind study. The fetal breathing index fell from 23% to 5.5% in the 30 minutes after membrane rupture. Fetal breathing movements were not observed during membrane rupture.

Fetal breathing activity occurs only rarely during labor. Maternal hypoglycemia, hypocapnia, or analgesia is not responsible. The onset of labor is probably associated with a marked change in the stage of the fetal CNS, possibly mediated by a change in circulating prostaglandin levels. Fetal apnea is normal during labor and has no adverse prognostic significance.

► [This study demonstrates that fetal breathing activity diminishes markedly during labor—in fact, even with amniotomy before the onset of contractions. Moreover, it is not stimulated by maternal hyperglycemia as occurs ante partum. Apparently something about parturition signals the fetus to cease breathing movements. The authors speculate that prostaglandins may be responsible, since prostaglandin inhibitors have been reported to stimulate breathing activities in the sheep.] ◄

Macrosomia—Maternal, Fetal, and Neonatal Implications. In a retrospective study, Houchang D. Modanlou, Wendy L. Dorchester, Anna Thorosian, and Roger K. Freeman[5-24] (Mem. Hosp. Med. Center, Long Beach, Calif.) evaluated a number of factors in 287 mothers of macrosomic (birth weight ≥ 4,536 gm) fetuses and 284 mothers of appropriate weight term-size fetuses. These variables included age, weight, medical history, past obstetric history, type of delivery, delivery complications, and pregnancy outcomes (table). The

(5–23) Obstet. Gynecol. 56:35–38, July 1980.

(5–24) Ibid., 55:420–424, April 1980.

COMPARISON OF MATERNAL, PATERNAL, AND FETAL FACTORS ASSOCIATED WITH THE
MACROSOMIC AND CONTROL GROUPS

	Macrosomic group ($N = 287$)		Control group ($N = 284$)		Value of P
	No.	Percent	No.	Percent	
Cesarean section	71	24.7	31	10.9	<0.005
Shoulder dystocia	22	7.7	1	0.4	<0.005
FHR monitoring	126	43.9	117	41.4	NS
Primiparous	72	25.1	131	46.5	<0.005
Grand multiparous (para >5)	12	4.2	5	1.8	NS
Diabetes mellitus	20	7.0	4	1.4	<0.005
Previous infant >4000 g	96	33.4	9	3.2	<0.005
Obesity (>15% above normal)	112	39.0	28	9.9	<0.005
Pregnancy weight >90 kg	37 ($N = 244$)*	15.2	4 ($N = 246$)	1.4	<0.005
Maternal age >35 years	17 ($N = 285$)	6.0	10 ($N = 283$)	3.5	NS
Paternal age >35 years	31 ($N = 254$)	12.2	25 ($N = 253$)	10.0	NS
Augmented labor	82	28.6	46	16.2	<0.005

NS, not significant.
*N is given in parentheses when records did not contain the information.

results of fetal monitoring were reviewed, as were the neonatal courses of the infants.

Macrosomia occurred in 1.3% of the deliveries over a 7-year period. There were 3 fetal and 1 neonatal deaths in the macrosomic group, for a perinatal mortality of 13.9/1,000. This is a lower rate than that found in other studies, but is almost twice the perinatal mortality rate of 7.0/1,000 in the controls. The difference is not significant, however.

The incidence of intrapartum fetal distress documented by monitoring was not significantly different in the macrosomic and control fetuses.

Cephalopelvic disproportion was the indication for cesarean section in a significantly higher proportion of macrosomic fetuses compared to controls.

A male to female ratio of 2.3:1 was observed in the macrosomic infants. Also, the number of macrosomic infants admitted to the neonatal intensive care unit was significantly higher. Increased morbidity in macrosomic neonates cannot be related to detectable intrapartum hypoxia prior to delivery, but, rather, is due largely to the traumatic aspects of delivery. It may be beneficial to identify the macrosomic fetus prior to delivery and to consider liberalizing the indications for cesarean section in these patients.

▶ [The results of this study of fetal macrosomia (defined here as a birth weight ⩾4536 gm) are similar to those of a recent report by Benedetti and Gabbe (1980 YEAR BOOK, p. 165) concerning predictive factors and risks. An interesting point is that macrosomic fetuses are not at increased risk for fetal distress in *labor*. The risk in this condition is associated with the delivery process.] ◀

Randomized Management of Term Frank Breech Presentation: Study of 208 Cases. Joseph V. Collea, Connie Chein, and Edward J. Quilligan[5-25] (Univ. of Southern California) conducted a pro-

(5–25) Am. J. Obstet. Gynecol. 137:235–244, May 15, 1980.

spective study of 208 women in labor at term with a single fetus in frank breech presentation. Elective section was performed in 93 instances; the other 115 patients were randomized to vaginal delivery. About 80% of women delivered infants weighing over 2,500 gm. Five women scheduled for cesarean section progressed rapidly in labor and were delivered vaginally without complications. Three women who had not undergone x-ray pelvimetry were delivered vaginally without incident. Fifty-two of the 112 women roentgenographed had inadequate pelvic measurements and were scheduled for cesarean section delivery, but 3 delivered vaginally without incident. Forty-nine women with normal measurements were delivered vaginally with no perinatal deaths. Eleven others required section for difficulty during labor.

There were no maternal deaths in this series, but postpartum morbidity occurred in 49.3% of the 148 women who were delivered by cesarean section. Only 4 women who delivered vaginally (6.7%) had postpartum complications. The rate of neonatal morbidity in infants delivered by cesarean section according to protocol was 6.1%. The rate for vaginally delivered infants was 16.3%.

From these findings it seems reasonable to allow vaginal delivery in carefully selected cases of term frank breech presentation. Both birth injuries in this study occurred during partial breech extractions complicated by the presence of a nuchal arm. The rate of maternal morbidity from cesarean section is striking. Selected frank breech presentations can be delivered vaginally with minimal risk for both mother and infant.

▶ [A preliminary report of this study was published a few years ago (Am. J. Obstet. Gynecol. 131:186, 1978; abstracted in 1979 YEAR BOOK, pp. 160–161). The additional patients do not change the earlier conclusions: If the pelvis is adequate and labor progress is normal, the term frank breech of moderate size can be delivered vaginally with safety; maternal morbidity is increased with cesarean section. Although oxytocin was used in this study for induction and stimulation of labor, we generally do not favor its use in breech presentations.] ◀

Minimal Brain Dysfunction in Children Born in Breech Presentation. An earlier study showed an association between breech presentation and reading and writing difficulties in children. Stefan Fianu and Ingemar Joelsson[5-26] sought to elucidate further the relation between breech delivery and the occurrence of minimal brain dysfunction (MBD). Of 274 prematurely delivered children, 136 had breech presentations. About 20% had hyperkinesia, learning disability, or both. Of 1,921 mature children, 963 had breech presentations. The rate of hyperkinesia and learning disabilities was 19% in the breech group and 4% in the vertex group. Reading and writing difficulties occurred in about 25% and 10% of cases, respectively, and speech disorders in 5% and 2% of these groups (Table 1). Disability was mostly confined to breech children delivered vaginally rather than by section (Table 2). There was a marked predominance of girls in the breech group.

Besides other causes, maturity at birth, trauma, and possibly even

(5–26) Acta Obstet. Gynecol. Scand. 58:295–299, 1979.

TABLE 1.—OCCURRENCE OF HYPERKINETIC SYNDROME, LEARNING DISABILITY, AND SPEECH DISORDERS IN TERM DELIVERED INFANTS

Group	Breech delivery No.	%	Vertex delivery No.	%
Hyperkinetic syndrome				
1. Impulsivity	242	25.1	68	7.1
2. Disorder of attention	241	25.0	57	5.9
3. Emotional lability	236	24.5	61	6.4
• All three symptoms combined	178	18.5	36	3.8
Learning disability				
1. Dyslexia	246	25.5	97	10.1
2. Dysgraphia	243	25.2	91	9.5
3. Dyscalculia	245	25.4	94	9.8
• All three symptoms combined	181	18.8	39	4.1
▪ *Hyperkinetic syndrome and learning disability combined*	134	13.9	17	1.8
Speech disorders	47	4.9	19	2.0
▪ *All three syndromes combined*	23	2.4	6	0.6
Total number of infants	963		958	

TABLE 2.—OCCURRENCE OF HYPERKINETIC SYNDROME, LEARNING DISABILITY, AND SPEECH DISORDERS IN INFANTS IN BREECH PRESENTATION BY MODE OF DELIVERY

Group	Vaginal delivery No.	%	Cesarean section No.	%
Hyperkinetic syndrome				
1. Impulsivity	239	27.6	3	3.1
2. Disorder of attention	239	27.6	2	2.0
3. Emotional lability	233	26.9	3	3.1
• All three symptoms combined	176	20.3	2	2.0
Learning disability				
1. Dyslexia	244	28.2	2	2.0
2. Dysgraphia	242	28.0	1	1.0
3. Dyscalculia	244	28.2	1	1.0
• All three symptoms combined	180	20.8	1	1.0
▪ *Hyperkinetic syndrome and learning disability combined*	133	15.4	1	1.0
Speech disorders	45	5.2	2	2.0
▪ *All three syndromes combined*	23	2.7	—	—
Total number of infants	865		98	

periods of asphyxia during delivery play significant roles in the occurrence of MBD. With correct management of deliveries, particularly in breech presentations, the obstetrician can substantially contribute to prevention of MBD.

▶ [This questionnaire-chart review study involves births of more than a decade ago. Despite these limitations, the results reported are disturbing. Although minimal brain dysfunction (MBD) was found in 20% of low birth weight infants whether delivered from vertex or breech presentation, a disproportionate share of non-low birth weight infants with breech presentations suffered from MBD as compared with their vertex presentation controls (14% vs 2%). Was this related to trauma or asphyxia at delivery or was it predetermined—ie, was the presentation breech because the baby was already abnormal? *Suggestive* evidence that the method of delivery may have been important is seen in Table 2—15% of infants with breech presentations delivered vaginally had MBD vs 1% of those infants delivered by cesarean section. Although there are many variables not controlled for in this study and one must, therefore, be careful in drawing conclusions, the issue is so important that we hope other workers will soon study the school performance of breech children as related to several perinatal factors, including their mode of delivery. One of us was a vaginally delivered term breech; the other thinks this explains many things!

Another possible infant complication of vaginal breech birth—temporomandibular joint (TMJ) injuries—is suggested by Grosfeld and colleagues (J. Oral Rehabil. 7:65, 1980). Evidence of TMJ injury on examination at age 4 to 6 years was found in 67.5% of infants born by breech with the classic Mauriceau maneuver compared with 50.7% of vertex controls. If only the more severe TMJ disorders were considered, the difference was more striking (48.2% vs 29.7%).] ◀

Hyponatremic Fits in Oxytocin-Augmented Labors. Water intoxication associated with oxytocin infusion has been reported frequently in varying clinical circumstances. P. McKenna and R. W. Shaw[5-27] (Birmingham, England) describe 3 patients who had seizures as a result of hyponatremia. Each was in spontaneous term labor and received conventional doses of oxytocin for augmentation of labor.

Woman, 18, a primigravida in good health, was admitted in spontaneous labor at 35 weeks' gestation. The membranes were ruptured at 3 cm cervical dilation. Oxytocin was started 2 hours later at 2 mU/minute, with the dosage increased stepwise to 10 mU/minute. The cervix was 9 cm dilated after 11 hours in labor, and remained at that level for 3 hours. Lower segment cesarean section then was elected, but the patient had a grand mal seizure that was controlled by intravenous diazepam. The blood pressure just before the seizure was normal, and there was no proteinuria. A 3.5-kg infant was delivered by lower segment cesarean section. Although a cyanotic attack and convulsion occurred 4 hours after birth, the infant's subsequent course was uneventful. The mother had received 5 L of 5% aqueous dextrose in 15 hours before the seizure, during which time the total urine output was 900 ml, 650 ml of it in the first 6 hours of labor. The total dose of oxytocin was less than 15 IU. The serum sodium level at the time of the seizure was 114 mM/L, the urea level was 2.8, and the potassium level was 3.3 mM/L. The patient recovered fully within 24 hours. An EEG obtained during the puerperium was normal.

The dosage of oxytocin did not exceed 15 IU in these cases, and the fluids were administered in a much shorter time than in previously reported cases. It is, however, not likely that the hyponatremia was merely a result of water intoxication. Treatment should be with normal saline rather than a diuretic, and hypertonic saline may be con-

(5-27) Int. J. Gynaecol. Obstet. 17:250–252, Nov.–Dec. 1979.

sidered. As a rule, no more than 2 L of 5% dextrose in water should be given in any labor, at least without medical reassessment of the patient. Some patients may be relatively susceptible to the effects of oxytocin.

▶ [Water intoxication associated with oxytocin administration usually occurs in situations where oxytocin is given for long periods of time in large volumes of electrolyte-free solutions. The duration of infusion was not remarkable in the cases described, but the amounts of 5% dextrose in water infused were striking. The problem can be avoided by infusing electrolyte solutions to women in labor, by increasing the concentration of oxytocin in the bottle rather than the amount of fluid administered, and by paying attention to the input and output sheet.] ◀

Increase in Cesarean Birth Rate. Sidney F. Bottoms, Mortimer G. Rosen, and Robert J. Sokol[5-28] (Case Western Reserve Univ.) point out that the threefold rise in the cesarean birth rate that has occurred in the United States in the past decade is a source of concern to both obstetricians and the general public. Maternal mortality from cesarean birth has become rare. Perinatal mortality is less than one third that reported three decades ago, and there is evidence that the selective use of cesarean section delivery can improve the prognosis for the fetus. Cesarean birth rates have long been high among infants with low birth weights. Older patients are more likely to have cesarean deliveries. Similarly, clinic patients are more likely today than in the past to have cesarean section delivery. In addition, more obstetric care today is provided by obstetricians, who perform cesarean sections more often than do nonobstetricians. Increased third-party payment of perinatal expenses may also be related to increased cesarean birth rates.

Changes in the cesarean birth rate pattern according to indication

PERCENTAGE OF INCREASE IN CESAREAN BIRTH RATE, ACCORDING TO INDICATION*

STUDY	INDICATION				ALL OTHER INDICATIONS
	DYSTOCIA	REPEAT	BREECH	FETAL DISTRESS	
	cesarean birth rate per hundred deliveries				
Hibbard	18.3	15.5	47.5	20.4	0.0
Haddad and Lundy	41.7	18.3	13.8	23.8	3.0
Gabert and Stenchever	22.6	28.0	−0.6	12.0	34.0
Hughey et al	50.9	18.9	15.1	4.2	11.3
Mann and Gallant	33.3	35.0	18.3	5.7	7.7
Mean increase	33.4	23.1	18.8	13.2	11.2

*As calculated according to the formula in the text.

(5–28) N. Engl. J. Med. 302:599–563, Mar. 6, 1980.

are shown in the table. Cesarean section for dystocia is the largest category, repeat cesarean births representing nearly 25% of the increase in such births. Changes in the management of breech presentation and the increased use of fetal monitoring procedures also are related to the increase in cesarean births. A selective approach could be used to reduce repeat cesarean section deliveries. There may also be safe means of modifying the management of dystocia so that cesarean birth rates will decline. These and other possible means of reducing cesarean birth rates have not received appropriate emphasis in the recent literature or in residency training programs.

▶ [This is a thoughtful analysis of the factors involved in the increased cesarean section rates in the United States. The following article reviews one year's experience of a particular hospital in more detail.] ◀

Cesarean Section: Contemporary Assessment. John R. Evrard, Edwin M. Gold, and Terrence F. Cahill[5-29] (Brown Univ.) report a 1-year retrospective study of cesarean section in 1977. Of 5,467 deliveries, 1,011 were by cesarean section, for a total rate of 18.5% and a primary rate of 13.4%. The leading indications were dystocia, breech presentation, malposition, and fetal distress (table). The mean maternal age was 25.3 years. Cesarean sections were done at 38 to 42 weeks' gestation in 75% of the patients. Nonelective repeat cesarean section was done on 322 women.

Postoperative complications occurred in 19.9% of patients. The complication rate was 24.3% for primary cesarean section and 10.2% for repeat procedures. Septic complications accounted for 75% of postoperative morbidity. Eighty-seven patients had serious septic sequelae related to the procedure. Three bladder injuries occurred, all in association with primary cesarean section. Severe postoperative bleeding occurred eight times, and 2 patients required hysterectomy. Elective sterilization by tubal ligation was carried out in 14.6% of patients.

INDICATIONS FOR CESAREAN SECTION

	Number	%	Multipara with previous vaginal delivery Number	%	Infants <2,500 gm Number	%
Repeat	322	100.0			22	6.7
Primary	689	100.0				
Dystocia*	267	38.8	34	12.7	5	1.9
Breech	103	14.9	32	31.1	14	13.6
Malposition	82	11.9	14	17.1	1	1.2
Fetal distress	78	11.3	17	11.8	12	15.4
Prolonged rupture—bow	33	4.8	6	18.2	9	27.3
Toxemia	26	3.8	4	15.4	13	50.0
Abruptio placentae	17	2.5	11	64.7	9	52.9
Placenta previa	14	2.0	10	71.4	9	64.3
Malpresentation	14	2.0	10	71.4	6	42.9
Diabetes	12	1.7	1	9.3	3	25.0
Other†	43	6.2	14	32.6	20	46.5

*Fetopelvic disproportion (246), uterine dysfunction (13), failure to progress (8).
†Previous genital surgery, intrauterine growth retardation, uterine anomaly, genital herpes, erythroblastosis, heart disease, failed induction, postmaturity.

(5–29) J. Reprod. Med. 24:147–152, April 1980.

Perinatal mortality was 21.2/1,000, compared to 14.1/1,000 for vaginal births. The rate for primary cesarean section was 26.7/1,000 births. The incidence of low birth weight infants was increased in the primary cesarean section group. Respiratory distress syndrome occurred in 10.3% of infants born by primary cesarean section and in 8% of those born by repeat cesarean section. Twenty-two perinatal deaths occurred, including 4 in infants with severe anomalies and 15 associated with a birth weight below 2,500 gm. Three neonatal deaths followed repeat cesarean section.

Most postoperative complications were related to sepsis. There was no indication that invasive fetal monitoring contributed to excess maternal morbidity. The trend toward increasing cesarean section deliveries raises questions concerning the risks and benefits of this procedure. Additional data from other institutions may help in resolving the risk-benefit status of cesarean section.

▶ [Because of differences in patient populations concerning the proportion of multiparas vs primiparas, low-risk vs high-risk patients, etc, it is not too helpful to compare cesarean section rates from one hospital to another. As obstetricians, our goal is to do the right thing for each patient rather than to target a particular cesarean section rate as being ideal. Because cesarean section rates have markedly increased over the past several years, the attention focused on this safe, but major, operation is appropriate. This nice review of one hospital's one year's experience highlights a problem. Dystocia (fetopelvic disproportion, uterine dysfunction, failure to progress) was the most common indication for primary cesarean section; 26% of these patients had radiologic evidence of disproportion but only 25% of the remaining patients who had cesarean section for this indication had an attempt at oxytocin stimulation. This suggests that the more traditional approach to abnormalities in the active stage of labor in the absence of disproportion (namely, the judicious use of intravenous oxytocin) may have obviated the need for abdominal delivery in some cases.] ◀

Influence of Scalp Sampling on Cesarean Section Rate for Fetal Distress. Today, many institutions are reporting a cesarean section rate of 15% or greater. In the 1950s, a rate of 5% to 7% was unusual. Richard W. Zalar, Jr., and Edward J. Quilligan[5-30] have reviewed the use of both continuous fetal heart rate monitoring and fetal scalp blood sampling in the management of high-risk patients at Women's Hospital, Los Angeles County-University of Southern California Medical Center, for 6–7 years. Experience in 1976, when there were 13,612 live births, was evaluated to determine how fetal scalp blood sampling might modify obstetric management. Fetal monitoring was performed in 4,978 labors, or 360 per 1,000 live births. If maternal pH was normal and fetal blood pH was 7.20 to 7.25, sampling was repeated within 30 minutes. If fetal blood pH was under 7.20 and maternal pH was normal, sampling was immediately repeated and the patient moved to the cesarean section room for surgery after confirmation was obtained.

Indications for cesarean section in 3 different years was compared in the table. The slight increase in total rate is explained almost entirely by a change in approach to breech presentation. No change in the rate of cesarean section for fetal distress was observed. Of the 1,019 primary cesarean sections in 1976, 134 were performed for fetal distress, in 92 cases because of changes in the fetal heart rate. A total

(5–30)   Am. J. Obstet. Gynecol. 135:239–246, Sept. 15, 1979.

INDICATIONS FOR CESAREAN SECTION

Indication	No.	1970* (Total No. of deliveries = 9,775) % Deliveries	% Primary	No.	1974* (Total No. of deliveries = 11,584) % Deliveries	% Primary	No.	1976 (Total No. of deliveries = 13,780) % Deliveries	% Primary
Cesarean section:	928	9.49		1,055	9.11		1,468	10.65	
Repeat	314	3.21		353	3.05		449	3.26	
Primary	614	6.28		702	6.06		1,019	7.39	
Malpresentation	134	1.37	21.8	262	2.26	37.3	375	2.72	36.8
Dystocia	322	3.30	52.4	238	2.06	33.9	426	3.09	41.8
Fetal distress	91	0.93	14.8	130	1.12	18.5	134	0.97	13.2
Placenta previa	37	0.38	6.0	43	0.37	7.1	64	0.46	6.3
Abruptio placentae	15	0.15	2.4	17	0.15	2.4	8	0.06	0.8
Miscellaneous	15	0.15	2.4	12	0.10	1.7	12	0.09	1.2

*Adapted from Hibbard, L. T.: Am. J. Obstet. Gynecol. 125:798, 1976.

of 258 patients had fetal scalp sampling. The indication was diagnosis or suspicion of late deceleration in 158 women. Eight-five percent of patients having fetal scalp sampling were not delivered by cesarean section for fetal distress. Compromised perinatal outcome in the group with birth weight over 2,500 gm was, with rare exceptions, confined to cases that were monitored, had indications for monitoring, or had identifiable prospective risk factors.

The incidence of cesarean section for fetal distress in the authors' institution is low and has remained low over the past 7 years. Fetal scalp sampling has prevented unnecessary cesarean section when the fetal heart rate tracing suggested distress. Infants with compromised perinatal outcomes were almost always monitored, had indications for monitoring, or had identifiable risk factors. The yield of monitoring the remaining two thirds of the population would appear to be small.

▶ [This study nicely demonstrates that the cesarean section rate for fetal distress need not be increased with electronic fetal heart rate monitoring, provided scalp sampling is available to aid in the evaluation of abnormal monitor tracings—85% of patients undergoing scalp sampling were *not* delivered by cesarean section for fetal distress. Nearly all depressed babies in this study had identifiable risk factors, had indications for fetal monitoring, or were delivered because of fetal distress.] ◀

Comparison Between Midline and Mediolateral Episiotomies.

Episiotomy is the most commonly performed operation in modern obstetrics, but there is much disagreement about the best incision to use. P. M. Coats, K. K. Chan, M. Wilkins, and R. J. Beard[5-31] compared the results of midline and mediolateral episiotomies at delivery and 3 months later in a prospective study of 407 primigravidas. Midline incisions divided 2 to 3 cm of the perineal tissues. Mediolateral incisions were carried from the midline to the right side of the anal sphincter for about 3 to 4 cm.

Division of the anal sphincter muscle and rectal mucosa injury complicated 11.6% of midline incisions and 2% of mediolateral incisions. Pain and need for analgesia were comparable with the two incisions. The perineum was less bruised with midline incisions, but

(5–31) Br. J. Obstet. Gynaecol. 87:408–412, May 1980.

the rates of wound breakdown were similar. No differences in pain were found 3 months after confinement. Patients who had midline incisions began intercourse significantly earlier. Cosmetic appearances were significantly better in the group who had midline episiotomies, and these scars had a softer texture.

Anal sphincter injury was more frequent after midline than after mediolateral episiotomy in this series, but no rectovaginal fistulas occurred. The ultimate quality of vaginal function is important in determination of the most suitable incision.

▶ [We applaud prospective, randomized studies of basic obstetric and gynecologic practices and procedures. The results reported here from England and Hong Kong are generally consistent with those of previous retrospective studies. Randomized assignment suffered, as some staff apparently refused to perform midline incisions when they were indicated by the study protocol (60% of the episiotomies were mediolateral rather than the expected 50%). Readers in the United States will find it interesting that midwives cut 57% of the episiotomies, but did not do the repairs, which were accomplished by medical students and obstetric residents. This split responsibility must explain the length of the mean interval from delivery to suture, which exceeded 30 minutes in both groups.] ◀

Management of Acute and Subacute Puerperal Inversion of the Uterus. Puerperal inversion of the uterus is an obstetric emergency with significant mortality. Peter Watson, Nicholas Besch, and Watson A. Bowes, Jr.[5-32] (Univ. of Colorado) encountered 18 cases of acute and subacute uterine inversion from 1969 to 1976, representing an incidence of 1 in 1,739 deliveries. Eight inversions were acute and 10 were subacute. All cases involved complete inversion with prolapse beyond the introitus. Controls included a group of patients of equal parity.

The study patients had a mean age of 22 years and a mean parity of 2. Mean infant weight was 3,269 gm. Three labors required oxytocin for augmentation, induction, or both. There were 4 forceps deliveries and 1 assisted breech delivery in the study group. There was no evidence of excessive traction on the cord at placental delivery. The

Fig 5–5.—Uterus lifted out of pelvis and directed with steady pressure toward umbilicus. (Courtesy of Watson, P., et al.: Obstet. Gynecol. 55:12–16, January, 1980.)

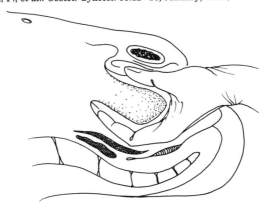

(5–32) Obstet. Gynecol. 55:12–16, January 1980.

maneuver used to reposition the uterus is shown in Figure 5–5. No uterine rupture or evidence of placenta accreta was found on manual exploration of the uterus. Seven patients were in shock, but in none was the degree of shock thought to be out of proportion to the blood loss. All patients but 2 received antibiotics, and no febrile morbidity was observed. The hospital stay was not prolonged. Inversion has not recurred.

Except for a past history of inversion or an antepartum ultrasound study showing a fundal placenta, there may be no reliable predisposing factors warning of a potential uterine inversion. Inversion can occur in patients of any parity. Prompt manual reinversion of the uterus will insure low morbidity and mortality from this rare but serious complication of the third stage of labor.

▶ [A nice review of an uncommon problem is presented here. Fundal implantation of the placenta coupled with traction on the cord prior to the separation of the placenta from the uterine wall seems to us to be the combination of factors involved in most cases.] ◀

6. Obstetric Analgesia and Anesthesia

Randomized Clinical Trial of the Leboyer Approach to Childbirth. Leboyer has suggested that the ideal birth takes place in a dark, quiet room, without sensory overstimulation. He suggested placing the newborn infant on the mother's abdomen and delaying clamping of the cord. The infant is to be gently massaged and placed in a warm bath. Many practitioners have objected to these suggestions. Nancy M. Nelson, Murray W. Enkin, Saroj Saigal, Kathryn J. Bennett, Ruth Milner and David L. Sackett[6-1] (McMaster Univ.) assigned 56 women to a Leboyer or conventional delivery and assessed the outcome with the use of a variety of clinical and behavioral measures. Women with low obstetric risk were included in the study. No perineal shave procedures, enemas or analgesics other than epidural analgesics were used in either group.

Twenty-eight Leboyer deliveries and 26 conventional deliveries were available for analysis. Twenty patients in each group were managed as planned. No differences in maternal or neonatal morbidity were noted and there were no differences in infant behavior in the first hour of life, at 24 and 72 hours post partum or at age 8 months. Maternal perceptions of the infants and of the birth experience were comparable, except that a mother in the Leboyer group was more likely to say at 8 months that the experience had influenced her child's behavior. Leboyer women had shorter active labors.

This trial failed to reveal clear-cut advantages of the Leboyer delivery method over conventional delivery. Controversial innovations in obstetric care can be evaluated in clinical trials that measure psychologic as well as physical outcome.

▶ [Although the sample size is small, this carefully designed and executed clinical study did not demonstrate differences in the neonatal period and at 8 months of age between infants delivered by the Leboyer method vs a gentle conventional delivery. These results are not surprising. Also not surprising is the finding that Leboyer mothers were more likely to think that their delivery experience had influenced their children's behavior.] ◀

Meperidine Disposition in Mother, Neonate, and Nonpregnant Females. The effects of pregnancy or immaturity on meperidine metabolism have not been fully clarified. B. R. Kuhnert, P. M. Kuhnert, A. L. Prochaska, and R. J. Sokol[6-2] (Case Western Reserve Univ.) used sensitive gas chromatographic techniques to compare the excretion and metabolism of meperidine by the mother, the neonate, and the nonpregnant female. Studies were done in 18 patients in labor, 8 nonpregnant females, and 30 neonates whose mothers had received meperidine during labor. Meperidine was given intravenously in doses

(6–1) N. Engl. J. Med. 302:655–660, Mar. 20, 1980.
(6–2) Clin. Pharmacol. Ther. 27:486–491, April 1980.

of 50 mg as needed to relieve pain. The pregnant patients received no other drugs during labor. In most instances pudendal anesthesia was induced with lidocaine at delivery.

Disappearance curves of meperidine from the plasma were similar for pregnant and nonpregnant females. No significant differences in kinetic constants were found. The amount of meperidine excreted and the pattern of metabolism were comparable in postpartum and non-pregnant subjects. Neonates excreted more parent compound than metabolite for the first two days, in contrast to adults. By the third day, neonates excreted more normeperidine than meperidine.

No major differences were found in this study in the ability of per-ipartum patients and nonpregnant females to clear or metabolize me-peridine. Although the neonate can N-demethylate meperidine to normeperidine, it cannot do so as effectively as the adult. A potential for pharmacologic effects exists for several days.

▶ [The results of this study indicate that metabolism and urinary excretion of meperidine do not seem to be affected by pregnancy per se, but may differ in newborns as opposed to adults. In newborns, the metabolism of meperidine to its demethylation derivative normeperidine appears to occur at a slower rate than in adults, presumably reflecting limited enzyme capabilities.] ◀

Human Fetal Oxygenation Following Paracervical Block. The etiology of postparacervical block fetal bradycardia is thought to involve hypoxia secondary to a decrease in placental blood flow and possibly a reflex-type mechanism. Laxmi V. Baxi, Roy H. Petrie, and L. Stanley James[6-3] (Columbia Univ.) measured fetal oxygenation continuously with a transcutaneous electrode to test the hypothesis that fetal heart rate changes that follow paracervical block (PCB) are secondary to fetal hypoxia. Studies were done in ten patients in uncomplicated normal labor at term. The PCB was induced with 200 mg of lidocaine. The fetal transcutaneous Po_2 (t_cPo_2) was monitored for 1 hour.

The mean t_cPo_2 before administration of PCB was 22.2 torr. A reduction began 5 minutes after administration of the block, and a maximum decline of 7.2 torr was observed at 11.5 minutes. Oxygenation remained at that level for about 3 minutes and then gradually returned to near baseline within about 30 minutes. The mean t_cPo_2 at 1 hour was 17.7 torr. Uterine activity declined after PCB administration and then increased; increases preceded the lowest t_cPo_2 values. Fetal heart rate variability was maximal at 7.5 minutes, and a loss of variability was observed at the time of the lowest t_cPo_2. Only 1 case of fetal bradycardia developed.

It appears that PCB analgesia tends to reduce fetal oxygenation to some degree. Usually no therapy is necessary. The severity of the fall in t_cPo_2 appears to be related to the analgesic effectiveness of the block. Paracervical block may be used in most term pregnancies when they are judged to be normal by modern fetal surveillance systems.

▶ [Transient fetal bradycardia after paracervical block has been recognized for at least 20 years, and a number of studies have led to the hypothesis that impaired uteroplacental blood flow is responsible. This report demonstrates transient lowering of trans-

(6–3) Am. J. Obstet. Gynecol. 135:1109–1112, Dec. 15, 1979.

cutaneously measured fetal Po_2 by about one-third over the period of 5 to 20 minutes after the block, suggesting strongly that the mechanism is hypoxic. The clinical significance of these data is unclear, but, as a minimum, it seems reasonable to limit the use of paracervical block to the totally normal term situation.] ◀

Diagnosis, Treatment, and Follow-up of Neonatal Mepivacaine Intoxication Secondary to Paracervical and Pudendal Blocks During Labor. Laura S. Hillman, Richard E. Hillman, and W. Edwin Dodson[6-4] (Washington Univ.) report findings in 7 newborn infants with seizures and depression due to intoxication with mepivacaine, seen over a 4-year period. The 6 survivors had follow-up and 4 over age 2 years have had psychologic evaluation.

Typically the prenatal course was benign and there was evidence of direct fetal injection at delivery. All pregnancies but one were uncomplicated and all deliveries were at term. In several cases, paracervical block had had little maternal effect. Fetal bradycardia did not follow injection of the anesthetic. All infants had punctures and scratches on the scalp. The four cord blood samples available showed a postnatal increase in mepivacaine concentration. Six infants were markedly depressed at birth and required active ventilation. They had decreased spontaneous movements, hypotonia and normal or increased reflexes. All had pupil or oculomotor reflex abnormalities. Seizure activity was tonic in 6 infants and occurred in 4 in association with apnea or hypoventilation. Exchange transfusion, gastric drainage or promotion of urine output was attempted in 3 infants. All 6 survivors who had follow-up were free of seizures without anticonvulsant therapy and have normal neurologic findings. One patient had a mild delay in expressive speech. Psychologic testing in the 4 older children gave normal findings.

These infants apparently were intoxicated by direct injection of mepivacaine. Gastric lavage and exchange transfusion were not very effective. Urine flow should be cautiously encouraged to promote renal clearance of the drug. Seizure control was not a major problem in these cases. The outcome was generally good. The prognosis in moderately severe cases of mepivacaine intoxication may be excellent if severe hypoxia is avoided.

▶ [This excellent article outlines the course of 7 infants intoxicated with local anesthetic agents given by paracervical or pudendal block, or both, almost certainly as a result of accidental direct fetal injection. Of course, prevention is vastly preferable to treatment but, if treatment becomes necessary, promotion of urinary excretion (fluid intake and perhaps diuretics) seems to be the most effective means. It is encouraging that all 6 survivors have developed normally.] ◀

Segmental Epidural Analgesia in Labor Related to Progress of Labor, Fetal Malposition, and Instrumental Delivery. Segmental epidural analgesia at the T10–T12 level relieves pain effectively in the first stage of labor. R. Jouppila, P. Jouppila, J.-M. Karinen and A. Hollmén[6-5] (Univ. of Oulu) examined the effects of segmental epidural analgesia produced with low doses of bupivacaine on duration of the stages of labor, frequency of fetal malposition and rate

(6–4) J. Pediatr. 95:472–477, September 1979.
(6–5) Acta Obstet. Gynecol. Scand. 58:135–139, 1979.

of vacuum extractions. One hundred parturients given segmental epidural analgesia were compared with 100 given no or conventional analgesia. The groups were matched for parity and induced or spontaneous labor. Each group included 77 primiparas; 39 in each group were induced with oxytocin and/or amniotomy. Epidural analgesia was induced with 4 ml of 0.5% bupivacaine when the cervix was about 3 cm dilated. About 50% of the control patients received pethidine for pain relief.

In primiparas the first stage of labor lasted significantly longer in the epidural group than in controls, but induction-delivery intervals were comparable. No significant differences in duration of the stages of labor were noted in multiparas. Fetal malpositions did not differ significantly in number between the epidural and control groups, and similar rates of vacuum extraction were observed. Five primiparas in the epidural group and 3 in the control group had uterine bleeding of over 500 ml in the third stage of labor. No significant differences in Apgar scores or birth weights were noted.

Segmental epidural analgesia at the T10–T12 level, given for pain relief during the first stage of labor, did not appear to disturb the normal progress of labor in this study, and did not increase the frequency of fetal malposition or that of instrumental delivery.

▶ [Segmental epidural anesthesia involves injection of small smounts of anesthetic agent to block only specific segments, as opposed to lumbar epidural or caudal in which all segments below a certain level are blocked. This study indicates that the segmental technique instituted as early as at 3 cm dilation of the cervix does not affect the course of subsequent labor, as evidenced by a lack of significant differences between epidural and control patients with respect to interval from instillation to delivery, duration of the second stage, or incidence of malposition. Lumbar (or full) epidural anesthesia given this early in the first stage, on the other hand, has been shown in other studies to lead to prolongation of the first and (particularly) the second stages and a greater frequency of persistent occiput transverse and posterior positions.] ◀

β-**Endorphin in Obstetric Analgesia.** The efficacy of β-endorphin, given intrathecally to patients with intractable pain from disseminated cancer, suggested its use as an obstetric analgesic agent that could not enter the fetal central nervous system. Tsutomu Oyama, Akitoma Matsuki, Takeo Taneichi (Hirosaki Univ.), Nicholas Ling, and Roger Guillemin[6-6] (Salk Inst. for Biological Studies, La Jolla, Calif.) evaluated β-endorphin in 14 women aged 18 to 32 years with expected normal vaginal deliveries. The 7 primiparas and 7 multiparas had had uncomplicated pregnancies. Synthetic β-endorphin was injected intrathecally in saline at the L3 or L4 interspace in a dose of 1 mg. It was preferably given when cervical dilatation was 3.5 to 5.0 cm.

The average cervical dilatation at the time of β-endorphin injection was 6.3 cm. The mean time from injection to delivery was 103 minutes. Labor pains disappeared completely in all patients within 3.5 minutes after β-endorphin injection, although a sense of pressure persisted. Uterine contractions were not depressed, and the fetal heart rate was not slowed. All 1-minute Apgar scores were over 8. Bleeding was considered to be unusually light. Normal blood gas values were

(6–6) Am. J. Obstet. Gynecol. 137:613–616, July 1, 1980.

found on analyses of umbilical venous blood immediately after delivery. Four patients had nausea and vomiting and 10 had headache after β-endorphin injection. No headache occurred when finer 24-gauge needles were used for intrathecal injections.

β-Endorphin is a normally occurring pituitary secretion that cannot penetrate to the fetal central nervous system. Intrathecal administration is necessary, with its attendant side effects. The optimal intrathecal dose of β-endorphin for use in obstetric analgesia remains to be established.

▶ [Endorphins are endogenously produced compounds discovered only recently that appear to have marked physiologic effects. β-Endorphin, secreted by the pituitary, has opium-like actions but does not cross the blood-brain barrier. In this study, intrathecal injection of synthetic β-endorphin produced rapid, complete, and prolonged analgesia for labor and delivery. Fetal effects were nil, which is expected since the agent should not gain access to the fetal central nervous system. The number of subjects (14) is small. Moreover, it is disquieting that nausea and vomiting occurred in 4 patients and headaches in 10.] ◀

Effect of Induction of General Anesthesia for Cesarean Section on Intervillous Blood Flow. Thiopental, the most widely used agent for intravenous induction of anesthesia at cesarean section, has several maternal cardiovascular effects, and it has been shown to reduce uterine blood flow in pregnant ewes. Pentti Jouppila, Jyrki Kuikka, Riitta Jouppila, and Arno Hollmén[6-7] (Univ. of Oulu) studied the effects of induction on intervillous blood flow in 10 healthy mothers at 37 to 41 weeks' gestation, with no signs of disturbance of the fetoplacental unit. The indication for section was a narrow pelvis in 7 women and previous section in 3. Patients received atropine and then 4 mg of thiopental per kg intravenously, followed by succinylcholine. Xenon-133 was injected during ventilation with pure oxygen. Anesthesia was maintained with 50% nitrous oxide in oxygen.

The mean intervillous blood flow was 131 ml per minute per 100 ml before induction and 84 during induction, a highly significant difference. The pulse rate tended to increase, and the mean blood pressure rose slightly. All pH values but one were above 7.30 during induction. The mean induction-delivery interval was 9.5 minutes. Acid-base balance was normal in all infants except 1, who showed signs of respiratory and metabolic acidosis. All neonates had Apgar scores of 7 or above.

Intervillous blood flow showed a highly significant decrease during induction of general anesthesia in this study. The infants were not depressed. The findings warrant further studies of the effects of different analgesic and anesthetic procedures on placental blood flow.

▶ [Previous studies and clinical experience have indicated that babies delivered by cesarean section under general anesthesia are nonacidotic and are in good condition at birth. Nevertheless, with the use of a xenon tracer technique, the present study suggests a significant fall in intervillous blood flow during induction. Further work along these lines involving both general and regional anesthesia should provide helpful information. As advances in technology permit more sophisticated measurements, we will probably learn that Apgar scores and even cord blood gas determinations do not tell us the whole story.] ◀

(6–7) Acta Obstet. Gynecol. Scand. 58:249–253, 1979.

Effects of Stopping Smoking for 48 Hours on Oxygen Availability from the Blood: Study on Pregnant Women. It is generally agreed that women who smoke should be advised to stop during pregnancy. Smoking reduces the amount of functional hemoglobin available due to carboxyhemoglobin formation; also, the increased affinity of hemoglobin for oxygen, caused by carbon monoxide, reduces the availability of oxygen from the blood. Judith M. Davies, I. P. Latto, J. G. Jones, Anne Veale, and C. A. J. Wardrop[6-8] (Welsh Natl. School of Medicine, Cardiff) assessed factors determining oxygen availability from the blood in 32 mothers in the last trimester of pregnancy. Eleven continued to smoke during the 48-hour study period, and 11 stopped smoking. The other 10 women were nonsmokers. The three groups were similar in age, weight, parity, gestational age, and clinical characteristics. Available oxygen was defined as the amount available to the tissues per dl blood, as assessed from the measured arterial oxygen tension, with an assumed mixed venous tension of 20 mm Hg.

Mothers who stopped smoking and those who did not stop smoked a mean of 43.9 and 44.9 cigarettes, respectively, in the 48 hours before the study. Those who continued smoking consumed fewer cigarettes than usual during the study period. All patients had normal hemoglobin concentrations. Initial carboxyhemoglobin values were much higher in the smoking mothers than in the nonsmokers, as was hemoglobin-oxygen affinity; however, total hemoglobin levels were also higher, and oxygen availability was not significantly reduced. In women who stopped smoking, the reduction in carboxyhemoglobin and the decrease in hemoglobin-oxygen affinity led to a significant 8% increase in available oxygen in 48 hours.

Improved oxygen transport should result from cessation of smoking for 48 hours, and this should be encouraged before elective deliveries. Even small improvements in oxygen delivery to the tissues may confer critical benefit on the fetus, especially during labor or on exposure to general anesthesia. The same considerations may apply to patients undergoing general anesthesia for all elective operations, particularly those with anemia.

▶ [Just 2 days without cigarettes resulted in a marked decline in carboxyhemoglobin concentration in these smokers in late pregnancy and in an increase in "available oxygen." The implications here are clear, especially concerning patients with upcoming repeat cesarean sections.] ◀

Antacid Pulmonary Aspiration in the Dog. It has generally been thought, since Mendelson's work, that pulmonary dysfunction after aspiration of gastric contents is caused by gastric acid. Oral antacid therapy has been suggested for subjects predisposed to aspiration, but the possibility that antacids themselves may injure the lungs has not been fully assessed. Charles P. Gibbs, Daniel J. Schwartz, James W. Wynne, C. Ian Hood, and Earlene J. Kuck[6-9] (Univ. of Florida) examined the effects of aspiration of antacid in dogs and compared the changes with those caused by the aspiration of sa-

(6–8) Br. Med. J. 2:355–356, Aug. 11, 1979.
(6–9) Anesthesiology 51:380–385, November 1979.

line solution and acid. Aspirates were delivered in a dosage of 1 ml/ kg to each lung through a catheter inserted through the endotracheal tube. Either saline, hydrochloric acid at a pH of 1.8, or antacid solution at a pH of 8.3 was delivered. The antacid used was Kolantyl Gel, a suspension of aluminum hydroxide and magnesium hydroxide. Other dogs received saline adjusted with sodium hydroxide to a pH of 8.3.

Mean Pa_{O_2} of saline-treated dogs fell from 81 to 60 torr at 10 minutes, whereas that of the alkaline saline-treated dogs fell from 83 to 58 torr. The fractional intrapulmonary physiologic shunt ($\dot{Q}_s/\dot{Q}_t$) increased in both groups, from 15% to 34% and from 16% to 42%, respectively, but returned to control levels by 4 hours. Acid- and antacid-treated dogs had more marked reductions in Pa_{O_2}, with abnormal levels persisting at 24 hours. The $\dot{Q}_s/\dot{Q}_t$ increased significantly more in these groups, from 14% to 66% in the acid-treated group and from 13% to 47% in the antacid-treated group. These changes persisted through 4 hours. The saline and alkaline saline aspirates produced little histologic change. The acid aspirate produced hemorrhage, exudates, and edema, which resolved within a month. The antacid aspirate produced a marked bronchopneumonia that persisted as a chronic inflammatory reaction after a month.

Antacids apparently can cause pulmonary damage when aspirated. The alkalinity of the solution was not the cause of damage in these studies. Further studies may lead to safer antacid preparations. Efforts to adjust the pH of gastric contents without the use of antacids also deserve study.

▶ [The consequences of the aspiration of gastric contents are related in part to the acidity of the aspirated material. Therefore, it seemed reasonable a few years ago to institute routine antacid administration to laboring patients in order to elevate the pH of the gastric contents. Our service and many others do this, thinking we are doing the right thing. Right? Not necessarily, according to this animal study. Aspiration of the antacid itself resulted in prolonged hypoxemia and marked histologic changes in the lung. The dose and gastric dispersion of the antacid must be important factors (currently we given 15 ml every 3 hours). We do not want to overemphasize the significance of this animal study, but it illustrates the need to be careful in extrapolating the results of laboratory experiments to clinical practice. Although alkaline saline solutions do not cause lung problems as do acid solutions, this does not necessarily mean that antacids are harmless when aspirated. By the same token, this study in dogs does not clearly indicate that our current clinical practice is unbeneficial.] ◀

Fatal Aspiration (Mendelson's) Syndrome Despite Antacids and Cricoid Pressure. Cesarean section is often done for delay in the first stage of labor. Mendelson, who described a syndrome following inhalation of gastric contents by anesthetized patients, suggested that irritation from the acid gastric juice could be prevented by antacid administration. R. M. Whittington, John S. Robinson and John M. Thompson[6-10] (Univ. of Birmingham) describe 2 patients who underwent cesarean section for failed labor without emptying of the stomach. Both women received antacid therapy preoperatively and cricoid pressure was applied; however, both patients died after inhal-

(6–10) Lancet 2:228–230, Aug. 4, 1979.

ing gastric contents during general anesthesia. Large volumes of fluid were found in the stomachs.

A primigravida aged 28 underwent cesarean section delivery because of slow progress in labor despite oxytocin infusion. Magnesium trisilicate was given preoperatively. The patient vomited when cricoid pressure was being applied during induction, before paralysis due to suxamethonium was apparent. She again vomited several liters of material at the end of operation. The patient died 3 hours later. Left tension pneumothorax, pulmonary edema with chemical pneumonitis and a normal stomach were found at autopsy.

Another patient, a healthy primigravida aged 25, was also treated with magnesium trisilicate preoperatively. Gastric fluid was aspirated from the pharynx during induction of anesthesia. This patient died 9 hours after undergoing cesarean section. At autopsy, a small amount of bile-stained fluid was found in the stomach. Death was due to acute pulmonary edema after inhalation of gastric contents.

It appears that acute gastric dilatation may develop during labor. Cricoid pressure and antacid therapy are not as effective in preventing Mendelson's syndrome as is commonly thought. Gastric emptying should be carried out either by forced emesis with apomorphine or with a gastric tube before obstetric anesthesia is induced.

▶ [These case reports are disconcerting. Death from aspiration occurred despite antacids and cricoid pressure. Maalox and cricoid pressure prior to intubation are prophylactic measures currently undertaken on our service in the hope of avoiding Mendelson's syndrome. Perhaps we are not doing as much as we think we are with these routines. In fairness, however, one of these patients was given a "light lunch" during labor and the problems in the other patient apparently occurred after extubation. Regional anesthetic techniques offer an advantage on this score, of course, as the patient is awake and her airway is protected.] ◀

7. Genetics, Teratology, and Drug Effects

PRENATAL DIAGNOSIS OF CONGENITAL MALFORMATIONS

MAURICE J. MAHONEY, M.D.

Associate Professor of Human Genetics,
Pediatrics, and Obstetrics and Gynecology,
Yale University School of Medicine

Introduction

A major congenital malformation is detectable in 2–3% of all babies either at the time of birth or during infancy. Many of these infants will have multiple anomalies, but in only a small number will an etiology for the defects be discovered. A few infants will have a demonstrable chromosome abnormality, but most will not and the malformation will be described only in terms of abnormal anatomy.

Although congenital anomalies are not uncommon in the population, most appear as first occurrences in a family and no prior suspicion of an increased risk for abnormal pregnancy outcome has existed. The sporadic nature of most malformations, the poor understanding of etiology, and the necessity for fetal visualization have combined to make prenatal diagnosis of these disorders challenging and difficult. Progress was initially slow, as compared to the in utero detection of chromosome abnormalities and inborn errors of metabolism, but has now begun to accelerate as tools for visualization have become available and processes for screening a larger proportion of pregnant women are being developed.

Several cogent reasons exist to pursue the diagnosis of fetal malformations. Important decisions about the management of a pregnancy inevitably follow a diagnosis. If information is available in the second trimester, parents may elect abortion because of serious fetal anomalies, or, alternatively, may use the time to prepare for the birth of a child with predicted problems. Decisions about delivery—method, place, and timing—become crucial as a pregnancy nears completion. Availability of necessary medical and surgical skills to give optimum care to a baby with a treatable malformation should be assured. Different plans would be made if the fetus had no hope of survival. For the future, when therapies have been developed for the fetus in utero, early diagnosis will have a high premium in certain disease states in order to preserve function.

Diagnostic Techniques

Whereas amniocentesis and the study of cultured amniotic fluid cells have been the primary modes of detecting chromosomal and metabolic errors, additional techniques have been necessary for suspecting and demonstrating the dysmorphic features of congenital malformations (Table 1). Prime among these are the measurement of α-fetoprotein (AFP) concentration in maternal serum and amniotic fluid and sonographic visualization of fetal anatomy. More invasive techniques for fetal visualization, amniography and fetoscopy, have also had limited application in special circumstances. The utility of each diagnostic method will be discussed after consideration of which pregnancies carry sufficient risk of a malformed fetus to warrant investigation.

Selection of At-Risk Pregnancies

Several factors in a family history, maternal medical history, or the course of the current pregnancy serve as signposts of a fetus with anomalies (Table 2). Attention to these factors allows selection of specific pregnancies for further investigation. In these instances, historical information and careful physical examination have their classic role of screening a large, mostly normal population to find the few individuals who warrant careful assessment.

TABLE 1.—TECHNIQUES USED IN THE DIAGNOSIS OF CONGENITAL MALFORMATIONS

Visualization of fetal anatomy
  Sonography
  X-ray (including amniography)
  Fetoscopy
Amniotic fluid studies
  α-Fetoprotein (AFP) concentration
  Amniotic fluid cell karyotype

TABLE 2.—FACTORS ASSOCIATED WITH CONGENITAL MALFORMATIONS

Family history
  Single gene (mendelian) disorders
  Previous child with malformations
  Prospective parent with malformations
Maternal history
  Diabetes mellitus
  Congenital heart disease
  Multiple miscarriages (see Table 3)
Hydramnios or oligohydramnios
Exposure to teratogens
Fetal chromosome abnormalities
Elevation of maternal serum α-fetoprotein (AFP)

An additional type of screening, dependent on a simple laboratory assessment during the pregnancy, is also being developed. Maternal serum AFP screening is the best example at present. The purpose of this type of screening is identical to that based on history and the course of pregnancy, ie, to select from among all pregnant women those who have a distinctly elevated risk of a fetus with anomalies and to investigate their pregnancies with special techniques.

FAMILY HISTORY

Certain malformation syndromes are caused by mutant genes inherited in classic mendelian patterns. The prior occurrence of one of these disorders in a key family member predicts a high chance of an affected baby and calls for careful genetic analysis of the pedigree and of the proband's diagnosis. Accurate genetic prediction and, with it, justification for prenatal diagnostic testing depend very greatly on accurate diagnosis. Careful physical examination, x-ray study, and pathologic examination of a previously born child, including stillborn or miscarried offspring, are often crucial to the intelligent planning and monitoring of a future pregnancy.

Examples of single gene, or mendelian, malformation syndromes include autosomal recessive Meckel syndrome, which usually has an encephalocele and often polydactyly as expression of the syndrome, and several skeletal dysplasias, such as diastrophic dysplasia or congenital osteogenesis imperfecta, in which severe shortening of limb bones is present during fetal life. Both phenotypically normal parents will be mutant gene carriers (heterozygotes) under these circumstances and face a 25% chance of an abnormal child in any of their pregnancies. The key affected individuals in recessive pedigrees are previous children. Parental consanguinity may also exist, especially if the disease state is rare.

Ectrodactyly (lobster claw deformity) and Holt-Oram syndrome (specific abnormalities of heart and upper extremities) are examples of autosomal dominant disorders. Key members of the pedigree are the parents and occasionally grandparents or siblings of the parents. If a prospective parent has an autosomal dominant disease (in which one mutant gene is sufficient to cause the syndrome), 50% of offspring are expected to show the disorder, with varying degrees of involvement. Sometimes a dominant disorder appears for the first time in a pedigree and neither parent, nor anyone else, shows any sign of the abnormality. Very often under these circumstances, the affected individual's disease was caused by a new mutation in one of the parents' sex cells, rather than having been inherited from a parent who carries the mutant gene. Recurrence in a subsequent pregnancy would be rare.

The important persons in an X-linked pedigree are a woman's sons, brothers, and maternal uncles or male cousins. If a woman can be shown to carry an X-linked gene, half of her sons are expected to have disease. Many cases of hydrocephalus due to aqueductal stenosis, when it occurs in boys, are due to a mutant X-linked gene.

Many malformation syndromes do not follow mendelian inheritance patterns, but empiric observations document increased recurrence in families. A local environmental factor or a compilation of relatively minor genetic and environmental factors in one or both parents explains some of these associations. If increased risk is recognized empirically and a prenatal diagnostic technique is available, subsequent pregnancies for these couples are appropriate candidates for study. The neural tube defects (spina bifida, anencephaly) follow this pattern.

MATERNAL HISTORY

Insulin-dependent diabetes in a mother has long been associated with fetal malformations. The major ones include caudal regression syndrome, with sacral agenesis and malformed lower extremities, neural tube defects, heart defects and renal abnormalities.[1] Some of these malformations can be diagnosed in the second trimester with the use of sonography or AFP measurements.

Women who have congenital heart defects have a considerably increased chance of malformations in their offspring, mostly heart malformations.[2] With more complicated heart defects in the mother, this chance may be as high as 5–10%. Whether this chance is higher for a mother with a heart defect than for a father, implicating teratogenic influences during the pregnancy, has not been answered. For either circumstance, a father or a mother with a defect, fetal echocardiography holds promise in the near future of detecting the very severe defects that have a poor prognosis postnatally.[3]

Repeated miscarriages identify couples who may have a balanced rearrangement of one member's chromosomes, eg, a translocation or an inversion, or may show mosaicism with two chromosomally different cell lines. Although the chance is small, less than 5%, that this would be true for a couple with more than one miscarriage, such a couple faces an increased chance of fetal malformations and once identified, should have the option of amniocentesis to determine the fetal karyotype in pregnancies that reach 16 weeks.

HYDRAMNIOS AND OLIGOHYDRAMNIOS

An abnormal volume of amniotic fluid is often associated with a malformed fetus. The pregnancy with a fetus that cannot swallow or cannot pass amniotic fluid into its intestinal tract very often shows hydramnios.[4] The fetus that does not contribute urine to the amniotic fluid, as in renal agenesis or an obstructed urinary tract, often is accompanied by oligohydramnios. Significant alterations of amniotic fluid volume in association with a fetal malformation occur only in the late second trimester or third trimester.[5] When hydramnios is found, about one fifth of fetuses will have a malformation.[6] Oligohydramnios is more difficult to quantitate, and comparable risk data are not available.

TABLE 3.—INDICATIONS FOR FETAL CHROMOSOME DETERMINATION BY AMNIOCENTESIS

Parental, especially maternal, age
Parent with balanced chromosome rearrangement
Previous child with a chromosome abnormality
Previous child with undiagnosed multiple anomaly syndrome
Indications to examine parents' chromosomes to aid decision about amniocentesis for fetal chromosome analysis:
Family history of Down syndrome if karyotype of proband unknown
Multiple miscarriages

EXPOSURE TO TERATOGENS

Several drugs and a few viruses are established human teratogens.[7] Satisfactory data about the teratogenic potential of most drugs and chemicals do not exist, however, although fears abound in our population. The same is true about the risks of irradiation. Only high levels of fetal exposure, ten rad or above, show effects that might lead to malformations via interruption of cell growth; even in these circumstances, most fetuses have no malformations.

The role of prenatal diagnostic techniques for pregnancies exposed to possible teratogens has not been well delineated as yet. Amniocentesis to examine chromosomes has not been useful. Ultrasound examination of the fetus might detect some malformations but would miss many, especially when several possible deformities were being sought instead of one specific one. When the likelihood of teratogenicity is only a few percent or the malformations expected are subtle, diagnostic procedures are more likely to give confusing, false positive information than true diagnostic information. Interpretations should be very cautious in these circumstances. It is expected that ultrasound examination will become more exact in coming years and, with the increased expertise, that greater numbers of exposed pregnancies will be appropriately studied.

FETAL CHROMOSOME ABNORMALITIES

Many malformation syndromes are due to abnormal chromosomes. Thus, determination of the fetal karyotype with the use of amniotic fluid cells is an indirect way of diagnosing these malformations. Experience of the past decade has generated recommended indications for determining a fetal karyotype.[8-10] These are listed in Table 3. The most common indication is increased maternal age, and most diagnostic programs offer amniocentesis to mothers at age 35 and older. There is some suggestion that a father's age, especially over 50 years, may contribute to risk, but this is not certain as yet. Parents with balanced chromosomal rearrangements, as mentioned above in the discussion of multiple miscarriages, should be offered prenatal diagnosis.

A previously liveborn or stillborn child who had a chromosome abnormality is an indication for amniocentesis in a subsequent pregnancy. If there is suspicion that the child might well have had an abnormality, because of the presence of multiple malformations, the subsequent pregnancies can be studied. If a relative other than an offspring of one of the parents has a chromosome abnormality, especially Down syndrome, it is possible that the parent carries a translocation chromosome predisposing his or her own children to Down syndrome. Karyotypes of the index patient or of the related prospective parent can answer this question of risk and help in the decision about prenatal diagnostic studies.

α-FETOPROTEIN AND NEURAL TUBE DEFECTS

α-Fetoprotein is the major plasma protein of the fetus during the first half of gestation. It is produced in the liver, circulates with the blood, and is excreted into amniotic fluid with the fetal urine. When a fetus has a major malformation through which this protein can leak into amniotic fluid (such as a neural tube defect), diagnosis can be made by measurement of amniotic fluid AFP concentration.[11]

α-Fetoprotein is also present in maternal serum. It is mostly fetal in origin and reaches maternal serum from fetal serum and amniotic fluid. During the second trimester when diagnostic measurements are made (15 to 19 weeks), AFP concentration in fetal serum and amniotic fluid are decreasing, with fetal serum concentration being much higher (1.5–2.5 mg/ml) than amniotic fluid concentration (2–20 μ/ml). At that same time in gestation, maternal serum concentration, which is much lower than amniotic fluid concentration, is increasing (20–100 ng/ml). These relationships are important and require accurate gestational age measurements, by ultrasound, and the avoidance of contaminating amniotic fluid with fetal blood during amniocentesis.

Pregnancies have an increased risk for neural tube defects if a previous child or one of the prospective parents has or had such a lesion. In North America this risk is about 2%, compared to the general population risk of 1 to 2 per 1,000. A previous child with hydrocephalus or some other close relative with a neural tube defect may cause some increased risk in addition.

Most babies with neural tube defects are born to families without a positive family history. Since an increased amniotic fluid AFP concentration very often leads to an increased maternal serum concentration, screening programs for all pregnant women who desire the test have been developed in Great Britain and are now appearing in North America; they are based on maternal serum. If protein concentration is elevated, there is a risk of approximately 10% that the fetus is affected.[12] Normal twins cause a serum elevation, and erroneous gestational age estimates may falsely suggest a serum elevation. For these reasons, an ultrasound examination is performed after an elevated serum concentration is found. If no explanation for the serum elevation is discovered, the woman has an amniocentesis to measure amniotic fluid AFP. This method of screening will detect about 80% of neural tube defects. Women with a positive family history for neural tube defect move directly to amniocentesis as the most accurate method for fetal diagnosis.

Five to ten percent of neural tube defects are not open to amniotic fluid and AFP cannot leak into the amniotic cavity. These closed neural tube defects, covered by skin or a thick membrane, will be missed by AFP measurement, although some may be diagnosed by ultrasound. Of open neural tube defects, 98% will be diagnosed by AFP measurement in amniotic fluid.[13]

A few other fetal malformations also lead to elevations of AFP. Of most significance are omphaloceles, most of which should be distinguishable by ultrasound. Occasional normal pregnancies have elevated amniotic fluid protein concentrations, and the introduction of fetal blood into amniotic fluid will falsely elevate the AFP concentrations. To make diagnosis as accurate as possible, expert ultrasound examination of the fetal head, spine, and abdomen should follow positive amniotic fluid studies to attempt visualization of a lesion, if present. Other ancillary tests with amniotic fluid are also being developed to aid accuracy of neural tube defect diagnosis. Most promising at this time is isoenzyme analysis of amniotic fluid acetylcholinesterases.[14] Neural tube defects, and some omphaloceles, have an extra isoenzyme. A proposed stepwise sequence for neural tube defect diagnosis is presented in Table 4.

Techniques of Fetal Visualization

SONOGRAPHY

Ultrasound technology and experience in fetal visualization are expanding one of the most rapidly advancing areas of prenatal diagnosis. Recent reviews document the several types of malformations that have been diagnosed and Table 5 lists most of them.[15, 16] Studies are currently in progress to provide normative anatomical data about the human fetus at various gestational ages, and fetal echocardiography is developing to provide physiologic as well as anatomical data.

Important caveats concerning current fetal ultrasonography should be stated. At present, only a few individuals have developed special skills in fetal examination, and diagnostic accuracy for most purposes is unknown. Also, the time during development when pathology is

---

TABLE 4.—STEPS IN PRENATAL DIAGNOSIS OF NEURAL TUBE DEFECTS

1. Maternal serum AFP measurement at 16–19 wk gestation (a screening test).
2. Ultrasonography if serum AFP elevated.
   Rule out twin pregnancies.
   Establish accurate gestational age.
3. Selection of women for amniocentesis and amniotic fluid AFP measurement. Two reasons:
   Family history of neural tube defects, or
   Elevated maternal serum AFP.
4. Additional diagnostic tests if amniotic fluid AFP concentration elevated.
   Detailed ultrasonography of fetal spine and umbilicus.
   Other amniotic fluid studies such as acetylcholinesterase isoenzymes.

TABLE 5.—PRENATAL DIAGNOSES
USING SONOGRAPHY

Neural tube defects
  Anencephaly
  Spina bifida
  Meningomyelocele
Hydrocephaly
Diaphragmatic hernia
Intestinal atresias
Tricuspid atresia
Cystic hygroma
Teratomas
Sacral agenesis
Short-limbed dysplasias
Osteogenesis imperfecta
Dysplastic kidneys
Renal agenesis
Infantile polycystic kidney disease
Omphalocele
Gastroschisis
Ectrodactyly

sufficiently defined for ultrasonic definition is not known for many malformation states or inherited defects (Figs 1 through 4).

X-RAY

Radiologic examination of the fetus has mostly been carried out in the third trimester. The skeleton can be well defined and amniography can outline the surface of the unborn baby. A few second-trimester examinations have led to diagnoses also. Concern about known hazards of radiation, albeit of low magnitude for such effects as genetic damage and oncogenic change, have limited the use of x-ray and

Fig 1 (left).—Fetal head at 20 weeks' gestation, showing normal head size but greatly dilated lateral ventricles *(arrow)* indicating hydrocephalus.
Fig 2 (right).—Cross section through fetal trunk at 21 weeks' gestation, showing vertebral body defect *(arrow)* of spina bifida.

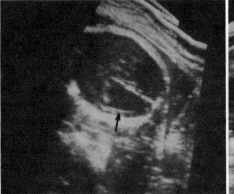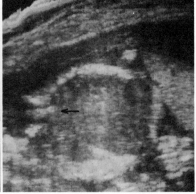

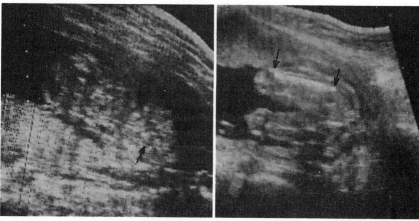

Fig 3 (left).—Mass *(arrow)* attached to fetal abdomen—an omphalocele.
Fig 4 (right).—Measurement of fetal femur length *(arrows)* at 17 weeks' gestation.

led to the current emphasis on ultrasound for anatomical definition. This would seem to be the appropriate course as we continue to search for any deleterious effects of diagnostic ultrasound.

FETOSCOPY

Direct visualization of the fetus is just developing as a clinical tool. It still carries a fetal mortality risk of about 5%. Limited areas of fetal anatomy (2–4 cm²) can be seen through a small-diameter fetoscope and a few diagnoses have been made.[15, 17] Fetoscopy has been most useful for fetal tissue sampling (blood and skin) and only a small number of diagnostic centers have developed clinical programs. Further experience with anatomical diagnosis is expected to occur slowly.

REFERENCES

1. Mills, J. L., Baker, L., and Goldman, A. S.: Malformations in infants of diabetic mothers occur before the seventh gestational week: Implications for treatment. Diabetes 28:292, 1979.
2. Whittemore, R., et al.: Results of pregnancy in women with congenital heart defects. Pediatr. Res. 14:452, 1980 (abstract).
3. Kleinman, C. S., et al.: Echocardiographic studies of the human fetus: Prenatal diagnosis of congenital heart disease and cardiac dysrhythmias. Pediatrics 65:1059, 1980.
4. Touloukian, R. J.: Intestinal atresia. Clin. Perinatol. 5:3, 1978.
5. Lind, T., and Hytten, F. E.: In Hodari, A., and Mariona, F. (eds.): *International Symposium on Physiological Biochemistry of the Fetus.* Springfield, Ill., Charles C Thomas, Publisher, 1972, p. 54.
6. Queenan, J., and Godow, E.: Amniography for detection of congenital anomalies. Obstet. Gynecol. 35:648, 1970.

7. Golbus, M. S.: Teratology for the obstetrician: Current status. Obstet. Gynecol. 55:269, 1980.
8. Antenatal Diagnosis: Report of a Consensus Development Conference Sponsored by the National Institute of Child Health and Human Development. NIH Publication No. 79-1973, 1979.
9. Golbus, M. S., and Stephens, J. D.: Prenatal diagnosis of chromosomal abnormalities and neural tube defects. Clin. Perinatol. 6:245, 1979.
10. Simpson, J. L.: Antenatal diagnosis of chromosomal disorders. Clin. Obstet. Gynaecol. 7:13, 1979.
11. Crandall, B. F., Lebherz, T. B., and Freihube, R.: Neural tube defects: Maternal serum screening and prenatal diagnosis. Pediatr. Clin. North Am. 25:619, 1978.
12. U. K. Collaborative Study on α-fetoprotein in relation to neural tube defects: Maternal serum α-fetoprotein measurement in antenatal screening for anencephaly and spina bifida in early pregnancy. Lancet 1:1323, 1977.
13. U.K. Collaborative Study on α-fetoprotein in relation to neural tube defects: Amniotic fluid α-fetoprotein measurement in antenatal diagnosis of anencephaly and open spina bifida in early pregnancy. Lancet 2:651, 1979.
14. Haddow, J. E., et al.: Acetylcholinesterase and fetal malformations: A modified qualitative technique for diagnosis of neural tube defects. Clin. Chem. (in press).
15. DeVore, G. R., and Hobbins, J. C.: Diagnosis of structural abnormalities in the fetus. Clin. Perinatol. 6:293, 1979.
16. Sabbagha, R. E.: Ultrasonic evaluation of fetal congenital anomalies. Clin. Obstet. Gynaecol. 7:103, 1980.
17. Elias, S.: The role of fetoscopy in antenatal diagnosis. Clin. Obstet. Gynaecol. 7:73, 1980.

Maternal Serum AFP Screening: Promise Not Yet Fulfilled is discussed by Henry L. Nadler and Joe Leigh Simpson[7-1] (Northwestern Univ.). The α-fetoprotein (AFP) concentration of amniotic fluid is a useful marker for the intrauterine detection of neural tube defects (NTD). Although the elevation is nonspecific, and is found in fetal death and other congenital malformations, its use in conjunction with ultrasonography permits about 90% of significant NTDs to be identified. Determination of amniotic fluid AFP levels is recommended in pregnancies at increased risk for NTD, and as a screening method where amniocentesis is done in the second trimester for other genetic indications. Although about 80% to 85% of all cases of NTD could be identified by routine maternal serum screening, the authors believe that routine screening is not warranted at present.

Values from immunologic assays of AFP vary between laboratories, and international standards are needed. Several pilot studies have shown elevated initial serum AFP concentrations in about 6% to 8% of all pregnant women at 15 to 19 weeks' gestation, and in 4% on repeat study. About half these findings can be attributed to incorrect gestational dating or multiple pregnancies. A small number of elevations appear to be related to low birth weight. The large number of false positive results involved in detecting NTDs require sophisti-

(7-1) Obstet. Gynecol. 54:333–334, September 1979.

cated follow-up facilities. Screening at present engenders substantial unnecessary parental anxiety.

Maternal serum AFP screening is a potentially valuable aid in determining fetal well-being. Carefully designed and controlled pilot studies are indicated, but mass screening is not recommended at present.

▶ [We agree with this editorial. Laboratory control problems, physician and patient inexperience, and the uncertain significance of elevated serum AFP levels in the face of normal amniotic fluid AFP levels all suggest that routine screening in the United States is "not warranted at the present time." We simply need more experience and more information before embarking on such a course.] ◀

Significance of Elevated Midtrimester Maternal Plasma α-Fetoprotein Values. Maternal plasma α-fetoprotein (AFP) measurements have been used primarily to detect fetal neural tube defects, but elevated midtrimester levels also are associated with intrauterine death, spontaneous abortion, perinatal death, low birth weight, and various other congenital malformations. David J. H. Brock, Lilias Barron, Pamela Duncan, John B. Scrimgeour, and Muriel Watt[7-2] (Western Genl. Hosp., Edinburgh) carried out a prospective trial of AFP determinations in 15,481 pregnancies at four hospitals over a 44-month period in 1975–78. The measurement of AFP was done by radioimmunoassay in venous blood collected at 15–22 weeks' gestation; the assay was repeated when the value was twice the median for the week of gestation.

A total of 667 women (4.3%) had plasma AFP values above two times the median. The outcome of pregnancy in these cases is shown in Table 1 and the outcome at higher plasma AFP cutoff levels in Table 2. A total of 378 patients had both AFP values above two times the median value. The proportion of "normal" singleton pregnancies declined rapidly at higher AFP cutoff values. At a cutoff of four times the median value, two thirds of pregnancies will end in spontaneous abortion, stillbirth, or neonatal death.

Counseling of women participating in AFP screening programs should be strongly influenced by the maternal plasma AFP levels, even if the ultrasonographic findings and amniotic fluid levels are normal.

▶ [This large experience in plasma AFP screening indicates that very high plasma AFP levels in the absence of multiple pregnancy or of elevated amniotic fluid AFP levels may well indicate something other than a normal pregnancy outcome. The plasma AFP value should influence the counseling of patients in such screening programs.] ◀

Comparison of Pregnancy Outcome After Amniocentesis for Previous Neural Tube Defect or Raised Maternal Serum α-Fetoprotein. A. P. Read, D. Donnai, R. Harris, and P. Donnai[7-3] (Manchester, England) sought to separate the effects of high maternal serum α-fetoprotein (AFP) values per se from those of amniocentesis by examining pregnancy outcomes in women undergoing amniocentesis because of a high AFP level or because of a history of neural tube defect in a previous pregnancy. There were 212 and 219 preg-

(7–2) Lancet 1:1281–1282, June 16, 1979.
(7–3) Br. J. Obstet. Gynaecol. 87:372–376, May 1980.

nancies, respectively, in these groups. Abnormal fetuses, low birth weight infants, and undesired fetal loss were significantly more frequent in the high-AFP group. A significant excess of male births was also observed in the group with high maternal serum AFP levels. A greater proportion of infants in this group weighed less than 2,500 gm at birth. When infants weighing less than 2,500 gm were omitted, males in the high-AFP group were still significantly lighter, but the group difference in birth weights for females was not significant.

Maternal serum AFP screening appears to be a particularly effective means of defining a group of high-risk pregnancies and of avoiding births of infants with neural tube defects. The greater fetal loss and lower birth weight associated with pregnancies characterized by high maternal serum AFP levels appear to be inherent features of these pregnancies rather than consequences of amniocentesis.

▶ [This is another study demonstrating the increased risk associated with elevated maternal serum AFP in the absence of a neural tube defect. The excess of male offspring in this situation (sex ratio, 1.37:1), which has also been reported by others, is curious.] ◀

Amniotic Fluid Acetylcholinesterase Isoenzyme Patterns in Diagnosis of Neural Tube Defects. The α-fetoprotein (AFP) level in amniotic fluid is widely used to identify neural tube defects, but occasional unaffected pregnancies produce falsely positive results. Paul K. Buamah, Lynne Evans, and A. Milford Ward[7-4] (Sheffield, England) determined acetylcholinesterase (AChE) isoenzyme patterns to learn whether the number of false positive results in normal pregnancies and after intrauterine fetal bleeding could be reduced. This enzyme is probably of CNS origin and may be secreted in large amounts into amniotic fluid in open neural tube defects.

Amniotic fluid was obtained by percutaneous amniocentesis from 140 normal pregnancies and 68 with various fetal abnormalities. The isoenzyme pattern of AChE was determined by flat-bed acrylamide gel electrophoresis. Samples from all 61 pregnancies with open neural tube defects yielded two bands that migrated into the gel, a slow-moving band A and a fast-moving band B. None of the samples from normal pregnancies or from those with other fetal abnormalities yielded band B. Four samples from nonneural tube defect cases complicated by exomphalos yielded the A and B bands, as did 3 from cases of intrauterine death. Only a single slow-moving band was seen in 8 normal pregnancy samples grossly contaminated by blood.

Qualitative demonstration of a fast AChE isoenzyme in amniotic fluid is a useful adjunct to the AFP assay in prenatal diagnosis of neural tube defects.

▶ [Elevated amniotic fluid acetylcholinesterase (AChE) levels have been previously described in association with open neural tube defects (1980 YEAR BOOK, p. 200). In the present study, a qualitative test for the presence of a fast-migrating AChE isoenzyme correctly distinguished normal from abnormal (neural tube defect, exomphalos, and intrauterine death). Testing of AChE may have a role in identifying the false positive amniotic fluid α-fetoprotein test result.] ◀

(7–4) Clin. Chim. Acta 103:147–151, Mar. 28, 1980.

Amniotic Fluid α-Fetoprotein Measurement in Antenatal Diagnosis of Anencephaly and Open Spina Bifida in Early Pregnancy is evaluated in the second report of the United Kingdom Collaborative Study of α-Fetoprotein in Relation to Neural Tube Defects by N. J. Wald and H. S. Cuckle[7-5] (Univ. of Oxford). Seventeen centers participated in a study of the efficiency of amniotic fluid α-fetoprotein (AFP) measurements as a means of diagnosing fetal open neural tube defects (NTDs) at 13 to 24 weeks' gestation. Data were obtained on 13,105 singleton pregnancies without fetal NTDs and on 385 with fetal NTDs. There were 222 cases of anencephaly, 152 of spina bifida, including 123 known open lesions, and 11 of encephalocele.

The proportion of unaffected pregnancies with amniotic fluid APF values equal to or greater than a given cut-off level increased with gestational age (Table 1), but similar percentages could be obtained by using different cut-off levels at different gestational ages. Using

TABLE 1.—OUTCOME OF PREGNANCY IN 667 WOMEN WITH PLASMA AFP VALUES ABOVE 2 TIMES MEDIAN (2M)

Outcome*	No. with both A.F.P.s above 2M	No. with only first A.F.P. above 2M
Anencephaly	28 *(7·4%)*	0
Open spina bifida	19 *(5·0%)*	0
Exomphalos	3 *(0·8%)*	0
Spontaneous abortion (<28 wk)	36 *(9·5%)*	6 *(2·1%)*
Twins	37 *(9·8%)*	7 *(2·4%)*
Stillbirth (≥28 wk)	5 *(1·3%)*	0
Neonatal death	5 *(1·3%)*	2 *(0·7%)*
Birth-weight <2·5 kg	39 *(10·3%)*	22 *(7·6%)*
"Normal" singleton	206 *(54·6%)*	252 *(87·2%)*
Total	378 *(100·0%)*	289 *(100·0%)*

*In classifying outcomes, each successive entry excludes those above it.

TABLE 2.—OUTCOME OF PREGNANCY AT HIGHER PLASMA AFP CUTOFFS

No. above plasma-A.F.P. in multiples of median

Outcome	Median×2·3	Median×3·0	Median×4·0
Anencephaly	28 *(11·3%)*	27 *(23·9%)*	19 *(27·5%)*
Open spina bifida	16 *(6·5%)*	12 *(10·6%)*	5 *(7·2%)*
Exomphalos	3 *(1·2%)*	2 *(1·8%)*	2 *(2·9%)*
Spontaneous abortion (<28 wks)	30 *12·1%)*	20 *(17·7%)*	18 *(26·0%)*
Twins	27 *(10·9%)*	12 *(10·6%)*	8 *(11·6%)*
Stillbirth (≥28 wk)	5 *(2·0%)*	3 *(2·7%)*	1 *(1·4%)*
Neonatal death	5 *(2·0%)*	5 *(4·4%)*	4 *(6·0%)*
Birth-weight <2·5 kg	26 *(10·5%)*	11 *(9·7%)*	6 *(8·7%)*
"Normal" singleton	108 *(43·5%)*	21 *(18·6%)*	6 *(8·7%)*
Total	248 *(100·0%)*	113 *(100·0%)*	69 *(100·0%)*

(7–5) Lancet 2:651–662, Sept. 29, 1979.

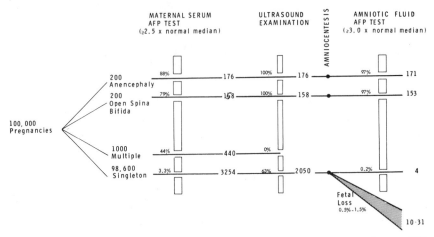

Fig 7–1.—Number of affected and unaffected pregnancies with positive maternal serum AFP and amniotic fluid AFP tests in 100,000 who are screened. (Courtesy of Wald, N. J., and Cuckle, H. S.: Lancet 2:651–662, Sept. 29, 1979.)

cut-off levels of 2.5 as the normal median at 13 to 15 weeks, 3.0 at 16 to 18 weeks, 3.5 at 19 to 21 weeks, and 4.0 at 22 to 24 weeks, 98% of cases of anencephaly and 98% of cases of open spina bifida gave positive results, as did 0.48% of unaffected pregnancies not associated with miscarriage. Seven positive results related to serious fetal malformation were excluded. The false positive rate was much lower in pregnancies with clear amniotic fluid samples (Table 2).

The findings are outlined in Figure 7–1. The false positive rate could be more than halved if all patients with positive results on blood-stained samples or borderline results on clear samples had repeat tests on fresh samples. Maternal serum AFP screening, which can detect about 80% of cases of open spina bifida, is likely to be the chief means of selecting women for amniotic fluid APF determinations.

▶ [This report of the large-scale British collaborative study of amniotic fluid AFP testing makes several important points. Different cutoff values are required at different gestational ages to minimize false positive results. Imminent miscarriage (often of a fetus already dead) and gross contamination of the amniotic fluid with blood will increase the chances of abnormally high AFP results. With clear fluid and continuing pregnancies, only about 0.3% of women with unaffected fetuses will have abnormal results. The possibility of using other diagnostic measures (rapidly adhering cells, amniography, gray scale ultrasound, etc) to further define these false positive results is not considered in the calculations.

The odds of having a fetus affected with open spina bifida in the face of an elevated amniotic fluid AFP value vary greatly according to the reason for the amniocentesis. If the woman was identified by serum AFP screening, the odds of an affected fetus are 18:1. If she did not have screening but previously had an infant with a neural tube defect, the odds are 5:1. If an unscreened woman underwent amniocentesis for some other reason, the odds are 1:2.

Amniocentesis is not without risk. According to Figure 7–1, the 153 fetuses with open spina bifida identified correspond with 10–31 fetal losses from the amniocentesis procedure itself. If one fourth of children born with open spina bifida survive to age 5 with severe handicaps and if this is the real target population, then the risk-benefit analyses get even more complex.] ◀

Anencephaly and Spina Bifida (ASB) and Retroversion. Because of a chance finding of frequent uterine retroversion in cases of anencephaly, Michael R. Buckley[7-6] (Ege Univ.) undertook a 3-year survey of 113 ASB births in Izmir, Turkey. Thirty-seven patients were recalled. Twelve patients were pregnant at recall. Twelve others had an anteverted or midposition uterus, 11 had a retroverted uterus, and 2 had an acutely flexed and levorotated uterus. The incidence of retroversion in a control group of 100 women was 18%, approximating the generally accepted normal rate of about 15%.

A significantly high rate of uterine retroversion has been discovered in mothers of ASB infants, but a causal relation is not proved. The pampiniform plexus of a retroverted uterus is often engorged. Venous congestion indicates back pressure on the endometrial vessels and presumably a fall in oxygen tension in the endometrium. Retroversion may exaggerate a deficiency in oxygenation due to the site of implantation or poor placentation, resulting in an increased risk of fetal abnormality. This could be checked by determining venous blood Po_2 in anteverted and retroverted nonpregnant uteri. Further studies may demonstrate a significant remediable factor in the cause of CNS defects and possibly of other birth defects.

▶ [Is this real? The suggestion here is that patients with previous deliveries of infants with open neural tube defects are more apt to have retroverted uteri than controls. The postulated mechanism concerns hypoxia related to vascular distortion caused by the abnormally (?) positioned uterus. We have always minimized the significance of uterine position in discussions with patients, likening it to eye color—some are brown and some are blue. Until or unless this finding is confirmed, we will remain skeptical.] ◀

Possible Prevention of Neural Tube Defects by Periconceptional Vitamin Supplementation. The well-known social-class gradient in incidence of neural tube defects suggests that nutritional factors may be involved in their etiology. Previous observations are compatible with the hypothesis that subclinical vitamin deficiency may contribute to the occurrence of these defects. R. W. Smithells, S. Sheppard, C. J. Schorah, M. J. Seller, N. C. Nevin, R. Harris, A. P. Read, and D. W. Fielding[7-7] report preliminary results of a study in which periconceptional multivitamin supplements were offered to mothers at increased risk of having infants with neural tube defects. Women who had had 1 or more infants with such a defect were admitted to the study. Most were from genetic counseling clinics. Study mothers received a multivitamin-iron preparation starting at least 28 days before conception and continuing to at least the time of the second missed period.

Only 1 of 178 infants-fetuses of fully supplemented mothers (0.6%) had a neural tube defect, compared with 13 of 260 infants-fetuses of unsupplemented mothers (5.0%), a significant difference. Control women had a recurrence rate entirely consistent with reported data; supplemented mothers had a significantly lower recurrence rate. Possible explanations include self-selection of low-risk women for supplementation, a factor other than vitamin supplementation, and an ef-

(7–6) J. Epidemiol. Community Health 33:297–298, December 1979.
(7–7) Lancet 1:329–340, Feb. 16, 1980.

fect of vitamin supplementation in reducing occurrence of these defects. The last is the most straightforward interpretation and the one consistent with circumstantial evidence linking nutrition with neural tube defects. The rate of spontaneous abortion was similar in the study and control groups.

▶ [Although the social-class gradient in the incidence of neural tube defects suggests a possible etiologic role for nutritional factors, these results seem almost too good. The members of the control group are not fully characterized in this preliminary communication, but in fairness, the recurrence rates they suffered are those generally quoted. Others are certain to study this important question. If this turns out to be real, which micronutrient(s) in the multivitamin preparation is (are) critical? If general adoption of periconceptional vitamin supplementation were to result in an eightfold reduction in neural tube defects, what would this do to the cost-benefit analyses of screening programs for these defects?

The vitamin supplement used did not contain zinc, defiency of which causes CNS malformations in the rat.] ◀

Central Nervous System Defects in Children Born to Mothers Exposed to Organic Solvents During Pregnancy. Organic solvents have received much attention as possible factors or cofactors in the etiology of embryotoxic effects in man. Peter C. Holmberg[7-8] (Helsinki) reports a 2-year study of mothers of children with congenital CNS defects and matched-pair controls, in which exposure to organic

EXPOSURE OF 14 MOTHERS OF CHILDREN WITH CNS DEFECTS AND OF 3 MOTHERS OF HEALTHY CHILDREN

—	Type of exposure	Solvents
Case		
1	Plastics manufacturing	Styrene; acetone
2	Leather industry	Denatured alcohol + dyes
3	Textile industry	Ethylene oxide; alkylphenol + dyes
4	Community services (laboratory)	Benzene; dichlormethane; methanol; ether
5	Cultural services (museum)	White spirit*
6	Plastics manufacturing	Styrene; acetone
7	Printing and publishing	White spirit
8	Rubber products manufacturing	Toluene; xylene; white spirit; methylethylketone
9	Metal products manufacturing	Petrol; denatured alcohol
10	Metal products manufacturing	Toluene
11	Leather industry	Denatured alcohol + dyes
12	Building	Toluene; white spirit
13	Handicrafts Husband	Styrene
14	at home	Mixed aromatic/aliphatic
Control		
1	Equipment manufacturing	Xylene, butanol
2	Community services (laboratory)	Mixed aromatic/aliphatic
3	Community services (surgery)	Halothane, ether

*Mixture of C7-9 aliphatic hydrocarbons.

(7–8) Lancet 2 :177–179, July 28, 1979.

solvents was defined as far as was possible. Information about exposure was obtained by interviewing the mothers, and sometimes by visiting their places of work.

A total of 132 children with congenital CNS defects were registered in 1976–1978; the final series included 120 patients plus matched controls. Mothers of children with defects had been exposed more often to organic solvents in the first trimester of pregnancy than mothers of controls. The difference was significant. Anencephaly was the most common defect. Twelve mothers had been exposed to organic solvents at work, and 2 had been exposed at home from their husbands' handicrafts. All 3 mothers of controls had been exposed at work. Aromatic hydrocarbons were the most common material in both groups (table). The two series did not differ substantially in parental age, drugs used, or infections during pregnancy. The proportions of subjects who worked during the first trimester also were the same. In 2 instances, earlier pregnancies with similar exposure to organic solvents had ended in spontaneous abortion. One mother was a diabetic.

The significantly greater number of mothers of children with defects who were exposed to organic solvents in the first trimester of pregnancy implies an association between this exposure and CNS defects in the children.

▶ [Studies in teratology are difficult to design and to interpret. This case-control study suggests that exposure to organic solvents in the first trimester is associated with an increased risk of CNS anomalies—11.7% of mothers of children with congenital CNS defects had such exposure vs 2.5% of mothers of control children. Because of the possibility of interviewer or patient bias and because of the uncertainties concerning other variables, one cannot draw firm conclusions from this study. Therefore, it is difficult to advise individual patients in this matter.] ◀

Reducing Birth Defect Risk in Advanced Maternal Age. The incidence of certain severe birth defects increases with maternal age. However, recent advances in fetal diagnosis, coupled with elective abortion, offer the older pregnant woman an opportunity to reduce this risk. To determine the magnitude of potential risk reduction, Marshall F. Goldberg, Larry D. Edmonds, and Godfrey P. Oakley[7-9] (Center for Disease Control, Atlanta, Ga.) reviewed the maternal age-specific incidence of infants born with one or more severe defects in data from the Metropolitan Atlanta Defects Program for 1968 to 1975 and from the National Center for Health Statistics (NCHS) for 1973 to 1975, with removal from analysis of anomalies that were preventable by currently available methods.

In the Atlanta data, the rate of selected major birth defects for women younger than age 35 years averaged 15 cases per 1,000 live births, whereas those for women aged 35 to 39, 40 to 44 and older than 44 years were 17, 31, and 76 cases per 1,000 live births, respectively. At age 30 years and older, chromosomal abnormalities contributed an increasingly larger proportion of the severe defects studied; no consistently similar trend was noted for anencephaly-spina bifida. Because of underreporting of malformations on birth certificates, the

(7-9) JAMA 242:2292–2294, Nov. 23, 1979.

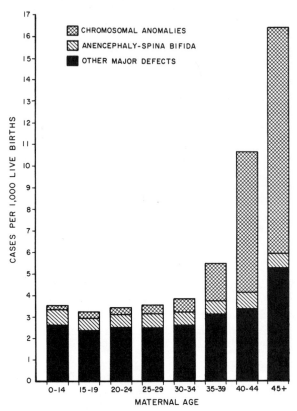

Fig 7–2.—Incidence of selected major birth defects by maternal age, National Center for Health Statistics, 1973 to 1975. (Courtesy of Goldberg, M. F., et al.: JAMA 242:2292–2294, Nov. 23, 1979; copyright 1979, American Medical Association.)

maternal age-specific incidence for defects obtained from the NCHS averaged 25% to 33% of those for Atlanta, but the data showed similar trends (Fig 7–2).

In the NCHS data, for women using fetal diagnosis and elective abortion, the estimated risk reduction was 46% (from 5.5 to 3.0 per 1,000 live births) for those aged 35 to 39 years, 68% (10.5 to 3.4) for those aged 40 to 44 years and 68% (16.5 to 5.3) for those aged 45 years or older. However, as shown in the Atlanta data, the risk was still higher for women aged 45 years or more than for those aged 34 years or less.

Through prenatal diagnosis and selective abortion of fetuses found to have chromosomal disorders or neural tube defects, women aged 35 to 44 years can lower risk of having an infant with a severe birth defect to a level experienced by women under age 35 years. Women aged 45 years and older can lower risk considerably, but only to a level twice as great as that for women aged 34 years or younger.

▶ [Amniocentesis for prenatal genetic diagnosis can now be considered an essential component of care of the gravida at high risk. Indeed, a New York court recently held a physician negligent for not advising a 37-year-old pregnant woman of the possibility of having an abnormal child. This analysis documents what is possible by such an approach—a 46% reduction in risk in women aged 35 or older of delivering a malformed infant, bringing the risk to the same range as that of younger women. It also points out the limitations, for, even assuming a 100% compliance in amniocentesis and a 100% abortion rate in affected cases, only 30% of live births of infants with chromosomal abnormalities and only 5% of those with any major defect would be prevented. Figure 7–2 demonstrates that the excess in birth defects with advanced maternal age involves principally chromosomal anomalies.] ◄

Enhanced Growth of Amniotic Fluid Cells in Presence of Fibroblast Growth Factor. Many amniotic fluid samples today are submitted for prenatal diagnosis, and some cultures grow slowly and need to be maintained for a long time. Richard P. Porreco, Christine Bradshaw, Siddhartha Sarkar, and O. William Jones[7-10] (Univ. of California, San Diego) investigated whether addition of fibroblast growth factor (FGF), a potent mitogen for mesodermal cells, to the standard method of processing primary amniotic fluid cultures would be advantageous. An FGF preparation purified from whole fresh frozen bovine brain was used. Amniocenteses were generally done at 16 to 19 weeks' gestation under ultrasonic control. The FGF, 1 μg/ml, was added to one of the two culture dishes of each sample.

At the initial harvest and at five scored metaphases, cultures incubated with FGF showed a 9-day advantage as a group compared with the untreated, paired control cultures. Less variability in growth was noted in FGF-treated cultures. All but 3% were harvested initially at 10 to 20 days, compared to only 48% of control cultures. Success was also noted in recovery of failing cultures treated with FGF.

Addition of FGF to the standard enriched medium used in amniotic fluid cell cultures has shortened processing times and provided more uniform growth in most cultures. The means by which FGF stimulates cell growth is not known. The mitogen may reduce the average length of the G_1 period of the cell cycle. Use of this approach in biochemical diagnosis merits further study.

► [The interval between the performance of a second-trimester genetic amniocentesis and the reporting of the results to the patient is generally 3 to 4 weeks on our service. This is clearly a time of high anxiety for the patient. This report suggests that fibroblast growth factor (FGF), a potent mitogen, can reduce this interval by a week or so, on the average. If this experience is confirmed by other laboratories, FGF will fill a useful role.] ◄

Amniotic Fluid Testosterone and Follicle-Stimulating Hormone Assay in Prenatal Determination of Fetal Sex. One indication for prenatal diagnosis by amniocentesis is carrier status for an X-linked disorder. Usually, diagnosis of an affected fetus is not possible, thus management decisions are based on determination of fetal sex by chromosome analysis of cultured amniotic fluid cells, a time-consuming and costly process. T. A. Doran, P. Y. Wong, L. C. Allen, and M. Falk[7-11] (Univ. of Toronto) describe the use of amniotic fluid testosterone and follicle-stimulating hormone (FSH) assays in prenatal sex determination.

Amniotic fluid samples were obtained by amniocentesis from 812

(7–10) Obstet. Gynecol. 55:55–59, January 1980.
(7–11) Am. J. Obstet. Gynecol. 136:309–312, Feb. 1, 1980.

patients at approximately 16 weeks' gestation; samples were then frozen and assayed for testosterone and FSH levels. The karyotype of the cultured amniotic fluid cells was used as the correct indicator of fetal sex.

Testosterone levels from male and female fetuses overlapped between 16.2 and 33.8 ng/ml. Thus, results in this zone could not be used to predict fetal sex directly. All results above 33.8 ng/ml were from male fetuses (218), whereas all results below 16.2 ng/ml were from female fetuses. Fetal sex could be assigned in all samples outside the overlap zone (45%).

Follicle-stimulating hormone levels were assayed in 353 samples (166 male and 187 female fetuses). Values from male and female fetuses overlapped between 7.6 and 10.9 mIU/ml. There were 23 results from male fetuses below 7.6 mIU/ml and 136 results from female fetuses above 10.9, allowing for sex assignment in the 45% of samples outside the overlap zone.

In the 353 instances in which both FSH and testosterone were assayed, fetal sex could be determined as long as one of the values fell outside the overlap zone; 71% of the samples could be so identified.

The testosterone-FSH ratio was calculated in an attempt to improve the diagnostic accuracy of the combined assay approach. The overlap zone for the ratio was 2.2 to 3.4. Of the male samples, 73% fell above the upper cutoff; of the female samples, 86% fell below the lower cutoff. Thus, 80% of all samples fell outside the overlap zone and in these the sex could be determined.

The testosterone-FSH ratio holds promise as a rapid biochemical screening tool in the prenatal diagnosis of fetal sex in X-linked disorders.

▶ [Earlier articles have described higher testosterone and lower FSH levels in second-trimester amniotic fluid with male than with female fetuses. Several reports have even been enthusiastic about the clinical usefulness of such measurements in sex determination. In this large series, only about half the measurements were diagnostic (ie, had values outside the overlap area) in the case of testosterone. By utilizing the ratio of testosterone to FSH, 80% of cases could be diagnosed. This is still not good enough for clinical application, but it might be feasible to use something like this as a primary approach and reserve the most costly and time-consuming chromosome cultures for the 20% in which they are necessary.] ◀

Amniotic Fluid 3,3′,5′-Triiodothyronine in Detection of Congenital Hypothyroidism. Fetal thyroxine metabolism differs markedly from that in extrauterine life. Concentrations of reverse triiodothyronine (rT_3) in amniotic fluid are much higher than corresponding values in maternal serum at 15 to 19 weeks' gestation, and this rT_3 may be of fetal origin and be of value in diagnosis of fetal thyroid dysfunction. Heddy Landau, Joseph Sack, Henriette Frucht, Zvi Palti, Drorith Hochner-Celnikier, and Ada Rosenmann[7-12] measured rT_3 concentrations in amniotic fluid in 2 pregnant women in an attempt to assess the thyroid function of the fetuses. Amniotic fluid rT_3 was measured in unextracted fluid with a radioimmunoassay kit.

The 2 women had previously given birth to infants with neonatal

(7–12) J. Clin. Endocrinol. Metab. 50:799–801, April 1980.

hypothyroidism. Repeated low concentrations of rT_3 in amniotic fluid of 20 to 64 ng/dl were found at 16 and 31 weeks' gestation in 1 case, but a normal infant was delivered. He is now aged 10 months and has no signs of hypothyroidism, without treatment. In the second case, amniotic rT_3 levels were well within the normal range for 15 to 19 weeks' gestation at 140 to 180 ng/dl, but a hypothyroid infant was born.

These findings suggest that amniotic fluid rT_3 determinations are not a reliable means of diagnosing intrauterine hypothyroidism. Low amniotic fluid rT_3 concentrations in a euthyroid fetus might be due to increased degradation of rT_3.

▶ [Previous work has indicated that amniotic fluid T_4 and T_3 levels do not reflect the thyroid status of the fetus and are therefore valueless in diagnosing fetal hypothyroidism. Because rT_3 seems to be the major thyroid hormone during fetal life, it has been hoped that amniotic fluid rT_3 might be useful. This report of 2 cases seems to dash that hope. In 1 case with very low amniotic fluid rT_3 levels at 16 weeks, the infant proved to be normal whereas in the other, amniotic fluid rT_3 levels were normal at midpregnancy but the infant was hypothyroid at birth.] ◀

Cigarette Smoking as Etiologic Factor in Cleft Lip and Palate. Decreased birth weights and increased perinatal mortality are associated with cigarette smoking during pregnancy, but few workers have found any definite effect of maternal smoking on fetal malformation rates. Anders Ericson, Bengt Källén and Peter Westerholm[7-13] carried out a case-control study of smoking habits in women who, in 1975, gave birth to infants with closure defects of the central nervous system or with cleft lip or cleft palate, or both. Each study infant was matched with 2 controls for time of delivery, maternal age and maternal parity. Data were available for 66 infants with cleft lip or cleft palate, 66 with closure defects and 261 controls. Significantly more women having cleft lip or cleft palate infants smoked compared to controls, but women having infants with closure defects had a normal smoking pattern. The findings were not attributable to patterns of drug use.

This study found a significantly increased rate of smoking among women who gave birth to cleft lip or cleft palate infants. Thus, maternal cigarette smoking may be one of many factors of importance in the etiology of these malformations. No other exogenous source of human malformations as important as cigarette smoking is apparent in Sweden.

Maternal Smoking Habits and Congenital Malformations: Population Study. Infants of mothers who smoke during pregnancy are more likely to be born small; also, increased perinatal mortality has been associated with maternal smoking. Dewi R. Evans, Robert G. Newcombe and H. Campbell[7-14] (Cardiff) examined the relationship between maternal cigarette smoking and congenital malformation in the offspring in a series of 67,609 singleton pregnancies during 1965–76. The overall incidence of congenital malformations was 2.8% in both smokers and nonsmokers. No significant differences were found

(7–13)   Am. J. Obstet. Gynecol. 135:348–351, Oct. 1, 1979.
(7–14)   Br. Med. J. 2:171–173, July 21, 1979.

in the rates of malformations according to the amount of smoking, except for neural tube defects. The rate of anencephaly increased with the degree of smoking. Neural tube defects were less frequent in non-smokers in social classes I and II. The rate of neural tube defects was very high in social classes IV and V, regardless of maternal smoking habits.

These findings suggest that maternal smoking does not have teratogenic effects on offspring, except for neural tube defects; even in these malformation the effect of smoking is modest at best. The population with the highest rate of neural tube defects in this survey was similar to that which is most likely to smoke, and to smoke heavily.

▶ [The relationship between maternal cigarette smoking and congenital anomalies is unclear. The case-control study from Sweden suggests an increased risk of cleft lip and palate in the offspring of smokers. The British survey of 67,609 pregnancies provides data that are consistent with this view although the differences lack statistical significance. The report from Cardiff suggests a relationship between smoking and neural tube defects, but this was not found in the Swedish study. Confounding factors (social class, alcohol use, etc) abound. This issue is sure to remain hazy.] ◀

Effects on Child of Alcohol Abuse During Pregnancy: Retrospective and Prospective Studies. R. Olegård, K.-G. Sabel, M. Aronasson, B. Sandin, P. R. Johansson, C. Carlsson, M. Kyllerman, K. Iversen, and A. Hrbek[7-15] (Göteborg) report a retrospective study of the children of 15 women who were or had been alcoholics and an extended retrospective study of 103 children of 30 such mothers. In addition, a prospective study was carried out in pregnant alcohol abusers seen in an 18-month period from 1977 to 1978.

Retrospective and prospective studies give an incidence of 1 fetal alcohol lesion per 300 deliveries. Half of the infants had the complete fetal alcohol syndrome. Perinatal and infant mortality was increased sevenfold to tenfold, and low birth weight was increased eightfold. Preterm deliveries (before 37 weeks' gestation) were increased threefold, small size for gestational age, 12-fold. Small size at birth correlated with reduced mental performance later in life. An intelligence quotient (IQ) below 85 was found in 58% of children, and an IQ below 70 in 19%. Cerebral palsy occurred in 8%. Follow-up of alcoholic women during pregnancy and appropriate treatment had a favorable effect on intrauterine growth when sobriety could be induced early in pregnancy. There was, however, no protection from functional brain disturbance as assessed by neurologic performance and evoked response electroencephalography.

Fetal damage from alcohol is now the most frequently occurring, but preventable, health hazard created by a noxious agent. An increased risk of cerebral palsy has not previously been described in children of alcoholic mothers. Effective measures must be found for halting the increasingly more frequent consumption of alcohol by young persons in order to protect fetuses from irreversible damage.

▶ [One fourth of the babies born of alcoholic mothers in the prospective portion of this study had fetal alcohol syndrome. Perinatal deaths and growth retardation were

(7–15) Acta Paediatr. Scand. (Suppl. 275):112–121, 1979.

frequent. The 5 mothers who stopped drinking in the early pregnancy delivered babies of normal birth weight. However, of these babies, the 3 who were tested had abnormal evoked response EEGs. The authors suggest that 1 of 300 newborns in Göteborg is damaged as a result of maternal alcohol ingestion.] ◄

Long-Term Propranolol Therapy in Pregnancy: Maternal and Fetal Outcome. S. C. Pruyn, J. P. Phelan, and G. C. Buchanan[7-16] (Naval Regional Med. Center, Portsmouth, Va.) reviewed the effects of propranolol therapy in 10 patients, 2 of whom delivered twice while using the drug. Fundal growth was poor in half the pregnancies, and 3 of these ended with the delivery of infants who were small for gestational age. The cesarean section rate was 41.6%, but only 2 cesarean sections were possibly drug related. One precipitous delivery occurred 30 minutes after an intravenous dose of propranolol. One intrauterine fetal death occurred. There was 1 case of premature membrane rupture. Three infants were hypoglycemic, 2 were jaundiced, and 1 each had bradycardia and polycythemia. All but 1 of the 11 surviving infants were at or below the 50th percentiles for weight and head circumference. The tendency toward growth retardation was confirmed when serial pregnancies in 5 mothers were assessed. Propranolol dosage could not be significantly correlated with infant weights.

Long-term propranolol therapy during pregnancy apparently leads to smaller-than-expected infants. The growth retardation appears to be symmetric. Whether these small infants are at an increased risk of physical or mental impairment remains to be seen. The use of propranolol in pregnancy should be carefully weighed, with benefits predominating over possible risks. Another form of therapy should be used if feasible. All pregnant patients on long-term propranolol therapy should be managed as having high-risk pregnancies.

► [Propranolol has come into very wide use for treatment of a variety of medical conditions—chronic hypertension, thyrotoxicosis, cardiac arrhythmias, and hypertrophic subaortic stenosis—and in previous editions of the YEAR BOOK we have expressed our concern with its chronic administration during pregnancy. This collection of 12 pregnancies in 10 patients is one of the largest series reported to date, and the results do not seem to confirm a number of previous risks suggested by earlier case reports. The one condition that did appear to be correlated with chronic propranolol therapy was fetal growth retardation, as nearly all infants were below the 50th percentiles for weight and head circumference and 3 of the 12 were frankly small for gestational age. An association between propranolol and fetal growth retardation suggested in previous reports has been confounded by the condition (ie, hypertension) for which the drug is usually given, but in this series only 1 of the 10 patients was hypertensive.] ◄

Placental and Mammary Transfer of Sulfasalazine. Sulfasalazine (SASP), which consists of sulfapyridine (SP) linked to a salicylate (SA) radical, is widely used as maintenance therapy for ulcerative colitis. Many patients are women of reproductive age, raising the question of to what extent the drug and its metabolites, particularly SP, reach the fetus and are present in breast milk. A. K. Azad Khan and S. C. Truelove[7-17] (Oxford, England) evaluated 5 patients with ulcerative colitis who became pregnant while on maintenance treatment with SASP. A dose of 0.5 gm 4 times daily was continued

(7–16) Am. J. Obstet. Gynecol. 135:485–489, Oct. 15, 1979.
(7–17) Br. Med. J. 2:1553, Dec. 15, 1979.

CONCENTRATIONS (µg/ml; MEAN ± SD) OF SASP AND ITS
METABOLITES IN MATERNAL SERUMS AND IN CORRESPONDING
CORD SERUMS, AMNIOTIC FLUID AND BREAST MILK

			Results in 5 cases			Results in 3 cases	
			Maternal serum	Cord serum	Amniotic serum	Maternal serum	Breast milk
SASP ..	..	..	7·3±4·0	4·2±3·0	0·6±0·5	8·8±1·9	2·7±1·8
Total-SP	..	..	10·6±4·6	11·0±4·0	16·0±8·9	19·0±3·1	10·3±1·6
Free-SP	..	..	6·7±4·1	4·6±3·0	8·6±5·6	13·8±4·0	6·5±2·2
SP-Gluc	..	..	0·0	0·4±0·2	0·6±0·9	0·1±0·2	1·6±2·8
Ac-SP ..	..	..	3·7±2·4	4·9±1·8	4·8±3·4	4·5±2·3	1·4±0·7
Ac-SP Gluc	..	..	0·5±0·3	0·6±0·5	1·9±0·7	0·6±0·4	0·8±1·0
Total 5-ASA ..	..	..	<0·5	<0·5	1·2+0·5	Not measured	Not measured

through pregnancy and the puerperium. It was found that SASP crosses the placenta (table); the mean concentration in cord serum was half that of maternal serum. An extremely low amniotic fluid concentration was found. Free SP concentrations were significantly lower in cord serum than in maternal serum. Both SASP and SP were found to pass into breast milk. The concentration of SASP in milk was about 30% of that in maternal serum, and that of total SP was about 50% of the maternal serum concentration.

No untoward effects of SASP on the fetus have been described. Both SASP and its metabolites do reach the fetus in concentrations not greatly different from those in maternal serum, presenting a theoretical risk of fetal complications. Concentrations of SASP and its metabolites in breast milk are much lower than those in maternal serum, making harmful side effects unlikely.

▶ [Concern has been raised from time to time about sulfasalazine (Azulfidine) treatment of the gravida with ulcerative colitis. We have usually dismissed these concerns, thinking that the drug is poorly absorbed. This study demonstrates that significant absorption and placental and mammary transfer *do* take place. The authors note, and we agree, that no adverse fetal effects have been found with quite extensive usage. Nevertheless, perhaps a systematic look at bilirubin levels in infants born to treated women is in order.] ◀

Serum Salicylate Levels and Right-to-Left Ductus Shunts in Newborn Infants With Persistent Pulmonary Hypertension. In persistent pulmonary hypertension of the newborn (PPHN), pulmonary arterial hypertension causes right-to-left shunting through a patent ductus arteriosus, foramen ovale, or both. Ronald M. Perkin, Daniel L. Levin, and Ronald Clark[7-18] (Univ. of Texas Health Science Center, Dallas) measured serum salicylate concentrations in newborn infants with a history of cyanosis or respiratory distress to determine whether maternal salicylate ingestion can cause intrauterine constriction of the ductus arteriosus in human infants. Tolazoline was infused in a dose of 1 mg/kg over 4 minutes as the systemic arterial pressure was monitored, and blood oxygen tensions were obtained. Salicylate concentration was measured in cord serums from 25 control term infants, 26 infants with cardiopulmonary disease but without a right-to-left ductus shunt, 6 infants with a ductus shunt, 5 with

(7–18) J. Pediatr. 96:721–726, April 1980.

PPHN and a right-to-left ductus shunt, and 6 with PPHN but no right-to-left ductus shunt.

Mean changes in PaO_2 with tolazoline were 70 mm Hg in infants with cardiopulmonary disease and a right-to-left ductus shunt and 2.2 mm Hg in infants with PPHN and a right-to-left ductus shunt. Infants with PPHN but no shunt had significantly higher serum salicylate concentrations than the other study groups. All 5 of the former infants responded to tolazoline infusion. All 4 infants with PPHN and a right-to-left ductus shunt who were studied responded to tolazoline. In only 2 of 6 cases of PPHN without a shunt was a history of maternal salicylate ingestion documented.

The findings, though not conclusive, suggest that use of aspirin and other nonsteroid anti-inflammatory agents should be considered to be potentially dangerous to the human fetus. Premature closure of the ductus arteriosus from maternal salicylate ingestion may be one cause of PPHN and may explain the absence of right-to-left ductus shunting in some infants with this syndrome.

▶ [Prostaglandins appear to play a major role in maintaining the patency of the ductus arteriosus during fetal life. Prostaglandin synthetase inhibitors have been shown to cause constriction or closure of the ductus in the fetus of several animal species and in the human newborn. This study compares salicylate levels in several groups of normal and abnormal infants studied during the first 48 or 72 hours of life. Significantly higher levels were found in those with pulmonary hypertension in the absence of ductus shunting compared with other conditions, which would be compatible with premature (ie, intrauterine) constriction or closure of the ductus due to maternal aspirin ingestion. There is no apparent explanation of why the infants with other forms of cardiopulmonary complications had salicylate levels that, while lower than those in infants with pulmonary hypertension and no right-to-left ductus shunting, were still higher than levels in completely normal infants. From the clinical point of view, these data argue for caution about the use of aspirin and other anti-inflammatory agents during pregnancy.] ◀

Subclinical Congenital Rubella Infection Associated With Maternal Rubella Vaccination in Early Pregnancy. Rubella virus vaccine, given to a susceptible pregnant woman, can cross the placenta and infect the fetus. No anomalies attributable to rubella, however, have been observed in liveborn infants of susceptible vacinees, and infants have had no serologic evidence of congenital infection. Gregory F. Hayden, Kenneth L. Herrmann, Elena Buimovici-Klein, Karen E. Weiss, Phillip L. Nieburg, and James E. Mitchell[7-19] report the cases of 4 clinically normal infants with serologic evidence of congenital rubella infection after maternal vaccination in early pregnancy.

Vaccine virus has been detected in abortion specimens from women vaccinated either inadvertently in early pregnancy or experimentally before scheduled therapeutic abortion. The rate of virus isolation in specimens from women known or estimated to have been rubella seronegative at vaccination was 19.8%. The incidence of rubella-specific IgM antibody in 30 infants of presumably susceptible vaccines was 10%. The rate of persistence of rubella hemagglutination inhibition antibody beyond age 6 months in this group has been 24%. Virus was

(7–19) J. Pediatr. 96:869–872, May 1980.

not isolated from the infant or placenta of any of 37 presumably susceptible vaccines. No infants of 68 presumably susceptible mothers have had clinical evidence of congenital infection or malformation attributable to rubella.

It is premature to conclude that there is no risk of malformation, although the estimated maximal risk of serious malformation attributable to rubella vaccine appears to be low. Rubella vaccine, in any case, is contraindicated in pregnancy. All women should be advised of the possible risk to the fetus if they conceive within 3 months after vaccination.

▶ [A number of earlier studies have documented that rubella virus can be isolated from the products of conception after vaccination in early pregnancy. This report confirms those observations by finding rubella-specific IgM antibodies in cord blood of 4 infants born at term to women vaccinated in the first trimester. Although the attenuated live virus clearly can cross the placenta to "infect" the fetus, according to the Center for Disease Control no infants born to 191 vaccinees, of whom 68 are known or presumed to have been susceptible, have exhibited clinical evidence of congenital infection or malformation attributable to rubella. Thus, although rubella immunization is contraindicated during pregnancy, the risk of untoward effects appears to be very small.] ◀

Origin of Chi 46 XX/46 XY Chimerism in Human True Hermaphrodite. A chimera is an individual having two or more cell types resulting from the fusion of different zygotes. The origin of whole body chimeras is often unclear, but may be determined by comparing markers in the cell lines of the chimera and the parents. Gordon Dewald, Morey W. Haymond, Jack L. Spurbeck, and S. Breanndan Moore[7-20] (Mayo Clinic and Found.) used chromosome heteromorphisms to study a true hermaphrodite who probably arose by fertilization of an ovum and its second meiotic polar body.

The patient was referred for chromosome analysis shortly after birth because of ambiguous genitalia. At laparotomy, a rudimentary unicornate uterus, fallopian tubes, and a streaklike gonad with oocytes were found on the left side and removed. The right side contained a fetal testis, vas deferens, and epididymis, which were also removed. Samples from the peripheral blood, skin, fetal testis, and ovarian gonad showed both 46 XX and 46 XY cells in all tissues. Chromosome analysis on the peripheral blood cells of the parents was also done.

Heteromorphisms of chromosomes 9, 13, 16, 21, and 22, and the Y chromosome, were useful in determining the origin of the chimerism. In the XY line of the infant, the Y and chromosomes 13 and 21 are of paternal origin, whereas the homologs are maternal. In the XX line, the paternal markers 9, 13, and 21 can be identified, as can the maternal markers 13 and 21. The maternal marker 16 and paternal marker 22 are not evident in either cell line of the patient.

Various blood group typings were also studied. In the Kidd antigen system, 70% to 80% of the cells were negative for Jk^a and 20% to 30% were positive. This is similar to the ratio of XX to XY cells in the patient's lymphocytes.

(7–20) Science 207:321–323, Jan. 18, 1980.

Mosaicism is unlikely because there are too many differences between the cell lines. Because there is a paternal and maternal haploid set of chromosomes in each of the cell lines, there were apparently two separate fertilization events. If the ovum and second meiotic division polar body derived from the ovum were each fertilized by a different sperm, the same maternal markers should be present in both cell lines of the chimera, as found in this case.

The paternal cytogenetic studies also indicate that two sperm were involved. The two cell lines had different chromosome 9 markers and sex chromosomes, but the same 22. Thus, random chromosome segregation in different gametogenic processes must have been involved.

The ovum second meiotic division polar body is produced at the time of fertilization and is in close proximity to the ovum, so that if both were fertilized, there would be an opportunity for cells from each zygote to mingle.

▶ [Although partial chimeras resulting from twin-twin or maternal-fetal transfusions of leukocytes are not difficult to understand, the mechanisms underlying the formation of whole body chimeras are not so clear. Using sophisticated techniques of chromosomal analysis, the authors of this report argue convincingly that in the case described the second polar body must have been fertilized by a second sperm and the two zygotes must have fused. Other whole body chimeras may result from other forms of zygote fusion.] ◀

8. Puerperium and the Newborn

Uncontrollable Postpartum Bleeding: New Approach to Hemostasis Through Angiographic Arterial Embolization. Extrauterine pelvic hematomas occur in about 0.1% of deliveries. Unless the site of bleeding is recognized early, repeated operative procedures, multiple blood transfusions and significant morbidity and mortality may result. Bryant J. Brown, Dennis K. Heaston, A. Marsh Poulson, Harvey A. Gabert, D. Edward Mineau and Franklin J. Miller, Jr.[8-1] (Univ. of Utah Med. Center) used angiographic arterial embolization in a woman, aged 22, with severe postpartum hemorrhage in whom three separate surgical procedures failed to reveal the source of bleeding, and standard surgical techniques, including bilateral ligation of the hypogastric arteries, did not produce hemostasis.

Fig 8–1.—Some pertinent pelvic collateral vessels. *IM,* inferior mesenteric artery; *SH,* superior hemorrhoidal artery; *MH,* middle hemorrhoidal artery; *SH,* middle sacral artery; *LS,* lateral sacral artery; *O,* obturator artery; *IE,* inferior epigastric artery; *CF,* common femoral artery; *MFC,* middle femoral circumflex artery; *SF,* superficial femoral artery; *DF,* deep femoral artery; *LFC,* lateral femoral circumflex artery; *SCI,* superficial circumflex iliac artery; *DCI,* deep circumflex iliac artery; *SG,* superior gluteal artery; *IL,* iliolumbar artery; *X,* point of internal iliac artery ligation. (Courtesy of Brown, B. J. et al.: Obstet. Gynecol. 54:361–365, September 1979.)

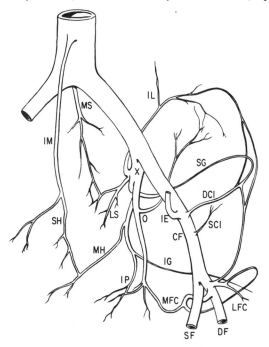

(8–1) Obstet. Gynecol. 54:361–365, September 1979.

TECHNIQUE.—An 18-gauge angiographic needle was placed in the right common femoral artery and then replaced with a no. 5 polyethylene catheter. With the use of fluoroscopy, the tip of the catheter was maneuvered over the aortic bifurcation, and angiograms of all pelvic vessels, including the hypogastric arteries distal to the ligature, were obtained. Selective injection of the left common iliac artery identified the site of bleeding as a vaginal branch of the left internal pudendal artery. The catheter was then advanced into the left middle femoral circumflex artery, which was supplying collateral flow into the internal pudendal system. A standard Gelfoam pad was cut into 2- to 3-mm fragments. About 30 to 35 of these were mixed with 5 ml of saline and 5 ml of contrast media and placed in a 10-ml syringe. Under fluoroscopy, small amounts of this material were repeatedly injected through the catheter into the collateral vessels. After this procedure, angiography showed occlusion of most of the collaterals and confirmed no further bleeding from this branch of the internal pudendal artery. The patient was discharged 8 days after embolization.

Hypogastric (internal iliac) artery ligation does not always control pelvic hemorrhage because extensive arterial anastomoses can provide efficient collateral circulation into the hypogastric system (Fig 8–1). Angiographic embolization should be considered prior to surgical intervention. This will permit direct catheterization of the hypogastric artery, identification of the hemorrhaging vessel, and specific vessel embolization. The 1 to 2 hours needed to obtain angiograms and perform embolization is less time than that often required for surgical control of bleeding. No significant complications of hypogastric embolization have been reported, probably due to the long course of the vessel and its easy accessibility.

▶ [Angiographic arterial embolization has again been shown to be effective therapy in intractable hemorrhage. Figure 8-1 demonstrates the extensive collateral circulation in the pelvis. Although we do not have firsthand experience with this technique, several recent reports have attested to its value.] ◀

Intramyometrial Prostaglandin $F_{2\alpha}$ ($PGF_{2\alpha}$) in Treatment of Severe Postpartum Hemorrhage. Tagaki et al. reported that intramyometrial prostaglandin $F_{2\alpha}$ therapy was effective in postpartum hemorrhage when other measures failed, but a subsequent report cast doubt on this finding. Mark M. Jacobs and Fernando Arias[8-2] (Washington Univ.) treated 3 patients who had severe postpartum hemorrhage due to uterine atony with intramyometrial injection of 1 mg of $PGF_{2\alpha}$, with excellent results. The agent was delivered transabdominally in all instances. Blood loss ceased within 1 to 2 minutes as strong uterine contractions took place. In 1 patient, clinical shock was rapidly reversed by $PGF_{2\alpha}$ administration. One patient had preeclampsia with abruptio placentae and defibrination, 1 had chronic hypertension and hypofibrinogenemia after cesarean section, and 1 had an apparently normal pregnancy.

Intramyometrial $PGF_{2\alpha}$ administration was a rapidly effective and safe treatment for severe postpartum bleeding in these patients. One patient had mild nausea and 1 had a moderate blood pressure elevation. More serious effects might result from inadvertent intravenous administration of the drug, but the extremely low dose used would

(8–2) Obstet. Gynecol. 55:665–666, May 1980.

probably endanger only the rare patient with uncontrolled asthma or severe hypertension. The procedure may be lifesaving when other treatments have failed. It may also be used in patients with moderate postpartum bleeding to avoid further blood loss and a need for blood replacement.

▶ [These 3 patients with acute and severe postpartum hemorrhage unresponsive to oxytocin, ergot agents, and uterine massage all responded promptly to intramyometrial $PGF_{2\alpha}$ injected transabdominally. Although 3 cases do not a therapeutic triumph make, the approach would surely seem to be reasonable prior to proceeding to operative management (internal iliac ligation or hysterectomy) or angiographic embolization.

Hertz and colleagues (Obstet. Gynecol. 56:129, 1980) reported a case of postpartum hemorrhage due to uterine atony that did not respond to usual ecbolic agents (oxytocin and ergot derivatives), but was corrected with vaginal PGE_2 suppositories.] ◀

Time-Related Peripartum Determinants of Postpartum Morbidity. Recent studies have focused on the identification of antepartum and intrapartum factors as determinants of postpartum infection. Among these factors are duration of labor, duration of ruptured membranes, number of vaginal examinations, length of time from the first vaginal examination to delivery, and duration of internal monitoring. Larry J. D'Angelo and Robert J. Sokol[8-3] (Case Western Reserve Univ.) prospectively studied these time-related factors as they relate to one another and to postpartum infectious morbidity.

Of the 101 patients evaluated, 70 delivered vaginally and 31 underwent cesarean section. Postpartum outcome was evaluated on the basis of fever index and diagnosis of endometritis or wound infection.

Of the 31 patients having cesarean section, wound infection or endometritis developed in 20 (65%). Endometritis developed in 2 patients having a vaginal delivery.

The results of this analysis indicate that, although several time-related events can be related individually to postpartum morbidity, when they are evaluated jointly by stepwise discriminant analysis, the only factor of significance is duration of labor. Although any of the time-related events may be associated with postpartum morbidity in isolation, these relationships may be mediated by their relationship in time to length of labor.

These findings may have important implications for patient management. Once the duration of labor was taken into account, other factors (length of internal monitoring, time from first vaginal examination to delivery, and number of vaginal examinations) were no longer significantly related to postpartum morbidity. Thus, it seems that intensive observation of high-risk patients during labor does not significantly contribute to the risk of postpartum morbidity and need not be avoided on this basis. Furthermore, labor duration might be a useful clinical consideration in selecting those cesarean section patients who would benefit from antibiotic prophylaxis.

▶ [Stepwise discriminant analysis of these data indicated that length of labor was the critical variable concerning postpartum infectious morbidity. The number of vaginal examinations and the duration of monitoring were related to infection, but only through their association with longer labors.] ◀

(8–3) Obstet. Gynecol. 55:319–323, March 1980.

Role of Anaerobic Bacteria in Postpartum Endomyometritis.
The exact role of anaerobes in female genital tract infections is unknown. Lawrence D. Platt, M. Lynn Yonekura, and William J. Ledger[8-4] (Univ. of Southern California) sought to clarify the role of anaerobes in postpartum endomyometritis. Twenty-five women with clinical evidence of this condition received metronidazole therapy. All were delivered vaginally and developed fever, uterine tenderness, and foul-smelling lochia after delivery, with no clinical evidence of infection elsewhere. Metronidazole was given by infusion over 1 hour in a dose of 13.6 mg/kg in bicarbonate-buffered aqueous dextrose solution, followed by 1.43 mg per hour. After fever was absent for 24 hours, metronidazole was given orally in a dosage of 250 mg every 6 hours to complete a treatment course of 10 days.

Sixty-seven anaerobic isolates were obtained from endometrial cultures in 24 women. Culdocentesis yielded similar findings. Paired transcervical endometrial and culdocentesis cultures were obtained from 23 patients, and 18 had at least one common anaerobic isolate. Twelve had two common isolates. Twenty-one patients were clinically cured by intravenous metronidazole therapy. Two failures were in patients who had organisms that were not susceptible to metronidazole. Another patient had difficulty with retained placental tissue.

Anaerobes have significance for patients with postpartum endomyometritis. Metronidazole provided a clinical cure in 84% of the patients in this study. The role of metronidazole in treatment of more serious pelvic infections is unclear. Needle culdocentesis is a convenient diagnostic procedure, but it does not indicate whether the organisms recovered represent the reality of the peritoneal cavity or contamination from the vagina. Prospective studies of direct and culde-sac sampling of the peritoneal cavity are needed in women undergoing elective postpartum tubal ligation.

▶ [This study provides new evidence that anaerobic organisms are involved in a substantial percentage of cases of puerperal endometritis. All patients tested had anaerobes isolated from endometrial cultures and 20 of 23 culdocentesis cultures were positive as well. From a clinical point of view, response was noted in 84% of patients treated with an agent known to have activity against anaerobic organisms but not against aerobic organisms. Metronidazole is not "approved" for this type of therapy, but perhaps it should be. In any event, it is probably important to use an agent with some antianaerobic activity as first choice. If there is no response, a specific agent (eg, clindamycin) should be added.] ◀

Prospective Evaluation of Combinations of Antimicrobial Agents for Endometritis After Cesarean Section. Cesarean section accounts for nearly 10% of births in many hospitals in the United States and is the chief risk factor for postpartum infection. P. Sen, J. Apuzzio, C. Reyelt, T. Kaminski, F. Levy, R. Kapila, J. Middleton, and D. Louria[8-5] (College of Medicine and Dentistry of New Jersey-New Jersey Med. School, Newark) evaluated the usefulness of cultures of amniotic fluid and the endocervix, taken through the internal os from the lower uterine segment, in determining risk factors for development of endometritis. Amniotic fluid or amniotic remnants

(8-4) Am. J. Obstet. Gynecol. 135:814–817, Nov. 15, 1979.
(8-5) Surg. Gynecol. Obstet. 151:89–92, July 1980.

were cultured after the infant was removed. No patient had infection at cesarean section, and none received antibiotics in the 2 weeks before operation. Patients who had diagnosed endometritis were treated with clindamycin in an intravenous dose of 600 mg every 6 hours until fever was absent for 48 hours, then with 150 mg orally every 6 hours to 10 days; or with 500 mg of cefazolin intravenously every 6 hours and then 1 gm of cephalexin orally every 6 hours to 10 days. Both groups also received gentamicin.

Clinical evidence of endometritis was present in 105 of the 236 patients studied. Seven had positive blood cultures. Endocervical cultures were positive in 52 infected and 61 uninfected patients. Amniotic fluid cultures were positive in 62 and 87 patients, respectively. The organisms recovered from the endocervix or amniotic fluid had no predictive value. Physician assessments of treatment outcome favored the clindamycin regimen. Among patients from whom both anaerobes and aerobes were recovered, all 6 given clindamycin and 3 of 7 given cefazolin did well.

The combination of clindamycin and gentamicin is quite effective in the treatment of endometritis that follows cesarean section. Cephalothin, cefazolin, and similar drugs should not be used for subdiaphragmatic infections, particularly if *Bacteroides fragilis* may be implicated. Such agents, however, may be useful for prophylaxis. A combination of clindamycin and an aminoglycoside is presently the regimen of choice for severe pelvic infections.

▶ [This article reemphasizes two points. First, cultures of the amniotic fluid or endocervix taken at the time of cesarean section do not reliably predict the development of endometritis. Second, if multiple-drug antibiotic therapy is used in treatment, at least one of the drugs should provide good anaerobic coverage.] ◀

Infections Following Classic Cesarean Section. The use of a classic cesarean section is traditionally thought to be associated with higher morbidity and mortality than when a low cervical transverse cesarean procedure is used. Jorge D. Blanco and Ronald S. Gibbs[8-6] (Univ. of Texas) compared the frequency and severity of infections occurring in patients following each of these surgical procedures from 1970 through 1977.

In all, 89 cesarean sections of each type were reviewed. The patients were matched for year of surgery, status of amniotic membranes, and status of labor. Morbidity was measured by standard morbidity criteria, source of infection, bacteremia, major complications, and length of hospital stay. Patients who received prophylactic antibiotics were not included.

The most common indications for classic cesarean section (group I) were transverse lie, previous classic cesarean section, and previous low cervical transverse cesarean section. The most common indications for low cervical transverse cesarean section (group II) were previous such procedures, breech presentation, and cephalopelvic disproportion.

Infection developed in 46 group I patients and 44 group II patients. There was no significant difference between the two groups with re-

(8–6) Obstet. Gynecol. 55:167–169, February 1980.

spect to site of infection. Types of infection included endometritis (34% in group I, 36% in group II), wound infection (6%, each group), urinary tract infection (9% in group I, 6% in group II), or pulmonary infection (3% in group I, 0% in group II).

In rates of standard morbidity, the two groups did approach a significant difference. In group I, 53% had standard morbidity, as compared to 39% of group II patients. However, some of the group I patients with standard morbidity did not have a specific diagnosis of infection or require treatment.

The data indicate that in the patients in this study, the incidence of operative site infection and of major infectious complications is comparable, regardless of type of cesarean section performed. However, none of the patients had prolonged rupture of membranes, nor were they infected at operation.

▶ [The results of this study suggest that the risk of infection after classic cesarean section may have been overestimated. Nonetheless, we are unconvinced because of our experience at the University of Iowa (J. Iowa Med. Soc. 69:52, 1979) where we see 2 or 3 patients each year referred because of very serious (and sometimes fatal) puerperal peritonitis because classic cesarean section was performed in the presence of actual or potential infection. In our practice, the use of the fundal uterine incision is exceedingly rare.] ◀

Control of Perinatal Infection by Traditional Preventive Measures. Leslie Iffy, Harold A. Kaminetzky, Jack E. Maidman, Janet Lindsey, and W. S. Michael Arrata[8-7] report a 9-year review of nosocomial infections that occurred at the University of Illinois Medical Center, Chicago, which serves mainly an indigent black population. More than 2,000 deliveries occur yearly in the obstetric division.

Strict asepsis and isolation have had dramatic effects on postoperative infection rates. Wound infection and endometritis have declined in frequency, as has the prevalence of gram-negative aerobes cultured from such infections, with rigidly enforced preventive measures and without the use of antibiotic prophylaxis. Adequate methods for accurately diagnosing anaerobic infection were not available at the time of the study.

All types of infection were substantially reduced by the introduction of strict preventive measures. Wound infections declined from a peak of 32% to an all-time low of 2%. Rates of obstetric and gynecologic infections were parallel throughout the survey period. The reduction in infection rates coincided with a decrease of about 25% in the perinatal mortality of infants who weighed more than 1,000 gm at birth. Other measures such as monitoring during labor and close antenatal follow-up were, however, instituted at the same time.

There is much evidence that physicians' education in infection control falls short of that of their predecessors and of current needs. It is apparent that, by implementing all traditional methods of asepsis, virtually all types of nosocomial infection can be controlled, and the increased prevalence of gram-negative infection observed in past decades can be reversed.

(8–7) Obstet. Gynecol. 54:403–411, October 1979.

▶ [As first pointed out by the writer of *Ecclesiastes,* there really is nothing new under the sun. This article documents the fluctuation of infection rates in response to a number of "old-fashioned" techniques of infection control such as isolation of infected patients, personnel policies to limit risk of cross-contamination, attention to principles of asepsis in examination and wound care, etc. Sixteen different factors, representing policies, procedures, or attitudes, were identified; it is impossible to even guess at their relative importance in reducing infection, but it seems clear that, in aggregate, they accounted for an impressive decline in infectious morbidity. Especially interesting is the parallelism in rates on obstetric and gynecologic services, lending further credence to the importance of these long-recognized, but frequently forgotten, principles.] ◀

Fatal Perineal Cellulitis from Episiotomy Site. Kirkwood K. Shy and David A. Eschenbach[8-8] (Univ. of Washington, Seattle) found that perineal cellulitis originating from an episiotomy incision resulted in 20% of the maternal mortality at affiliated hospitals in 1969 to 1977. Necrotizing fasciitis was present in 2 cases and clostridial myonecrosis in 1. Only 3 cases of episiotomy-related maternal mortality were found in a review of the recent literature; 2 of the deaths were caused by necrotizing fasciitis.

Woman, 23, a primigravida, was delivered of a 3,459-gm infant at 41 weeks' gestation by a midline episiotomy with caudal anesthesia. A 1-cm tear over the right ischial spine was repaired with gut sutures. Increased perineal pain was noted on the second postpartum day, and an area of induration was noted in the right labia majora and gluteal region. The episiotomy was opened on the third postpartum day. No hematoma or rectal mucosal involvement was noted. A drain was placed, and ampicillin was given intravenously. A clostridial species was isolated from a culture, and the patient deteriorated rapidly. Intravenous chloramphenicol and hyperbaric oxygen therapy were administered, but intravascular coagulation and hemolysis developed, followed by pneumothorax and hypotension. The patient died on the sixth postpartum day. Extensive cellulitis and myonecrosis typical of *Clostridia perfringens* infection were found both at the episiotomy site and in the posterior pelvic wall musculature.

Episiotomy infections have potentially severe and even fatal consequences. Severe extensive infections with systemic manifestations call for deep tissue culture, optimal antibiotic therapy, and excision of necrotic tissue. In superficial fascial infections, surgical exploration may be necessary to rule out necrosis. Infection may spread along fascial planes from the perineum to the anterior abdominal wall or onto the thigh and buttock. Exploration is indicated if edema or erythema extends beyond the immediate area of the episiotomy, severe systemic manifestations are present, or the infection does not resolve after 24 to 48 hours of antibiotic therapy. Myonecrosis is most commonly due to *C. perfringens* infection, but it can result from neglected necrotizing fasciitis that invades deep fascia.

▶ [These cases are similar to those described by Ewing et al. (Am. J. Obstet. Gynecol. 134:173, 1980). Tissue necrosis was more common in these patients than in those in the series of Ewing et al. Whether or not the problem is always infectious is unclear and, if it is, what the offending organisms are is unknown. Vascular volume depletion is common. Why have these severe episiotomy problems only recently come to our attention?] ◀

(8–8)   Obstet. Gynecol. 54:292–298, September 1979.

Vulvar Ectopic Breast Tissue Mimicking Periclitoral Abscess

is reported by Keith O. Reeves and Raymond H. Kaufman[8-9] (Baylor College of Medicine, Houston). A recent review of 18 cases of vulvar ectopic breast tissue in the English literature did not mention this complication.

Woman, 29, gravida 3 and para 3, reported a painful vulvar mass 2½ weeks after a normal delivery. The mass had begun to enlarge about the time of full milk production on postpartum day 5. An exquisitely tender, 3 × 4-cm solid mass was seen just to the left of the clitoris. Drainage yielded a milky fluid, and pain immediately resolved. The mass enlarged again in the next 48 hours as the patient continued to nurse her infant. An extremely tender mass was again present 8 days later, and the patient had a temperature of 38.3 C. The mass was excised without difficulty, and the patient became afebrile within 24 hours. Histologic study of the specimen showed ectopic breast tissue with lactational changes.

This rare lesion should be included in the differential diagnosis of painful vulvar lesions that appear to be abscesses, particularly in postpartum patients.

▶ [Ectopic breast tissue can occur in the vulva. Just as axillary ectopic breast tissue often enlarges with lactation, so too, as demonstrated by this patient, can its vulvar counterpart. This entity should be remembered when one evaluates a painful vulvar lesion in the early puerperium.] ◀

Acute Deep Vein Thrombosis (DVT) after Cesarean Section.

Pregnancy and certain gynecologic operations are considered to be risk situations for development of thromboembolic complications. A. Bergqvist, D. Bergqvist, and T. Hallböök[8-10] (Skövde, Sweden) determined the frequency of DVT after cesarean section in 169 consecutive patients, with the use of the noninvasive diagnostic method of strain gauge plethysmography. Ninety operations were done on an emergency basis. Ten emergency patients and 5 of those operated on electively received blood transfusions. General anesthesia was administered with thiomebumal sodium, suxamethonium chloride, pethidine, and diazepam. Epidural analgesia was with bupivacaine and mepivacaine, often supplemented with diazepam.

Three cases of postsectional DVT (1.8%) were observed. One patient had bilateral thrombosis. All 3 patients had had emergency operations. None received estrogens. Follow-up plethysmography done about 2 months later showed progression in 1 case and resolution of the changes in 2. A DVT developed in 1 patient during pregnancy, and the patient was given subcutaneous heparin from the 15th week. There was no evidence of progression after the cesarean section; the patient received dextran 70 during and after surgery. A biphasic venous emptying pattern was observed in 26 (33%) of 79 patients examined preoperatively, indicating obstruction of venous outflow by the pregnant uterus.

The low rate of postsectional DVT indicates that prophylaxis against thrombosis is not necessary. The use of elastic compression stockings with graded pressure is a practical method of prevention for these low-risk subjects.

(8–9) Am. J. Obstet. Gynecol. 137:509–511, June 15, 1980.
(8–10) Acta Obstet. Gynecol. Scand. 58:473–476, 1979.

► [Lower extremity deep vein thrombosis was diagnosed in 1.8% of patients screened after cesarean section. This figure is much lower than the 10–20% noted after gynecologic operations. Routine anticoagulation (with low-dose heparin, for example) does not appear to be indicated in patients undergoing cesarean section.] ◄

Relationship of Newborn Serum Prolactin Levels to Respiratory Distress Syndrome and Maternal Hypertension. Newborn infants with respiratory distress syndrome (RDS) have been found to have subnormal cord blood concentrations of prolactin. D. S. Grosso, C. P. MacDonald, J. E. Thomasson, and C. D. Christian[8-11] (Univ. of Arizona) examined the relation between RDS and prolactin concentrations in cord blood in a series of 782 newborn infants. Maternal blood was sampled in 233 cases. Median maternal age was 23.5 years, and median gestational age was 38 weeks. Cesarean section delivery was carried out in 22% of cases. Of the 66 infants with RDS, 44 were delivered vaginally. Preeclampsia was diagnosed in 109 patients, and 7 of these patients delivered infants who developed RDS.

Serum prolactin concentrations rose markedly with increasing gestational age. At 30 to 33 weeks' gestational age, prolactin values were significantly lower in infants with RDS. Serum prolactin concentrations were higher in infants of preeclamptic mothers than in those of normotensive mothers at gestational ages of 39 weeks or less, but not at 40 to 42 weeks. Serum prolactin values in RDS infants of preeclamptic mothers were at least as high as in non-RDS infants or normotensive mothers and approximated the values in the non-RDS, preeclamptic group.

Prolactin may be involved in promoting lung maturation, but it would be only one of a number of hormonal or other factors that influence pulmonary development. The cause of elevated prolactin concentrations in infants of preeclamptic mothers is unknown, but stress may be a factor, as may duration of labor. Further studies are needed to determine whether prolactin acts directly on the fetal lung through an effect on pulmonary metabolism or indirectly through interaction with other endocrine factors.

► [These findings are consistent with several recent reports suggesting that prolactin may be involved in lung development in the fetus. At 30 to 33 weeks' gestational age, lowered prolactin levels in cord blood correlated with risk of RDS, a relationship that did not apply at 34 weeks and beyond. Another finding of this study is the higher cord prolactin levels in preeclamptic as opposed to normal pregnancy, which offers a potential explanation of the generally lower incidence of RDS with gestational hypertension. Maturation of the fetal lung is a complex process and one probably subject to multiple influences; glucocorticoids have received the most attention, but there is reason to suspect that other hormones—prolactin, estrogen, and thyroid, to name but a few—are involved as well.] ◄

Mode of Delivery and the Lecithin-Sphingomyelin Ratio. The mortality from hyaline membrane disease is increased in infants born by elective cesarean section. P. Callen, Sheila Goldsworthy, Linda Graves, D. Harvey, Heather Mellows, and Christine Parkinson[8-12] (Queen Charlotte's Maternity Hosp., London) determined the amniotic fluid and pharyngeal L/S ratios in three groups of infants born at term: 20 delivered vaginally after elective induction of labor, 20

(8–11) Am. J. Obstet. Gynecol. 137:569–574, July 1, 1980.
(8–12) Br. J. Obstet. Gynaecol. 86:965–968, December 1979.

delivered by elective cesarean section, and 14 delivered by cesarean section after spontaneous onset of labor. Elective deliveries were done at 38 weeks' gestation or later. Amniotic fluid was sampled by intrauterine catheter or by needle aspiration at the time of section delivery.

No significant difference in amniotic fluid L/S ratios was found between the two elective delivery groups. Pharyngeal aspirate values were significantly higher in infants born after induction of labor than in the elective section group. Infants born by cesarean section after labor had begun had higher pharyngeal aspirate L/S ratios than both of the other groups, even excluding the 2 with respiratory distress syndrome (RDS). A higher proportion of non-RDS infants in the elective section group had pharyngeal aspirate L/S ratios below 2.5.

Some factor present in labor may stimulate release of lung surfactant from alveolar cells into the alveoli, making it detectable in pharyngeal fluid aspirated at birth. Surfactant release appears to be stimulated in the hours before birth. A significant relation was found in the present study of term infants between length of labor and increase in the L/S. ratio.

▶ [Whether cesarean delivery per se increases the likelihood of RDS is controversial, but a number of studies over the years have suggested a correlation. These findings that term infants born either vaginally or abdominally after labor had higher pharyngeal aspirate L/S ratios than those delivered by elective cesarean section suggest that labor or something associated with it (cortisol?) leads to increased surfactant synthesis and thus to some degree of protection against RDS. It may be of importance that the induction-vaginal delivery group (group A) mostly had conditions thought by some to lead to accelerated lung maturity (hypertension, intrauterine growth retardation, etc) and this characteristic, rather than the manner of delivery, might have been responsible for the results. This concern is minimized, however, by the similarity of amniotic fluid L/S ratios in the vaginal delivery and elective cesarean section groups and by the finding that the highest value of all occurred in the group with cesarean section after at least 4 hours of labor.] ◀

Accuracy of Prenatal and Postnatal Assessment of Gestational Age. A certain date of the last menstrual period in a woman with regular cycles is accepted as the most accurate estimate of gestational age. Measurement of the biparietal diameter by ultrasound is being increasingly used in routine antenatal care. Postnatally, physical and neurologic criteria or maturity are used to assess the gestational age of the newborn infant. Deborah Mitchell[8-13] (Guy's Hosp., London) used these methods to assess the gestational age at delivery of 20 neonates, and compared the results with gestational ages calculated from the date of the last menstrual period. The method of Dubowitz et al. was used to assess maturity after delivery. Singleton infants were evaluated within a few hours after birth. The coefficient of correlation for ultrasound biparietal diameter and last menstrual period estimates of gestational age was 0.884. The coefficient for the Dubowitz scoring system and last menstrual period estimates of gestational age was 0.413.

Biparietal diameter measurement correlated much more closely with the gestational age as estimated from the date of the last men-

(8–13) Arch. Dis. Child. 54:896–897, November 1979.

strual period than did the Dubowitz scoring method in this series. When accurate last menstrual period data are not available, ultrasound biparietal diameter measurement early in pregnancy is the most reliable means of assessing gestational age. This method is particularly suitable for sick neonates, who should be handled as little as possible.

▶ [There was a better correlation between gestational age determined by reliable last menstrual period data and second-trimester ultrasound than by the Dubowitz scoring system and last menstrual period. There certainly must be a biologic variation in maturity as determined by neonatal examination that is not exclusively dependent on the length of time spent in utero. It is of interest that the Dubowitz score suggested the same length of gestation as last menstrual period calculation in 1 case, longer gestation in 4 cases, and shorter gestation 15 times. This tendency for neonatal examination to "undercall" gestational age is consistent with our experience.] ◀

Birth Weight and Gestational Age in Children With Cerebral Palsy or Seizure Disorders. Jonas H. Ellenberg and Karin B. Nelson[8-14] (Natl. Inst. of Health) examined the relation of prenatal growth and duration of gestation to the risk of cerebral palsy (CP) and seizure disorders in a population having follow-up to age 7 years. The population consisted of about 54,000 children in the Collaborative Perinatal Project of the National Institute of Neurological and Communicative Disorders and Stroke, born at 12 urban teaching hospitals between 1959 and 1966. Whites and blacks each represented 46% of the group, with the rest chiefly Puerto Rican.

Both low birth weight and short gestation increased the risk of CP. Immature small infants were at higher risk of CP than infants small for dates at term. The latter had a significantly increased risk only of spastic diplegia. Spastic diplegia was present in 30% of children with CP. Most children with CP were of normal birth weight and term gestational age. Afebrile seizures among children without CP were more frequent in infants weighing 1,500 to 2,500 gm and at 37 weeks' or more gestational age than in other groups, but the increase was not significant. Nearly 70% of children with seizure disorders but without CP were well grown.

Except where cerebral palsy and seizure disorders coexist, these conditions differ in their relation to birth weight and gestational age. Low birth weight and short gestation were important risk factors for CP in the population studied, but these characteristics were uncommon. Low birth weight, preterm birth, and smallness for dates at term were not significantly related to the risk of seizure disorders in children without CP.

▶ [Seizure disorders in the absence of cerebral palsy were not more common at age 7 years in low birth weight or premature infants in this study. The risk of cerebral palsy increased with both shorter gestation and lighter birth weight. The highest *rate* occurred in infants of very low birth weight (<1,500 gm), but these infants accounted for only 9% of the total number of cases of cerebral palsy. About two thirds of the children with cerebral palsy weighed more than 2,500 gm at birth.] ◀

Relation Between Apgar Score and Subsequent Developmental Functioning. C. Kreisler, S. Levin, A. Klutznik, M. Mintz, A.

(8–14)   Am. J. Dis. Child. 133:1044–1048, October 1979.

Aviram, and V. Insler[8-15] sought to relate differences in functioning in various developmental areas at ages 6 to 18 months to differences in newborn condition as reflected by the 5-minute Apgar score. A total of 252 randomly selected infants (140 boys) aged 6 to 18 months were evaluated medically, neurologically, and developmentally. Instrumental intervention had been necessary in 29% of deliveries.

No difference in developmental quotient was found between infants with low Apgar scores (LAS) of 1 to 6 and those with high Apgar scores (HAS) of 7 to 10, but LAS infants aged 12 to 18 months consistently showed better performance than those aged 5 to 8 months. No such tendency was seen in the HAS group. Of the 29 LAS infants, 42% were delivered by vacuum extraction. Apgar scores were low in half of these deliveries and in 3% of spontaneous deliveries. No influence of forceps delivery alone was apparent. Fetal distress had occurred in 59% of LAS infants and 15% of the HAS group. Only 34% of infants with fetal distress, however, had LAS. No significant relation was found between fetal distress and subsequent developmental functioning.

Apgar scores, on the whole, are an inaccurate means of evaluation. They are influenced by habits and attitudes of obstetric personnel and by various environmental factors. The Apgar score was of no prognostic value with respect to future development in this study. Many adverse perinatal influences can be overcome or compensated for by proper medical and family care and through the process of maturation.

▶ [The prognostic significance of the Apgar score is a complex issue. Data from the Collaborative Perinatal Project indicated a significant correlation, albeit a relatively weak one, between low 5-minute Apgar scores and various impairments in development. In the study presented by Kreisler et al., however, no relationship with developmental quotients at age 6 to 18 months was found. Perhaps the number of subjects was too small or the measurement not sufficiently discriminatory. In any event, there does not seem to be a strong correlation, and this should be kept in mind when counseling parents of depressed infants.] ◀

Neonatal Asphyxia.—*I. Relationship of obstetric and neonatal complications to neonatal mortality in 38,405 consecutive deliveries.*— Asphyxia contributes greatly to neonatal and perinatal mortality. Hugh M. MacDonald, John C. Mulligan, Alexander C. Allen, and Paul M. Taylor[8-16] (Univ. of Pittsburgh) assessed those perinatal risk factors that might be reliable predictors of neonatal asphyxia in a series of 38,405 consecutive live births that occurred between 1970 and 1975. A total of 447 infants had neonatal asphyxia, for an overall rate of 1.16%. The incidence was indirectly related to gestational age and to birth weight. Asphyxia occurred in 9% of preterm infants and in 0.5% of infants at over 36 weeks' gestational age.

Among term infants, neonatal asphyxia was significantly more frequent in ward patients, blacks, infants of unmarried mothers, and infants of diabetic and toxemic mothers. Among preterm infants, these factors were not associated with a higher rate of asphyxia. In both groups, breech delivery and growth retardation were associated

(8–15) Int. J. Gynaecol. Obstet. 17:620–623, May–June 1980.
(8–16) J. Pediatr. 96:898–902, May 1980.

with an increased incidence of asphyxia. Maternal age per se was unrelated to an increased risk of asphyxia. Cesarean section by itself was not an apparent causative factor. Neonatal survival declined with decreasing gestational age and birth weight and with neonatal asphyxia in all birth weight and gestational age categories. The only obstetric factor associated with significantly higher mortality among asphyxiated infants was socioeconomic status. Neonatal mortality was greater among private than among ward infants. Among neonatal factors, growth retardation, hyaline membrane disease, hypothermia, and neonatal seizures were associated with greater mortality, but hypoglycemia, hyperkalemia, and hypocalcemia were not.

Degree of prematurity was by far the most important predictor of mortality among infants asphyxiated at birth in this series. Efforts to provide optimal obstetric care to women whose pregnancies have reached 36 weeks and whose gestations are identified as being at high risk should significantly reduce both the incidence of asphyxia and neonatal mortality.

II. Neontal mortality and long-term sequelae.—Mulligan, Michael J. Painter, Patricia A. O'Donoghue, MacDonald, Allen, and Taylor[8-17] determined the incidence and extent of developmental abnormalities among survivors of neonatal asphyxia, defined as a delay of over 1 minute in onset of spontaneous respiration at birth. Asphyxia occurred in 1% of 13,221 live-born infants weighing over 500 gm at birth in 1970 and 1971. Of the 133 asphyxiated infants, 75 (56%) survived the neonatal period. Survival was directly related to gestational age. Sixty-five survivors were available for assessment at a mean age of 4.8 years.

Twelve survivors (18.5%) had major sequelae. Nine had both neurologic and intellectual impairment. Five children were seriously impaired and will probably never function independently. One child with severe spastic quadriplegia and hydrocephalus died at age 18 months. Six children had mild abnormalities at follow-up. The overall median Stanford Binet score was 108; 15% of children were intellectually impaired. The outcome could not be related to prenatal complications associated with acute or prolonged stress. Severe sequelae were not associated with fetal malnutrition, hypothermia, or hypoglycemia. Postasphyxia seizures were related to poor outcome. Although survival was related to gestational age, both the incidence and the severity of impairments were similar in mature and premature infants.

The most common neurologic abnormalities among survivors of neonatal asphyxia in this series were spastic diplegia and choreoathetosis. Postasphyxia seizures were associated with a high incidence of severe sequelae. Control or, preferably, prevention of seizures appears to be important in management of postasphyxia infants.

▶ [These two articles concerning neonatal asphyxia describe associated obstetric factors and predictive factors concerning survival and subsequent neurologic sequelae. Not surprisingly, the prevalence of asphyxia was inversely correlated with gestational age at delivery. Prematurity was the most important predictor of mortality in as-

(8–17)   J. Pediatr. 96:903–907, May 1980.

phyxiated neonates as well. When survivors only (56% of the asphyxiated infants) are viewed at a mean age of 4 years 10 months, 18.5% had major neurologic-intellectual sequelae. The presence or absence of sequelae was unrelated to birth weight, gestational age, or a variety of neonatal complications. Neonatal seizures, however, did correlate with poor outcome.

These two articles do not support the contention made by some that perinatal asphyxia is an all-or-nothing phenomenon, ie, that the outcome is either death or intact survival. The uncertainty of prognosis in an individual patient is illustrated by the fact that 12 of the 65 children evaluated had an IQ⩾130.] ◄

Pathogenesis of Neonatal Hyperbilirubinemia After Induction of Labor With Oxytocin. The association between oxytocin-induced labor and neonatal hyperbilirubinemia has been attributed to hepatic glucuronyltransferase immaturity, anoxic liver damage, enhanced placentofetal transfusion, increased red blood cell fragility, and mechanical damage to red blood cells. Peter C. Buchan[8-18] (St. James's Univ. Hosp., Leeds, England) found that fetal erythrocytes are less deformable after oxytocin-induced labor than after spontaneous labor, and he investigated the effect of oxytocin on red blood cell deformability in vivo and in vitro. Studies were done on 95 healthy neonates, 40 delivered after spontaneous labor and 40 after induction by amniotomy and intravenous oxytocin administration. The other 15 infants were delivered by elective cesarean section. The average dose of oxytocin was 4,500 mU. Labor lasted 6 to 14 hours in the study group. Analgesia was achieved with intramuscular meperidine injection.

The hematologic and biochemical findings are presented in the table. No significant differences were found between the spontaneous delivery and and the section groups, but infants born after oxytocin-induced labor had decreased packed cell volumes and plasma haptoglobin concentrations and increased plasma bilirubin and lactate dehydrogenase values. A significant reduction in the red blood cell deformability index was also observed. Plasma osmolality was reduced in this group. In vitro studies showed a time- and dose-related effect of oxytocin on red blood cell deformability.

Red blood cell destruction is increased during oxytocin-induced labor. Decreased deformability of red blood cells leads to accelerated hemolysis. The total dose of oxytocin used for induction should be kept to a minimum. The use of phenobarbital or antipyrine ante partum to activate fetal hepatic glucuronyltransferase and increase the ability of the neonate to eliminate bilirubin has been suggested, but it would be more logical to prevent hyperbilirubinemia by reducing the dose of oxytocin than to treat it with potentially toxic drugs.

► [Several reports in recent years have considered the association between neonatal hyperbilirubinemia and oxytocin-induced labor. The issue of the induction vs the oxytocin as the causative factor has not been completely resolved. This study is consistent with the view that oxytocin is the culprit. Presumably oxytocin results in swelling of the fetal erythrocytes, with a subsequent decrease in deformability and increased hemolysis. If this is the case, one would expect hyperbilirubinemia with oxytocin-*stimulated* labors as well, and there are studies that suggest this is not so (1978 YEAR BOOK, p. 201). Perhaps this discrepancy relates to differences in dosage or in length of administration of the oxytocin. It would be of interest to measure erythrocyte deformability

(8–18) Br. Med. J. 2:1255–1257, Nov. 17, 1979.

MEAN (±SE) HEMATOLOGIC AND BIOCHEMICAL VALUES* IN CORD BLOOD FROM INFANTS DELIVERED BY ELECTIVE CESAREAN SECTION AND AFTER SPONTANEOUS AND OXYTOCIN-INDUCED LABORS (NUMBERS OF INFANTS GIVEN IN PARENTHESES)

Cord blood	Elective caesarean section	Spontaneous labour	Oxytocin-induced labour	P value† (oxytocin-induced v spontaneous labour)
Packed cell volume	0·52 ± 0·012 (15)	0·53 ± 0·013 (40)	0·47 ± 0·014 (40)	<0·001
Erythrocyte deformability index (ml/min)	0·83 ± 0·03 (15)	0·81 ± 0·04 (40)	0·61 ± 0·06 (40)	<0·001
Plasma bilirubin concentration (µmol/l)	31 ± 1·2 (15)	33 ± 1·3 (40)	38 ± 1·5 (40)	<0·001
Plasma haptoglobin concentration (g/l)		0·091 ± 0·024 (25)	0·023 ± 0·006 (25)	<0·01
Plasma lactate dehydrogenase activity (IU/l)		223 ± 8 (25)	346 ± 25 (25)	<0·001
Plasma osmolality (mmol/kg)	286 ± 4 (15)	290 ± 6 (40)	277 ± 6 (40)	<0·001

*Conversion of SI to traditional units: packed cell volume, 1.0 = 100%; plasma bilirubin, 1 µM/L ≈ 0.06 mg/100 ml; plasma osmolality, 1 mM/kg = 1 mOsm/kg.
†Derived with Student's t test.

in cord blood after labors induced by amniotomy and by prostaglandins and after labors of spontaneous onset that were stimulated with oxytocin.] ◄

Diagnostic and Prognostic Value of Retinal Hemorrhages in the Neonate. The incidence of retinal hemorrhage in newborns is estimated to be between 2.6% and 50%. However, the etiology of retinal hemorrhage and its relationship to the course and management of labor are disputed. S. Levin, J. Janive, M. Mintz, C. Kreisler, M. Romem, A. Klutznik, M. Feingold, and V. Insler[8-19] examined whether the course of pregnancy and management of delivery affected the incidence of retinal hemorrhage and whether the incidence of such hemorrhages could be reduced by fetal monitoring. The infants had physical and psychologic examinations at 6 to 18 months of age to assess the prognostic value of retinal hemorrhage.

Within 24 hours of delivery, 410 infants were examined. In addition to the ocular examination, a general examination was carried out with particular emphasis on neurologic status.

The incidence of retinal hemorrhage was 37.3%; 123 neonates were affected bilaterally. There was no correlation between incidence of retinal hemorrhage and maternal age, parity, maternal diabetes, sex of the newborn, birth weight, mean Apgar score at 5 minutes, presence of cord complications, gestational age, use of electronic monitoring during labor, use of oxytocin for induction of stimulation of labor, type of anesthesia or analgesia, or the occurrence of fetal distress.

Although the difference was not statistically significant, retinal hemorrhage was more common among infants born in the occiput posterior position as compared to those born in the occiput anterior position.

There was a correlation between length of the first stage of labor and incidence of retinal hemorrhage. Of 28 infants born to mothers in whom the first stage of labor was under 1 hour, only 1 had retinal hemorrhage, whereas 42.2% of the infants born to mothers whose first stage of labor lasted from 1 to 11 hours had retinal hemorrhage.

The incidence of retinal hemorrhage was higher in infants having both meconium-stained amniotic fluid and late decelerations, compared to the nondistressed group.

The mode of delivery also influenced the incidence of retinal hemorrhage. Neonates delivered by cesarean section had significantly lower incidences of retinal hemorrhage than those delivered vaginally. The use of forceps seemed to lower the incidence of retinal hemorrhage, compared to normal or vacuum extraction deliveries, although the differences were not significant.

Assessment of the infants at 6 to 18 months of age showed no correlation between the occurrence of neonatal retinal hemorrhage and the child's later development.

These data suggest that examination of the ocular fundi of the newborn for retinal hemorrhage is of limited diagnostic and prognostic value.

▶ [Retinal hemorrhages were more common after vaginal delivery (39%) than after

(8–19) Obstet. Gynecol. 55:309–314, March 1980.

cesarean section (12%). Apart from this finding, retinal hemorrhages did not relate to antepartum or intrapartum complications, Apgar scores, or developmental tests at 18 months of age. Newborn retinal hemorrhages are common and apparently without diagnostic or prognostic importance.] ◄

Iatrogenic Hazards of Neonatal Intensive Care in Extremely Low Birth Weight Infants. There has been excessive enthusiasm in neonatal pediatrics in the introduction and use of innovations in management that are accompanied by unforeseen hazards. V. Y. H. Yu, P. H. Hewson, and E. Hollingsworth[8-20] (Melbourne) reviewed present practices in the intensive care of 55 infants weighing less than 1,000 gm at birth, who were cared for in 1977 and 1978. Mean birth weight was 830 gm, and mean gestational age was 26 weeks. Overall neonatal survival was 60%; it was 67% for infants weighing over 750 gm and 44% for the lighter infants. Umbilical artery catheters were inserted for various purposes. If base was required, a slow infusion of bicarbonate at 2.8% or less was given over 2 to 3 hours. Fresh breast milk was fed where possible. Parenteral nutrition was used before establishment of enteric feeding.

All infants but 2 received oxygen therapy, and 81% had a Pa_{O_2} above 100 mm Hg at some time. Retrolental fibroplasia was diagnosed in 1 surviving infant. All infants but 1 received alkali therapy. Intraventricular hemorrhage occurred in 8 of 14 infants with hypernatremia and in 8 others. Morbidity from umbilical artery catheterization was 29%, but none of the complications contributed to mortality in this series. Late cholestatic jaundice developed in 2 infants, both of whom had periods on no oral feeds lasting longer than 10 days. Forty-two infants received phototherapy, and 9 of them required exchange transfusion. Fifty infants received antibiotics during the nursery stay. Eight infants had over 30 x-rays. Three of 4 infants with postnatally acquired cytomegalovirus infection were probably infected by transfused blood.

Current nutritional management can lead to hyperglycemia, hypocalcemia, and hyponatremia. Iatrogenic factors may contribute to the occurrence of necrotizing enterocolitis, patent ductus arteriosus, and cholestatic jaundice. Present neonatal intensive care practices require ongoing scrutiny, and great caution is indicated in introduction of new procedures. Concern has been raised regarding the excessive noise level of incubators and also separation of the infant requiring high-technology support from the family and its effect on parent-infant bonding.

► [Modern neonatal intensive care has led to a remarkable improvement in prognosis for the infant with very low birth weight. In this report, survival was 67% in infants weighing 751–1,000 gm and 44% in those weighing 501–750 gm, figures undreamed of a few short years ago but currently standard for first-class neonatal intensive care units. Yet, few blessings are unmixed. The main message is that the techniques of neonatal intensive care may cause complications themselves. This certainly does not mean that such things as oxygen therapy, umbilical catheterization, and blood sampling should be abandoned, but there is a need, as the authors point out, for continuing scrutiny of care practices and caution about introduction of "new advances."] ◄

(8–20) Aust. Paediatr. J. 15:233–237, December 1979.

Effects of Early Mother-Infant Contact Following Cesarean Birth. The exact limits of the "maternal sensitive period" during which maternal-infant contact is necessary for bonding to begin have not been clearly defined, but it appears to be the first 12 hours after birth. Muriel S. McClellan and William A. Cabianca[8-21] examined the effects of early mother-infant contact on the perceptions, attitudes, and behavior of 40 mothers who delivered infants by cesarean section in 1978 and 1979. They were multiparas who had repeat cesarean sections with spinal anesthesia and delivered healthy infants. Some mothers held their infants in the recovery room, alternating between skin-to-skin contact and visual contact with the infant in a nearby warmer. Controls had only brief contact with their infants in the first 12 hours after birth.

Group differences in maternal perceptions of the infants and maternal behavior were significant. Early-contact mothers appeared to have significantly more positive perceptions of their infants on the first or second postpartum day, but perceptions of the infants at age 1 month did not differ significantly. Early-contact mothers exhibited more caretaking behavior both in the postpartum period and when the infant was aged 1 month.

The findings support the concept of a maternal sensitive period for attachment to the child. Mothers undergoing cesarean section delivery seem to be affected in this period similarly to mothers who deliver vaginally. Hospitals should adopt procedures that encourage mother-infant contact after cesarean section delivery.

▶ [The concept of the importance of early mother-infant contact in the bonding process has gradually gained acceptance, and many hospitals now permit and even encourage it. However, we suspect that in most instances the practice is limited to normal vaginal birth. With cesarean delivery, most obstetricians probably feel that the mother must be whisked away to the recovery room and most pediatricians want to whisk the infant to the neonatal intensive care unit, in both cases for prolonged and careful observation because of their respective high-risk status. This report describes a study of repeat cesarean section in which patients were randomly assigned to early (and fairly extensive) contact or brief (less than 5 minutes) contact. Those who had early contact exhibited significant differences in various aspects of "mothering," effects similar to those previously noted with vaginal birth. Of course, in many cesarean sections the clinical circumstances will not permit attention to such matters. For example, the woman sectioned for hemorrhage from placenta previa or abruption is likely to need intensive intraoperative and postoperative care and the infant delivered by emergency cesarean section for fetal distress will likely require resuscitation and immediate care. However, where possible, we should provide the same opportunities for maternal-infant contact for cesarean section patients as we do for those who deliver normally.] ◀

Hats for the Newborn Infant. The mortality of newborn infants is markedly reduced if they are kept warm. The brain of the newborn infant is a major heat-producing organ. Strothers and Warner found that a close-fitting woolen hat lined with Gamgee (Vernaid gauze and cotton tissue) provides measurable thermal protection in a cool environment, as opposed to a stockinette hat. D. M. Chaput de Saintonge, K. W. Cross, M. K. S. Hathorn, Sheila R. Lewis, and J. K. Stothers[8-22] (London) studied the effects of heat insulation in a prospective con-

(8–21) Obstet. Gynecol. 56:52–55, July 1980.
(8–22) Br. Med. J. 2:570–571, Sept. 8, 1979.

trolled trial of hats in 211 infants, 107 of them exposed to overhead radiant heaters. Only 30 of these infants had been normally delivered. In the infants not subjected to radiant heat, body weight, initial rectal temperature, hat application, the environmental temperature, and the duration of exposure while naked influenced the rate of fall in rectal temperature in the first 30 minutes.

Gamgee-lined hats should be routinely used to minimize heat loss, especially in small infants exposed at birth, during operations, and during investigations necessitating prolonged exposure. The hat could, however, be dangerous if left on when an infant is placed in an incubator that is providing a thermoneutral environment.

▶ [In neonates not exposed to a radiant heater, a woolen hat helped maintain body temperature. Although radiant heaters are the rule in delivery rooms, this sort of adjunct may be of value in the "birthing room." Although one could argue which is more "natural," a bonnet has the advantage of being more familiar.] ◀

Of Human Bonding: Newborns Prefer Their Mothers' Voices. Human responsiveness to sound reaches sophisticated levels by birth, but the role of maternal voice discrimination in formation of the mother-infant bond has been unclear. Anthony J. DeCasper and William P. Fifer[8-23] (Univ. of North Carolina, Greensboro) found that an infant under age 3 days can discriminate his or her mother's voice and will work to produce her voice in preference to that of another female. Studies were done in 10 neonates, 5 of each sex. Tape recordings were made of the voices of the mothers reading a story, and infant responses were estimated from recorded activity in sucking on a nonnutritive nipple. Each infant could produce either its mother's voice or the voice of another woman by sucking on the nipple.

Infants learned how to produce their mothers' voices and did so more often than they produced control voices. A sucking burst terminating an interburst interval equal to or greater than the baseline median produced only the mother's voice. An increase in the proportion of interburst intervals capable of producing the mother's voice was observed. The findings were confirmed when the experiment was repeated in 16 female neonates, using a different discrimination procedure involving 4-second tones of 400 Hz.

Newborn infants have auditory competence adequate for discriminating individual speakers. Their general sensory competence may permit other maternal cues, such as odor and manner of handling the infant, to serve as supporting bases for discrimination and focal preference. Prenatal auditory experience may also be a factor. The perceptual preferences and proximity-seeking responses of some infrahuman infants are profoundly affected by auditory experience before birth. The present findings suggest that the period shortly after birth may be important in initiation of infant bonding to the mother.

▶ [This fascinating study presents evidence that infants within the first 3 days of life recognize, as reflected in suckling behavior, their own mother's voice. Moreover, they seem to prefer, and actually work to produce, the voice of their mothers over that of another woman. The title of the article is a catchy play on another title: *Of Human Bondage,* by Somerset Maugham (who was, incidently, a physician).] ◀

(8–23) Science 208:1174–1176, June 6, 1980.

Prolactin Secretion during Prolonged Lactation Amenorrhea.
Lactation amenorrhea is a widespread phenomenon among mammals,
but the physiologic processes by which lactation inhibits reproductive
activity in women are poorly defined. B. A. Gross and C. J. East-
man[8-24] measured the serum prolactin level in both lactating amenorrheic and menstruating women, as well as in women who had
weaned their infants. In addition, the prolactin response to suckling
was examined during prolonged lactation amenorrhea. Basal studies
were done on 4 lactating mothers with return of menses and on 6 who
had weaned their infants and resumed regular cycles. Suckling studies were done at 5–66 weeks post partum in 18 lactating mothers.
Four were evaluated after 1 menstrual period and the rest during
prolonged lactation amenorrhea.

Basal serum prolactin levels 5–9 weeks post partum were significantly higher than at 14–26 weeks. Mean prolactin levels in amenorrheic lactating women were significantly higher than prolactin levels in menstruating, lactating women (33.8 vs 20.2 µg/L). The latter
group had higher levels than women who had weaned and resumed
menstruation. Women who were fully breast-feeding had higher prolactin levels than those who were partially breast-feeding their infants. Suckling evoked a rise in serum prolactin in most amenorrheic
and menstruating women, but responses were variable. Responses in
amenorrheic women were significant up to 26 weeks post partum, but
not thereafter. The peak level, and time of the peak in relation to
suckling, varied considerably among individuals.

Prolactin secretion is increased in women with prolonged lactation
amenorrhea, although the marked variability of individual suckling
responses may obscure the importance of prolactin secretion in the
postpartum period. Daily measurements may be necessary to evaluate the role of prolactin in lactation amenorrhea.

▶ [The importance of prolactin in the initiation of lactation and its maintenance during
the first 2 or 3 months of breast-feeding has been demonstrated clearly, but prolactin's
role during prolonged lactation is questionable. This study found evaluated hormonal
function in patients who continued nursing for more than a year. Basal levels and
response to suckling, while falling off after a few months, remained elevated throughout. Moreover, among those with prolonged lactation, prolactin secretion was higher
in amenorrheic than in menstruating subjects, suggesting that prolactin is involved in
lactation amenorrhea. The influence of diet on prolactin levels in lactating women is
examined in the following article.] ◀

**Influence of Maternal Diet on Plasma Prolactin Levels Dur-
ing Lactation.** Plasma prolactin levels remain high throughout lactation in developing countries, but soon return to nonpregnant values
in most western societies. Child feeding patterns are not likely to
fully explain this difference. P. G. Lunn, A. M. Prentice, S. Austin,
and R. G. Whitehead[8-25] attempted to learn whether plasma prolactin
levels during lactation respond to changes in the maternal diet.
Thirty women in England and 119 in Gambia were evaluated.
Plasma prolactin was measured by radioimmunoassay.

In most women in England, prolactin levels fell to nearly normal

(8–24) Aust. N.Z. J. Obstet. Gynaecol. 19:95–99, May 1979.
(8–25) Lancet 1:623–625, Mar. 22, 1980.

by 12 weeks after parturition. In Gambia the levels increased during this period, followed by a gradual decline; however, mean values still remained above nonpregnant levels after 18 months of breast-feeding. At 12 weeks, the mean prolactin levels of Gambian women were 5–6 times higher than in women in England, despite similar milk output in the two groups. Prolactin levels continued to rise longer during the wet season in Gambia, when food intake generally is lower, than in dry periods. Dietary supplementation for 4–8 weeks in the last part of the dry season further reduced plasma prolactin levels at all stages of breast-feeding. Studies in Zaire indicated that menstruation did not return until the plasma prolactin fell below 860 μU/ml and that such levels were reached earlier after parturition in women given supplements.

Prolonged high prolactin levels in undernourished mothers may ensure milk synthesis when the food intake is limited, by preferentially channeling nutrients toward the breasts. The lower levels associated with improved maternal nutrition may shorten the period of postpartum infertility despite prolonged breast-feeding. The contraceptive effect of prolactin may protect against new pregnancies where food is less readily available, and any nutritional program designed to improve the lot of lactating mothers and their infants should consider the possible need for some artificial form of birth control.

▶ [These interesting observations suggest an effect of maternal nutritional status on plasma prolactin levels during lactation. Presumably well-nourished English women had lower prolactin levels than did presumably poorly nourished Gambian women. Moreover, levels in Gambian mothers were lower during seasons of better diet than during those of poorer diet. Teleologically, perhaps the woman of poor nutritional status "needs" more prolactin in order to support milk production in the face of nutritional adequacy. Moreover, relative hyperprolactinemia during lactation might explain a more marked contraceptive effect of breast-feeding in developing countries than among industrialized societies. However, one overriding question remains: What could possibly be the mechanism?

A related study by Canto and colleagues (Int. J. Gynaecol. Obstet. 17:437, 1980) found similar results. The levels of FSH, LH, and prolactin were measured during lactation in urban and rural Mexican women. Only prolactin differed—levels averaged 38.1 ng/ml in rural subjects and 20.4 ng/ml in urban women.] ◀

Nutritional Composition of Milk Produced by Mothers Delivering Preterm. The use of human milk for feeding preterm infants has received increasing attention in recent years because it is highly digestible, has a unique protein composition, and offers immunologic protection against infection. It may not, however, provide adequate amounts of protein and minerals for rapidly growing preterm infants. Steven J. Gross, Richard J. David (Duke Univ.), Linda Bauman, and R. M. Tomarelli[8-26] (Wyeth Labs., Radnor, Pa.) compared the nutritional composition of milk produced by mothers delivering at 28 to 36 weeks' gestation with that of milk produced by mothers delivering at term. Milk was sampled 3, 7, 14, 21, and 28 days post partum from 18 mothers with term infants and 33 with preterm infants.

Lactose concentrations were significantly lower in preterm than in term milk in the first month of lactation. No significant differences in

(8–26) J. Pediatr. 96:641–644, April 1980.

fat concentrations were observed. Protein concentrations were significantly higher in preterm milk throughout the first month of lactation. Protein concentrations decreased with progressing lactation in both groups. Caloric concentrations were similar in the two types of milk. Sodium and chloride concentrations were significantly higher in preterm than in term milk. Concentrations of potassium, calcium, phosphorus and magnesium were comparable in preterm and term milk samples.

The cause of differences in composition of milk from the two groups of mothers is unclear. Although the differences may be of little biologic or clinical importance, slower growth has been noted in preterm infants fed pooled mature human milk than in those fed a cow's milk formula. Milk produced by the mother of the preterm infant in the first postpartum month, with higher protein, sodium and chloride concentrations, may be a more appropriate nutrient for the preterm infant than pooled mature breast milk.

▶ [This study found a higher density of some nutrients, specifically protein, sodium, and chloride, along with a lower concentration of lactose, in lactating mothers delivering prior to term compared with those giving birth at term. Contents of energy and other nutrients did not differ significantly. There is currently great interest in feeding human milk to premature infants because of its apparent anti-infectious properties.These results would suggest that the best choice is milk from the infant's own mother for nutritional as well as for immunologic reasons. It is somewhat unfortunate that the study design involved manual expression of milk from women delivering prematurely whereas the term mothers nursed their babies, so it is not altogether certain whether the differences reflect gestational duration at delivery or collection technique.

Generally similar results were reported by Scanler and Oh (J. Pediatrics 96:679, 1980), who compared composition of milk from mothers of premature infants with pooled donor milk. The former had significantly higher levels of nitrogen and calcium, although the differences tended to disappear after 2 weeks of lactation.] ◀

Effects of Vitamin C, Vitamin B₆, and Vitamin B₁₂ Supplementation on Breast Milk and Maternal Status of Well-Nourished Women.

Effects of Vitamin C, Vitamin B_6, and Vitamin B_{12} Supplementation on Breast Milk and Maternal Status of Well-Nourished Women. Changes in maternal diet can influence the nutrient level of breast milk, especially with regard to the water-soluble vitamins. M. Rita Thomas, Joanne Kawamoto, Sharon M. Sneed, and Randi Eakin[8-27] (Univ. of Utah) evaluated the effects of vitamin supplements and diet on the vitamin C, B_6, and B_{12} content of breast milk and maternal blood levels in 17 women at 1 and at 6 weeks post partum.

Diets in 10 women were supplemented with Natalins, a multivitamin and multimineral preparation; 7 received no supplementation. Dietary records were kept for 4 days at 1 and 6 weeks. Milk samples were collected from 5 to 7 days and from 43 to 45 days post partum.

The mean dietary intake of vitamin B_6 was less than 60% of the recommended daily allowance for lactating women. At 43 to 45 days post partum, the nonsupplemented women consumed 34% of the recommended daily allowance and the supplemented group ingested 44%. Milk concentration of vitamin B_6 was significantly lower in the nonsupplemented group at 5 to 7 days post partum than in the sup-

(8–27) Am. J. Clin. Nutr. 32:1679–1685, August 1979.

plemented group at that interval post partum. The concentration of pyroxidine in the milk of the nonsupplemented group increased significantly by 43 to 45 days post partum, so that the difference between the two groups was no longer significant.

All women in both groups consumed more than the recommended daily allowance of vitamin C. The unsupplemented group ingested twice the recommended daily allowance and the supplemented group three times the recommended amount. The plasma vitamin C level in women not receiving supplements was significantly lower than in the supplemented group at 7 days, but not at 6 weeks, post partum.

Dietary intake of vitamin B_{12} in the nonsupplemented women was 71% of the recommended daily allowance at 1 week post partum and 53% at 6 weeks. All serum values of vitamin B_{12} were normal in all women. Milk levels of vitamin B_{12} were not significantly different between the two groups at 5 to 7 days post partum. By 6 weeks the levels of vitamin B_{12} had decreased in both groups. The nonsupplemented group had a significantly lower level of vitamin B_{12} in the milk at 6 weeks as compared to the 1 week postpartum level; the level was also significantly lower than that of the supplemented group at 6 weeks.

It appears that for healthy, well-nourished women with a history of short-term oral contraceptive use, concentrations of vitamins B_6, B_{12}, and C in milk and maternal status can be maintained by diet alone. None of the milk values or maternal blood levels measured was less than published norms for vitamins C, B_6, and B_{12}.

▶ [Levels of water-soluble vitamins in milk generally correlate with maternal blood levels, which in turn reflect maternal intake. Thus, it is possible to increase milk content by maternal supplementation. This study of vitamins C, B_6, and B_{12} notes a modest (and, in the case of vitamins B_6 and B_{12}, a statistically significant) elevation in milk levels in supplemented over nonsupplemented patients. However, all of the values determined in this population of presumably middle-class Texas mothers were within accepted norms, so it is unclear whether there is any benefit from maternal supplements during lactation. We regard vitamin supplements as unnecessary—but a reasonable option—for the breast-feeding mother whose diet is adequate.] ◀

Resurgence of Nutritional Rickets Associated with Breast-Feeding and Special Dietary Practices. "Nutritional rickets" is a disease caused by inadequate exposure to sunlight. Dietary vitamin D is essential only when there is inadequate exposure of the skin to ultraviolet irradiation, resulting in decreased calcium absorption, hypocalcemia, hyperparathyroidism and skeletal changes. Deborah V. Edidin, Lynne L. Levitsky, William Schey, Nives Dumbovic, and Alfonso Campos[8-28] (Chicago) encountered 10 cases of nutritional rickets in a 10-month period. Several recent reports of nutritional rickets in breast-fed infants have appeared. The American Academy of Pediatrics statement of 1977, addressing changing nutritional trends and high-risk dietary patterns, makes no clear statement about vitamin supplementation of the breast-fed infant.

These cases are associated with low calciferol intake due to unsupplemented breast-feeding, dietary manipulation, or fad diets. Expo-

(8–28) Pediatrics 65:232–235, February 1980.

sure to sunlight is minimal because of protective clothing or unsafe neighborhood conditions, prohibiting outdoor activities. Many of the authors' patients had rickets when receiving only unsupplemented breast milk. Special diets may be used because of poverty, religious beliefs, or misguidance. Oral calciferol in a daily dose of 5,000–10,000 IU reversed the biochemical, radiologic and clinical features of rickets.

The authors do not wish to discourage breast-feeding, but pediatricians should review their patients' nutritional status and, if a child is being breast-fed or is on a restricted or unusual diet, questions should be asked about supplementation of the child's diet as well as the diet of siblings. A history of lack of immunizations should alert the physician to review the dietary practices in effect. Many families may be amenable to counseling and revision of such practices.

▶ [This collection of 10 cases (and an eleventh as an addendum after the paper was submitted) of rickets in breast-fed infants seen during a 10-month period at Michael Reese Hospital, Chicago, is especially pertinent in view of current infant feeding practices. Many pediatricians feel that the breast-fed infant should receive supplemental vitamin D unless there is ample exposure to sunlight. Several years ago, Lakdawala and Widdowson (1978 YEAR BOOK, p. 211) described a water-soluble form of vitamin D present in substantial quantities in human milk, but its biologic activity was not defined. This article suggests that its antirachitic properties are minimal.] ◀

Lack of Protective Effect of Breast-Feeding in Congenital Hypothyroidism: Report of 12 Cases. It has been postulated that breast-feeding decreases or delays the clinical effects of hypothyroidism in infants with primary hypothyroidism. Jacques Letarte, Harvey Guyda, Jean H. Dussault, and Jacqueline Glorieux[8-29] compared 12 breast-fed and 33 bottle-fed hypothyroid infants, seen since 1974, with respect to clinical, biochemical, radiologic, and psychologic status. Anthropometric parameters at referral and biochemical values, including plasma thyroxine, triiodothyronine, and thyroid-stimulating hormone concentrations, did not differ significantly. Bone maturation was identical in the two groups of infants, and the groups had similar psychologic performances at age 1 year. No differences were observed on the Griffiths developmental test.

Breast-feeding appears not to protect against the deleterious effects of congenital hypothyroidism or to prevent its appearance. Other explanations must be sought for infants said to have developed clinical and biochemical features of congenital hypothyroidism when breast-feeding was discontinued.

▶ [It has been claimed that human milk contains sufficient thyroid hormone to protect against hypothyroidism but this study indicates otherwise. There were no differences between breast- and bottle-fed hypothyroid infants in clinical, biochemical, radiologic, or psychologic status. With the increasing use of routine screening, congenital hypothyroidism, which occurs in approximately 1 in 5,000 births, will be recognized more frequently. Based on this study, infants so identified will require thyroid supplementation regardless of the method of feeding.] ◀

Propylthiouracil in Human Milk: Revision of a Dogma. Treatment of lactating women with antithyroid drugs is considered to be contraindicated because of a potential antithyroid effect on the suck-

(8–29) Pediatrics 65:703–705, April 1980.

ling infant, but withdrawal of antithyroid therapy after delivery is often inconvenient. Jens P. Kampmann, Klaus Johansen, Jens Mølholm Hansen, and Jeppe Helweg[8-30] examined the excretion of the antithyroid drug propylthiouracil (PTU) in human milk. Concentrations in nine euthyroid healthy lactating women, aged 21 to 34 years, were evaluated 1 to 8 months after delivery. Two women were given PTU for Graves' disease. The PTU concentration was determined in serum and milk every 30 minutes for 4 hours after oral administration of 400 mg of PTU. An infant whose mother received 200 to 300 mg of PTU daily was studied for 5 months.

The mean serum PTU concentration reached 7.7 μg/ml at 90 minutes and fell to 3.9 μg/ml 4 hours after drug administration. The mean concentration in milk reached 0.7 μg/ml at 90 minutes and fell to 0.5 μg/ml at 4 hours. The mean total PTU excreted in milk in 4 hours was 99 μg, or 0.025% of the ingested dose. No changes in serum thyroxine, TSH, or triiodothyronine-resin uptake were noted in the infant of the PTU-reated mother.

It is concluded that lactating mothers on PTU therapy should continue nursing, if they wish, with close supervision of the infant.

▶ [The standard teaching has been that women receiving PTU should not breast-feed their infants. This study suggests that the standard teaching is overly cautious. The levels of PTU in breast milk were only about 10% of the maximum maternal serum levels, and the calculated daily dosage received by a nursing baby is very small (the equivalent of 3 mg/day to a 70-kg adult). It therefore seems reasonable to permit a patient taking PTU to nurse her baby if she wants to. Periodic evaluation of the infant's thyroid status would offer reassurance to both the mother and the physician.] ◀

Relactation: Study of 366 Cases. Mothers separated from their infants by premature birth or illness may later wish to initiate or resume breast-feeding when milk production has decreased or ceased. Kathleen G. Auerbach and Jimmie Lynne Avery[8-31] (Univ. of Nebraska, Omaha) evaluated methods of preparation and the factors affecting the infant's response in the relactation situation among women with a median age of 26 at the time of relactation. Relactation followed untimely weaning in 174 cases, birth of a low weight infant in 117, and hospitalization of the mother, infant, or both because of illness or injury in 75. The chief reasons for the decision to relactate were benefit to the infant, opportunity to nurture through breast-feeding, and the mother-infant relation.

Most mothers increased their fluid intake in preparation for relactation, and nearly half also increased the amount of dietary protein taken. Half the subjects used an oxytocin nasal spray to enhance the milk ejection reflex. Infant suckling and breast massage with nipple-rolling exercises were the chief means of nipple stimulation. The infant's willingness to suck at the breast decreased as extrauterine age increased, but willingness improved over time in each relactation situation. Most women in all groups supplemented their own milk supplies for some period. The Lact-Aid Nursing Supplementer and a nursing bottle were frequently used for this purpose. Nursing pat-

(8–30) Lancet 1:736–738, Apr. 5, 1980.
(8–31) Pediatrics 65:236–242, February 1980.

terns were quite similar to normal nonscheduled breast-feeding. Nearly half the infants were weaned in the second half of the first year of life.

Relactation may be viewed as one way to enhance the mother-infant relation. It may not, however, always be a sure means of providing a complete milk supply to the infant. Three fourths of mothers in this series evaluated their relactation experience positively. Most stressed the importance of nursing to the mother-infant relation; milk production was less often a goal.

▶ [This article describes the results of a questionnaire survey of 366 women who relactated—ie, who instituted or reinstituted breast-feeding after a lapse of at least one week. The reasons for relactation cited as most important were strengthening of the maternal-infant relationship and nutritional and emotional benefits to the baby, whereas physical benefits to the mother were regarded as of least importance. To quote directly from the discussion section: "The majority of respondents repeatedly emphasized that breast-feeding is as much nurturing *at* the breast as it is nutrition *from* the breast."] ◀

PART TWO

PRIMARY CARE AND PUBLIC HEALTH

9. Primary Care and Public Health

Smoking and Health: Role of the Obstetrician and Gynecologist is discussed by Robert M. Kretzschmar[9-1] (Univ. of Iowa). Obstetrician-gynecologists are primary-care physicians for many women. As such, they have the responsibility to provide comprehensive care and to inform the patient so that she can make enlightened decisions regarding her health. The opportunity also exists for obstetrician-gynecologists to influence women's health care behavior, including their attitudes toward smoking.

Cigarette smoking has been associated with cancer of various organs, coronary artery disease, chronic bronchitis, and emphysema. However, smoking is an addictive behavior that is difficult to stop.

Although the number of adult male smokers is decreasing, the number of women who smoke has increased, so that women and men are now smoking at about the same rate. The amount of tobacco smoked by young women has also increased dramatically.

Deaths from lung cancer are rising sharply among women. In 1979 it was estimated that more women would die from lung cancer than from gynecologic cancers. If smoking trends in women remain the same over the next 30 years, there could be over 100,000 deaths among the female population from lung cancer.

Obstetrician-gynecologists have been instrumental in public education about other health-related topics such as uterine cancer, but have made few efforts to educate patients about lung cancer. Over 70% of women under age 35 deny being informed by their physicians about the hazards of smoking.

It has been estimated that 50% of pregnant women smoke. The association of lower birth weight infants born to smoking mothers is well known, but the long-term effects of low birth weight are unclear and require further investigation. Other obstetric complications (eg, pregnancy wastage) may also be linked to smoking.

The health hazards of smoking and taking oral contraceptives, especially in later childbearing years, should also be stressed. Women over 40 years of age who use the pill should not smoke and vice versa.

Health professionals must participate actively in an antismoking education effort on several fronts. Approaches can include self-education, education of other health professionals, patient education, and community involvement.

▶ [Kretzschmar has made a timely and thoroughly appropriate statement. Whatever the government calls us, obstetrician-gynecologists are primary-care physicians to women. Improving health in the United States is more a matter of altering behavioral choices than of achieving technologic breakthroughs. Cigarette smoking is a perfect example. Kretzschmar suggests that lung cancer will soon displace breast cancer as

(9–1) Obstet. Gynecol. 55:403–406, April 1980.

the leading cancer killer of women. It is important for us to encourage our patients to quit the weed. It has been suggested that women are more willing to stop smoking during pregnancy "for the baby" than they are in the nonpregnant state. We should take advantage of this willingness.] ◄

Effects of a Swimming Training Regimen on Hematologic, Cardiorespiratory, and Body Composition Changes in Young Females. Although trained female swimmers have physical and physiologic features distinguishing them from nonathletes, little is known of the specific effects of swim training on young females. Alfred W. Stransky, Ronald J. Mickelson, Corey Van Fleet, and Ronald Davis[9-2] (Rochester, Mich.) attempted to isolate the effects of a swimming conditioning program on females participating on a high school competitive swim team. Thirty students were studied, including 16 competitors and 14 controls, with respective mean ages of 15.8 and 15.9 years. The training regimen averaged 12,806 yards per week for 7 weeks, in an average of 4 sessions a week.

Lean body weight (LBW) was significantly greater in competitors than in controls, but differences in body weight and percent body fat (BF) were not significant (table). Maximal breathing capacity was greater in the trained group. Increases in mean corpuscular volume and hemoglobin values were significant at the 5% level in the trained group. Maximal oxygen uptake and maximal ventilation on exercise were significantly increased in the competitors. Maximal heart rate for the experimental group and all maximal values for the control group were unchanged.

Lean body weight was the only significant body composition variable affected by swim conditioning in this study. A swimming program designed for women can produce physical and physiologic changes distinguishing trainees from nonswimmers. The contribution

PRE-POST COMPARISONS FOR BODY COMPOSITION MEASUREMENT
FOR EXPERIMENTAL AND CONTROL GROUPS

Variables	Pre mean	Pre SD	Post mean	Post SD	Pre-post mean diff.	SE diff.	t
Experimental Group N=16							
A. Weight (kg)	59.4	9.2	58.6	8.4	—.8	1.6	1.70
B. % BF	21.9	3.8	19.8	3.3	—2.1	1.5	2.11
C. LBW (kg)	46.0	5.2	46.7	5.3	.7	1.0	2.91†
Control Group N=15							
A. Weight (kg)	57.9	6.2	58.6	6.6	1.9	.7	1.26
B. % BF	21.7	3.2	21.4	3.1	—.4	1.4	.94
C. LBW (kg)	45.2	4.4	45.9	4.5	.7	1.6	1.52

*Significant at 5% level of confidence.
†Significant at 1% level of confidence.

(9–2) J. Sports Med. Phys. Fitness 19:347–354, December 1979.

of training can be better defined through studying world-class swimmers undergoing intense training.

▶ [This article and the following one relate to the phenomenal interest in women's athletics. In this article, an intensive swimming training program produced changes in body composition and hematologic and cardiorespiratory function. Particularly noteworthy are the body composition effects noted in the table—decrease in body fat and increase in lean body weight. The former was not statistically significant, perhaps due to the indirect (ie, measurement of skin-fold thickness) method of estimation.

Decrease in body fat that accompanies intensive physical training is thought to account for the high incidence of menstrual irregularity observed in females who engage in active sports and other forms of exertion, such as ballet dancing. In this regard, Webb and associates (J. Sports Med. 19:405, 1979) surveyed female athletes (participants in basketball, gymnastics, track and field, swimming, and rowing) who competed at the Montreal Olympic games. Most (59%) reported menstrual changes, most commonly oligomenorrhea, amenorrhea, hypomenorrhea, or decreased length of menses, during their competitive seasons. Additionally, menarche did not occur until after age 17 in 43%.] ◀

Women's Injuries in Collegiate Sports: Preliminary Comparative Overview of Three Seasons. Kenneth S. Clarke (Univ. of Illinois, Urbana-Champaign) and William E. Buckley[9-3] (Pennsylvania State Univ.) reviewed injuries to collegiate women athletes reported to the National Athletic Injury-Illness Reporting System in its first 3 years of operation between 1975 and 1978. The high injury rate in women athletes could not be attributed to inferior health supervision. Dissimilarities in injury patterns were more numerous between various women's sports than between comparable men's and women's sports. Women's athletic injuries appeared to be essentially sport related, rather than sex related. Differences were observed between men and women participating in the same sports with respect to sites of injury and nature of injuries at various sites.

Further reports on women athletes' injuries should be delimited to respective sports. Attention should be given to patterns of injury within a given sport and shifts in patterns, so that practical preventive measures may be devised, implemented, and subsequently evaluated. Current injury patterns that may be associated with inadequate preparation for training and competition may be shifting to patterns associated more with the intensity of competition. Periodic multiple-variable studies are needed to demonstrate any changes in the influence of interacting factors on patterns of athletic injuries.

▶ [This analysis of athletic injuries indicates a general similarity in type and incidence of injuries sustained by women and men in comparable sports. The only very striking differences seems to be in injuries to the lower extremity in sports characterized by running and jumping; average annual rates per 100 cases in men and women, respectively, were 5.4 vs 19.0 in gymnastics, 7.2 vs 11.1 in track and field, and 14.3 vs 16.2 in basketball.] ◀

Female Dyspareunia. Most women who are sexually active experience coital discomfort at some time. John A. Lamont[9-4] (McMaster Univ.) reviewed 230 patients with dyspareunia seen from January 1972 to June 1978. Dyspareunia was defined as encompassing all coital pain occurring in females.

Each patient was assessed for intrapersonal (intrapsychic), inter-

(9–3) Am. J. Sports Med. 8:187–191, May–June 1980.
(9–4) Am. J. Obstet. Gynecol. 136:282–285, Feb. 1, 1980.

personal (relationship), and physical factors that might play an etiologic role in the problem. Dyspareunia was the chief complaint in 74.8% of the patients; other major complaints included dysmenorrhea, premenstrual tension symptoms, pelvic and abdominal pain, fertility control or infertility, menstrual irregularity, depression, and tension headaches.

The evaluation of each patient included menstrual, obstetric, and contraceptive history. The patient profile included questions about family and religious influences, sexual knowledge, history of sexual trauma, sense of body image, and sexual experience and attitudes. If the patient was involved in a relationship, the level of her communication skills and presence of support systems were assessed. General physical and pelvic examinations were done, with efforts made to involve the patient.

The goal was to identify the primary underlying cause of pain, although the etiology often encompassed more than one category. The treatment strategy was aimed at alleviating the dyspareunia. Physical causes were treated with the appropriate medical or surgical techniques. When indicated, individual or conjoint marital and sexual therapy was offered.

Most patients were in their 20s and were married. The duration of symptoms was less than 2 years for most, but 9 had experienced ongoing or recurrent symptoms for over 10 years. Of the 230 patients, 81 had never experienced comfortable coitus. Vaginismus was observed in over 50% of all patients during the pelvic examination.

The primary source of the problem was believed to be intrapersonal in 43%, interpersonal in 27%, and physical in 30% of the patients. Intrapersonal problems, identified in 100 women, included fear of sex-related activity, of pain, and of intimacy; trauma; ignorance of physiology, of sexual experience, and of partner; anxiety and guilt; and belief in the concept of sex for reproduction only.

Interpersonal problems, when relationship conflicts seemed directly related to the presenting symptoms, were identified in 62 patients. These conflicts involved areas such as family size and planning, relationship priorities, and sexual practices or preferences.

Physical abnormalities were identified as the primary source of discomfort in 68 patients and as a contributing but secondary factor in 22.

Treatment was successful in 69% of patients in the intrapersonal category, but 26% refused treatment. The corrected success rate was 93.2%. Of the 62 women with interpersonal problems 17 (27.4%) were successfully treated and 43 (69%) refused treatment. The success rate among those treated was 89.4%. Patients with physical problems had an 82.4% rate of successful treatment, with 9 patients refusing treatment, giving a corrected success rate of 94.9%.

▶ [This is an interesting description of one physician's extensive experience with the symptom of dyspareunia. Nearly one third of patients were felt to have a primary physical cause, and physical factors were regarded as secondary problems in 10% more. Not surprisingly, the best chance of successful treatment was in those cases with an organic basis. The worst prognosis was in women in whom the symptom was regarded as indicative of interpersonal difficulties with the sexual partner.] ◀

Female Orgasm: Role of Pubococcygeus Muscle. Orgasm remains a neurophysiologic event, but just what constitutes the efferent response has not been clearly defined in men or women. There also is confusion regarding afferent stimulation. Benjamin Graber and Georgia Kline-Graber[9-5] (Univ. of Nebraska, Omaha) attempted to determine whether there is any relationship between the physiologic state of the pubococcygeus muscle and the presence or absence of female orgasm. The findings in 291 women seen at a sexual therapy clinic in 1972–75 were reviewed. Of these, 153 were not orgasmic with either noncoital or coital stimulation, whereas 114 were orgasmic with noncoital stimulation only. Twenty-four women were orgasmic with both types of stimulation. All but 1 of the latter group had psychosexual pathology, presenting with marital, medical, or psychiatric problems. One was a nondysfunctional partner of a male with a sexual problem.

The pubococcygeus muscle was evaluated with a pressure-sensitive device inserted in the vagina. Women who achieved both coital and noncoital orgasm had significantly better muscle strength than those who achieved only noncoital orgasm. Both groups had better muscle strength than women who were unable to achieve orgasm by any means. No significant group differences were found for age, length of foreplay or intercourse, or age at onset of masturbation. Both coitally anorgasmic groups had intercourse more often than the coitally orgasmic group. The coitally and noncoitally orgasmic groups had the most pregnancies.

Encouraging women to use resistive exercises to improve the pubococcygeus muscle facilitated the achievement of coital orgasm by coitally anorgasmic women and also permitted women already coitally orgasmic to achieve coital orgasm more easily and frequently. This major circumvaginal muscle may be impaired physiologically in women who are unable to achieve orgasm.

▶ [Pubococcygeal muscle function differed between orgasmic and anorgasmic women with sexual dysfunction in this study. If these findings are confirmed, a logical next step would be to assess the value of Kegel's exercises in the therapy of anorgasmic sexual dysfunction in those women with decreased pubococcygeal strength.] ◀

A Prospective Psychologic Study of 50 Female Face-Lift Patients. Many plastic surgeons believe that postoperative depressions are more frequent after face-lifts than after other esthetic procedures. Marcia Kraft Goin, R. W. Burgoyne, John M. Goin, and Fred R. Staples[9-6] (Univ. of Southern California, Los Angeles) evaluated the psychologic status of 50 female face-lift patients before and after surgery with semistructured psychiatric interviews and psychologic tests. The Minnesota Multiphasic Personality Inventory (MMPI) and the Beck Depression Scale were used, as well as the Fundamental Interpersonal Relationship Orientation-Behavior scale. All patients but 1 were treated in the office operating room after being given local anesthesia. Major complications totaled only 6%.

Most patients were pleased with the physical outcome of surgery. The MMPI results indicated that this was a relatively normal group.

(9–5) J. Clin. Psychiatry 40:348–351, August 1979.
(9–6) Plast. Reconstr. Surg. 65:436–442, April 1980.

Seven patients (14%) were thought to have some evidence of clinical depression preoperatively. Postoperatively, 27 patients (54%) exhibited clinical evidence of psychologic disturbance. Eight continued to be depressed for several weeks, and 7 first became depressed 2 to 3 weeks postoperatively and depressed for several weeks. These patients were more likely than the others to have shown preexisting depression or have a high depression-scale score on the MMPI. Patients with delayed depression had higher scores on the psychasthenia and social introversion scales of the MMPI. These were the only patients whose depression was in any way related to disappointment with the results of surgery. Many patients, especially those who wished an improved self-image, improved psychologically after surgery. Disturbance was less likely for those who wished to retain a job or advance in their careers.

Depressive reactions are frequent in postoperative face-lift patients. Preoperative depression does not necessarily contraindicate the procedure. A desire to improve self-image or to advance in a career is a reasonably reliable predictor of psychologic improvement after face-lift surgery.

▶ [Over half of these women undergoing face-lift operations experienced some type of depressive reaction postoperatively, and in half of these the depression lasted for several weeks. Not surprisingly, the likelihood of depression correlated with depression-proneness detectable on preoperative interview or psychologic testing. On the other hand, a substantial percentage of patients were improved psychologically after the operation (ie, 28% felt increased self-esteem).] ◀

Hepatitis After Transfusion of Frozen Red Cells and Washed Red Cells. The consensus of reports on posttransfusion hepatitis is that the use of frozen or washed red blood cells virtually eliminates the problem. R. K. Haugen[9-7] (Holy Cross Hosp., Fort Lauderdale, Fla.) has not, however, had such a favorable experience with the use of these cells. A high-glycerol, mechanical-freeze system is used to process red blood cells collected in citrate-phosphate-dextrose solution. A total of 31,125 units of blood and blood products were transfused over 52 months, an average of 4 units to each recipient; 56 cases of hepatitis occurred. In 37, the recipient had received only frozen and/or washed red blood cells. Posttransfusion hepatitis was of the non-A, non-B type in 95%. Commercial blood accounted for 30% of the donor base in the first 4 years and was involved in 44 cases of hepatitis. Elimination of commercial blood from the donor base led to a fall in the incidence of hepatitis from 2.1 to 0.3 per 1,000 transfusions (table).

These findings support the view that a safe donor base is the best available protection against transmission of infectious disease by blood. The findings of Alter et al. in chimpanzees indicate that the use of frozen red blood cells will not prevent transfusion-induced hepatitis. The present observations do not support the use of either frozen or washed red blood cells for the prevention of posttransfusion hepatitis caused by hepatitis B virus or hepatitis of the non-A, non-B type.

▶ [A few years ago, the suggestion was made that frozen or washed packed red blood

(9–7) N. Engl. J. Med. 301:393–395, Aug. 23, 1979.

TRANSFUSION-INDUCED HEPATITIS IN RELATION TO USE OF FROZEN RED CELLS, WASHED RED CELLS, AND COMMERCIAL BLOOD

YEAR	TOTAL TRANSFUSIONS*	FROZEN RED CELLS %	WASHED RED CELLS %	FROZEN & WASHED RED CELLS %	COMMERCIAL BLOOD %	HEPATITIS CASES	INCIDENCE PER 1000 TRANSFUSIONS
1975	6536	14	28	42	32	10	1.5
1976	6784	45	37	82	38	14	2.0
1977	6634	44	46	90	38	14	2.1
1978	8055	19	70	89	17†	17	2.1
1979 (1st 4 mo)	3116	15	78	93	0	1	0.3
Total	31,125						

*Includes 1,295 units of fresh-frozen plasma and 1,316 of platelet concentrate.
†No commercial blood purchased after Aug. 1, 1978.

cells were not associated with posttransfusion hepatitis. Not so, according to this study. The source of blood (commercial vs volunteer donor) is again demonstrated to be an extremely important factor. It is not surprising that in this era of screening donors for hepatitis B surface antigen, most cases of hepatitis were of the non-A, non-B variety.] ◄

Consolidation of Hospital Obstetric Services: Is It a Reality?
Warren H. Pearse[9-8] (American College of Obstetricians and Gynecologists, Chicago) reports the findings of a survey of hospitals with maternity services in the United States, carried out in the course of overall manpower planning studies to examine the widespread belief that the number of hospitals with maternity services has declined. Data obtained in an American Hospital Association survey of hospitals for 1973 to 1977 were analyzed.

Despite efforts at regional planning of maternity services and consolidation of small hospital units, the number of United States hospitals with maternity services has increased each year since 1973. Only two states show a significant reduction in hospitals performing fewer than 500 deliveries annually. The average number of annual deliveries per hospital is 728, and no state has achieved an average as high as the 1,500 called for in national guidelines for health planning.

The impact of attempts to consolidate obstetric services has been minimal or nonexistent in most states to date.

▶ [Although consolidation of obstetric services in the United States has been recommended as a means of improving care and lowering costs, the suggestion is a controversial and politically sensitive one. Thus far, not much has happened.] ◄

(9–8) Obstet. Gynecol. 54:330–332, September 1979.

PART THREE

GYNECOLOGY

10. Operative Gynecology

URINARY INCONTINENCE

Douglas J. Marchant, M.D.

Professor of Obstetrics and Gynecology, and Director,
The Cancer Center of Tufts-New England Medical Center, Boston

Introduction

The diagnosis and treatment of urinary incontinence remain controversial. Postgraduate courses dealing with this subject appear at almost every national meeting of gynecologists and urologists. Many free-standing courses are offered in the United States and abroad, and a new national society, the Gynecologic Urology Society, held its first meeting in the fall of 1980.

A number of sophisticated diagnostic techniques are available and have produced an entirely new vocabulary, eg, inappropriate detrusor activity, functional urethral length, urethral pressure profile, etc. In contrast, previous reviews have emphasized operative technique, including the more than 100 operations that have been recommended for the cure of urinary incontinence.

This continuing and occasionally intense interest in urinary incontinence is difficult to explain. Perhaps it is due to our frustration in attempting to understand the physiology of micturition and, as a result, the inability to diagnose correctly and treat disorders of urination, including anatomical stress incontinence.

Urinary incontinence can be classified as (1) anatomical stress incontinence, (2) urgency incontinence (sensory or motor), (3) inappropriate detrusor contractions, or incontinence caused by loss of tissue integrity (vesicovaginal or ureterovaginal fistula). Disorders of micturition are difficult to diagnose; however, the surgical technique involved is relatively simple. Total incontinence due to loss of tissue integrity is relatively easy to diagnose but surgically difficult to correct. Taken together, they require a thorough understanding of female urology and exceptional surgical skill. Neither disorder occurs often in the daily practice of urology or obstetrics and gynecology. Medical malpractice claims continue to request large compensations for complications of treatment, including damage to the bladder and ureter. In this presentation, I shall attempt to put these issues into perspective and make recommendations based on an understanding of the pathophysiology involved.

History

The term "stress incontinence" was first used by Sir Eardley Holland. A survey of the literature indicates that recommendations for treatment were suggested as early as 1864.[1] Medical management consisted of a variety of physical maneuvers, including a foot bath of cold water and cold hypogastric douches followed by aromatic baths and vaginal douches. Schatz suggested injections of sterile water into the spinal theca and the epidural space. The first surgical procedure, although it was not directed to the anterior vaginal wall or urethra, was suggested by Neveu in 1880. He recommended ligating the prepuce of the clitoris and painting the external meatus of the urethra with collodion.[1] Perhaps he had observed the involuntary loss of urine with orgasm? Beginning in the 1900s, a number of operations were recommended, including excision of various portions of the vaginal wall and even rotation of the urethra. In 1901, Kelly described his now-famous plication of the vesical neck.[1] During the next 80 years, various operations were introduced, some utilizing the vaginal approach alone or combined with hysterectomy and others employing a sling either of fascia or artificial material; later, a retropubic approach, first described by Marshall, Marchetti, and Krantz,[1] was also used. To date, well over 100 different surgical procedures have been recommended to control involuntary loss of urine, attesting to the ineffectiveness of any one.

Anatomy and Physiology of Continence

An acceptable theory of micturition has yet to be devised. There is increasing interest in the role of the sympathetic nervous system, and a number of newer techniques have been advocated to evaluate detrusor and urethral function. It is clear that disorders of urination, except those related to loss of tissue integrity, cannot be considered solely in anatomical terms. Recommendations concerning the analysis of stress and urgency incontinence and, in particular, inappropriate detrusor activity must be considered in light of our present lack of knowledge of the precise function of this complex elastrohydrodynamic system. Because we do not have an acceptable theory of the physiology of micturition, recommendations for treatment must be based on incomplete understanding of the problem—no doubt the reason for the number of different surgical approaches to the problem and the wide variation in reported successful results.

Whereas the anatomy of continence and the description of the function of the base of the bladder and female urethra are subject to revision, a few general statements can be made. Because the urinary bladder and urethra arise from common mesenchymal tissues, the muscular layers of the bladder and urethra are identical. The outer and inner layers are continued along the urethra, the inner layer becoming the longitudinal layer and the outer layer forming a somewhat circular arrangement of smooth muscle surrounding the entire urethra. It has been suggested that this "circular" arrangement may be responsible for the resting pressure or closure pressure in the urethra, closure pressure being the difference between the simultaneously measured bladder pressure and the maximal urethral pressure. These concepts will be described in greater detail in the following sections. It has been suggested that alterations in the circular arrangement of these muscles provide a more oblique path that results in a lower resting pressure and eventually involuntary loss of urine. There is little argument that in the continent woman the bladder and urethra respond to increases in intra-abdominal pressure. The portion of the urethra *below* the urogenital diaphragm is not affected by changes in intra-abdominal pressure. Therefore, for the patient to be continent, the upper urethra or bladder neck must be positioned to respond to these increases in intra-abdominal pressure. If the bladder neck descends to the level of the urogenital diaphragm, and is not affected by changes in intra-abdominal pressure, incontinence results. In addition to the location of the bladder neck, there is considerable controversy concerning the importance of the so-called posterior urethrovesical angle, that is, the angle at which the base of the bladder joins the urethra. Loss of the posterior urethrovesical angle results in funneling of the bladder base, the anatomical prerequisite for the first stage of voiding. The continent patient therefore must have a bladder neck located in a position that responds to increasing intra-abdominal pressure, a posterior angle that prevents funneling and the first stage of voiding, and a circular arrangement of the smooth muscle surrounding the urethra that provides sufficient closure pressure.

When we move from the area of anatomy to that of physiology or pharmacology, we are faced with a variety of conflicting theories. The bladder not only expels urine under voluntary control, it also stores urine. These two paradoxical functions are coordinated by a nervous system that must act as a biologic computer. Unfortunately, as Turner-Warwick has succinctly put it, "Our present knowledge and understanding of the central and peripheral pathways and the mechanisms of neuromuscular control leave nearly everything to be desired."[2] It is clear that passive collection and active expulsion of urine are under voluntary control. Histochemical studies have revealed adrenergic nerve endings concentrated in the bladder base and proximal urethra.[3] The exact role of these receptors is poorly understood despite a voluminous literature on the subject. Perhaps this is due to the complexity of the interactions of the catecholamines.[4] The initial reaction of catecholamines is influenced by a number of conditions. They must reach the target cells, interact with membrane-bound receptors, and trigger biochemical changes within the cells. A number of events can influence these reactions. There may be changes in catecholamine availability at the receptor sites, in receptor function, and in cellular events themselves. All of these affect the biologic response. To complicate matters, it now appears that epinephrine and norepinephrine are cleared through mechanisms that are modulated by β-adrenergic receptors but not α-adrenergic receptors.[4] It is not clear, however, whether catecholamines are cleared through β-adrenergic receptors themselves, or whether they are cleared through systems regulated by β-adrenergic receptors.[4] A sustained decrease in catecholamine release is associated with an increased number of adrenergic receptors in the target cells and an increased response to catecholamines. Conversely, a sustained increase in catecholamines is associated with decrease in the number of receptors and in responsiveness.[4]

It has been shown that prostaglandins are released during nervous stimulation of the bladder and may cause increased detrusor activity. Studies on the effect of norepinephrine and isoproterenol on in vitro detrusor muscle contractility and cyclic AMP content provide evidence that cyclic AMP and enzymatic pathways related to cyclic nucleotide metabolism are present in dog detrusor muscle. Further studies involving manipulation of the cyclic nucleotide system may provide an explanation of clinical detrusor dysfunction.[5]

The use of bromocriptine has produced improvement in patients with detrusor instability.[6] This may be due to a decrease in the level of circulating prolactin which reduces the production of prostaglandin or to the action of bromocriptine as a dopamine agonist, thus reducing detrusor activity either by modulating adrenergic transmission or by a direct action.[6]

The complexity of the pharmacology of micturition precludes any definitive statement concerning the role of the α- and β-adrenergic receptors. However, the following sequence of events is suggested by the available knowledge. There is a precipitous drop in urethral pressure prior to a detrusor contraction. This drop is due both to skeletal muscle relaxation and sympathetic blockade. The drop in pressure can be caused by skeletal muscle paralysis with the use of curare or by the administration of α-blocking agents such as phentolamine (Regitine). The proportional effect of each is not known.[3] Anatomical studies have indicated that muscular continuity is not required to produce this drop in pressure, and it is probably due to a reflex phenomenon.[3] It has been suggested that this response is mediated through the parasympathetic nervous system via acetylcholine acting on α- and β-receptors located in the bladder base, proximal urethra, and fundus. Acetylcholine affects adrenergic nerve endings locally and facilitates the release of noradrenaline. The response is mediated by noradrenaline activating the receptor that is not occupied. It has been shown that the *concentration* of adrenaline is important in mediating this response, ie, low concentrations relax, whereas high concentrations of these catecholamines contract the same region.[3]

Urination therefore is the result of the interaction of a complex series of events. Clearly, there is voluntary control at the highest cerebral levels. The infant voids by utilizing the stretch reflex in response to bladder filling. Voluntary control is achieved by "toilet training" that results in an inhibition of this reflex. Any neurologic condition that affects cerebral function may result in involuntary loss of urine due to reactivation of the stretch reflex. This may occur after a cerebrovascular accident. In other patients, there is simply a gradual loss of awareness of the need to inhibit this reflex.

In order to void, the diaphragm is fixed, the abdominal muscles are contracted, and the pelvic floor is relaxed. These are large striated muscles under voluntary control. Immediately after these maneuvers or possibly as a consequence of them, there is a drop in urethral pressure. This is followed by a detrusor contraction and expulsion of urine. Urination ceases when the bladder is empty, or the stream can be voluntarily interrupted by contraction of the pubococcygeus.

It is clear that disorders of urination may result from a variety of alterations in these hydrodynamic events. Disorders that affect skeletal muscle, the spinal cord, the cerebral cortex, or the complex interaction between α- and β-receptors may result in involuntary loss of urine. In the following section we will discuss the diagnostic methods for evaluation of bladder and urethral function. It should be remembered, however, that the study of isolated urodynamic events presents serious difficulties because the information obtained is the *end product* of a series of reactions, many of which have only recently been described and are presently incompletely understood. Recent articles have described urodynamic measurements and alterations in function that have resulted in recommendations for treatment. It is clear from the discussion of the physiology of micturition that such measurements may not reflect the true cause of incontinence and therefore the treatment may be inappropriate.

Diagnostic Procedures

Several methods have been introduced to evaluate cystourethral function. They may be grouped under the following headings: (1) anatomical measurement, (2) urethral dynamics, (3) endoscopy, and (4) urologic radiology.

Much of the gynecologic literature has concentrated on the evaluation of the operative procedure rather than the indications for surgery. However, a review of the recent urologic literature reveals a number of sophisticated evaluation techniques and experimental and clinical studies of the pharmacology of micturition.[2] The physician must strike a balance between the overzealous use of diagnostic instrumentation and the complicated descriptions of operative techniques, which emphasize surgical skills rather than clinical judgment. It is important to point out that a good history and physical examination plus sound clinical judgment may provide the best basis for choosing proper treatment.

ANATOMICAL MEASUREMENTS

Several articles appearing in the urologic literature have emphasized the anatomical length of the urethra. Instrumentation is available that measures anatomical length before and after surgery. It has been suggested that the lengthening of the urethra associated with retropubic suspension of the urethra is the important determinant of continence. Most authorities now believe that the *functional* length of the urethra is more important.[7] This will be described in greater detail under the heading "Urodynamics."

The degree of anatomical relaxation is often mentioned as a consideration in choosing appropriate treatment for anatomical stress urinary incontinence. In essence, this is a determination of the posterior urethrovesical angle. The position of the urethra relative to the base of the bladder may be exaggerated with the so-called Q-tip test. The lubricated Q-tip is placed into the urethra. In the normal situation, the Q-tip points downward. With anatomical stress incontinence and with straining there is a reversal, with the Q-tip rotating anteriorly and actually pointing upward.[8]

In my opinion, one should not rely too heavily on anatomical features. A number of patients are quite continent with what appears to be a relatively short urethra anatomically and complete loss of the posterior urethrovesical angle with straining. It should be remembered that a second- or third-degree cystocele *exaggerates* the posterior urethrovesical angle and more often results in retention or overflow incontinence.

URODYNAMICS

Cystometry using either fluid or gas (carbon dioxide) permits evaluation of the threshold of detrusor reflex and the ability of the patient to suppress the reflex on command. Carbon dioxide has the advantage of rapidly distending the bladder; however, the reproducibility and interpretation of carbon dioxide cystometry has been challenged.[9] When carbon dioxide is used, the volumes at which an individual patient perceives the first bladder sensation and the desire to void are extremely subjective and variable. Also, the amplitude of a detrusor contraction varies depending on the amount of leakage of carbon dioxide around the catheter. The failure of carbon dioxide cystometry to provide quantitatively reproducible data casts some doubt on its effectiveness and appropriateness in evaluating disorders of micturition. It has been suggested that liquid cystometry may yield more reproducible results, at least under the present operating conditions.

Two abnormalities of detrusor function have been reported using cystometry: (1) detrusor hyperreflexia or detrusor dyssynergia, which is defined as a reflex contraction that the patient cannot suppress on command, and (2) detrusor areflexia, which is secondary to denervation or injury. Bladder denervation is suggested if there is a pressure elevation of 15 to 20 cm H_2O after the administration of bethanecol (Urecholine) on a repeat cystometric study. Cystometry can be a rather complicated procedure depending on electronic instrumentation, or a relatively simple procedure utilizing a catheter and a water monometer. Liquid cystometry with electronic equipment provides a record of baseline pressure and detrusor activity. Most patients describe a sense of filling and fullness and finally the urge to void. The volumes at which these changes occur vary. The tonus limb of the cystometrogram has been divided into three distinct phases. The first phase represents the resting bladder pressure, which normally is approximately 5 cm H_2O. Secondly, smooth muscle accommodation is normally recorded as a straight line, with the first desire to void at approximately 200 ml. The third phase is a relatively rapid rise in pressure reflecting the inability of the inelastic collagen fibers of the bladder wall to stretch. Changes in the slope of the second phase and the volume at which the final stage occur on the cystometrogram have clinical significance. A shift to the left of the second phase suggests a hypertonic bladder; a shift to the right or a delay in the third phase suggests an atonic bladder.

The resting bladder pressure may be elevated in patients with chronic infection, prior operations, or anxiety. However, the accommodation phase remains relatively normal. Patients with emotional problems may demonstrate inappropriate detrusor activity throughout the second phase of the tonus limb. The voiding pressure is obtained by asking the patient to void with the catheter in place. Forty to 50 mm Hg is the normal voiding pressure and it should return promptly to the baseline. Continued unstimulated detrusor contractions may indicate neurologic dysfunction.

There are various techniques for performing cystometrics. The simplest is the introduction of a catheter and the use of a large burette that is successively filled with 50-ml volumes of saline. If the bladder can be filled only once or twice, a hypertonic bladder is suspected. If continued filling occurs, a hypotonic bladder may be present. At the other extreme, advanced electronic instrumentation using gas or liquid and appropriate transducers and strain gauge amplifiers may be used to provide a permanent record of bladder function. These advanced methods have their limitations. The failure of carbon dioxide cystometry to provide quantitatively reproducible data casts some doubt on its appropriateness. Also, the term "resting pressure" is not applicable to gas cystometry. Some investigators have used direct electrourethrocystometry, which simultaneously records pressure in the bladder and proximal urethra, and measurement of pressure in the abdomen with a rectal balloon. This is considered to be the most accurate technique for the evaluation of bladder function. Some form of cystometry is essential for the complete evaluation of the patient with incontinence; however, the limitations of the technique used should be carefully scrutinized in any interpretation of the data.

URETHRAL PRESSURE PROFILE

This is a record of pressures generated throughout the urethra and obtained by means of a recording catheter withdrawn through the urethra at a predetermined rate. The pressure curve generated provides a measurement of the initial bladder pressure and the "functional" length of the urethra. Closure pressure is the difference between the bladder pressure and the maximum urethral pressure. This is usually 50 to 100 cm H_2O. With appropriate instrumentation, the functional and total length of the urethra can be measured. The functional length begins at that point where urethral pressure exceeds bladder pressure and continues until the pressure returns to the recorded bladder pressure. In normal patients this varies between 3 and 5 cm. The most sophisticated equipment uses a catheter with four channels and two balloons to record intravesical and intraurethral pressures simultaneously. The resulting recording illustrates intra-urethral and intravesical pressure, and with the use of appropriate electronics, the closure pressure.[8]

UROFLOWMETRY

There are a number of sophisticated techniques to measure urine flow through the urethra.[8] Unfortunately, in the female, because of the anatomy, none is very accurate. In the male, appropriate equipment can be placed around the penis and the flow rate measured directly. If a patient can void 20 to 25 ml per second, there is usually no obstruction. Abnormalities in flow rate are rather clear-cut in the male. The urologist often observes the male patient voiding and with considerable accuracy predicts prostatic enlargement. Unfortunately, disorders of micturition in the female cannot be viewed solely in anatomical terms.

ELECTROMYOGRAPHY

Sphincter electromyography has been recommended by several investigators. Although it is valuable in patients with neurologic dysfunction, there are problems with the technique, and interpretation is difficult. The electromyogram is obtained by inserting needle electrodes into the sphincter muscles and combining this with gas or water cystometry.[8]

URETHROSCOPY

The urethra is inspected with the female urethroscope and the use of carbon dioxide rather than liquid. When carbon dioxide is utilized, there is a dynamic assessment of the urethra. Minor alterations in the urethra and the presence or absence of a urethral diverticulum can be visualized with this technique. The anatomical length of the urethra can be noted and the diameter calibrated. Inspection of the bladder mucosa is best performed with the fore-oblique cystoscope. This will reveal the presence or absence of acute or chronic infection, ulceration, or fistulas. The location of the urethral orifice in relation to the trigone is noted and, when the instrument is withdrawn, the presence or absence of stress incontinence in the lithotomy position may be observed. Instrumentation is available, using carbon dioxide, that permits direct cystometric and urometric tracings as the bladder and urethra are observed.

RADIOLOGIC STUDIES

The most obvious radiologic study is the intravenous pyelogram. This, of course, is essential when there is loss of tissue integrity and a fistula is suspected. It is of questionable value in patients with anatomical stress incontinence. It should always be obtained in patients with marked cystocele or prolapse because the ureters may be obstructed and could be damaged during a surgical repair.

One of the most lingering controversies in female urology regards the appropriateness of a static cystourethrogram (chain cystogram).[10] The cystogram has been recommended for a number of years and represents an attempt to correlate anatomy with degree of function. Basic requirements for this test are contrast material, a metallic chain to mark the urethra, and proper anterior and posterior and lateral films. The films should not be exposed during voiding but should be taken in the lateral view with the patient straining. The reliability of this technique depends on the clarity of the films and the accuracy of the measurements recorded by the radiologist. The normal cystogram shows a posterior urethrovesical angle and a normal degree of inclination of the urethra. Abnormalities reported include loss of the posterior urethrovesical angle and loss of the angle combined with the downward and backward rotation and descent of the urethra and bladder neck. Green has suggested a classification of the cystourethrogram that indicates simple loss of the posterior urethrovesical angle, and rotation and descent with the downward and backward rotation of the urethra and bladder neck. For the former, that is, type I, he advises a vaginal approach and for the latter, type II, a retropubic suspension. Drutz et al. have challenged the role of the static cystourethrogram; in a recent article they stated, "After analyzing our own data, we have concluded that there is no role for the static cystourethrogram in the investigation of female incontinence. Both micturition and incontinence are dynamic phenomena and require urodynamic and not static measurements of assessment."[11] A middle-of-the-road approach has been taken by Hodgkinson: "In these times of technical advancements, there is hardly any reason to eliminate a procedure that has the possibility of adding to our knowledge and efficiency in diagnosis and treatment of a condition that is managed with such unpredictable results as stress urinary incontinence. In order to improve results of treatment of stress incontinence, patients should receive as thorough a preliminary study as possible. In addition to being valuable in this respect, colpocystourethrography (chain cystogram), by graphically demonstrating the anatomical changes wrought by various operative procedures, is useful as a teaching aid for residents."[12]

Anatomical alterations may be the inevitable result of childbearing and the normal loss of tissue support with aging. Perhaps, therefore, the most useful application of cystography is the anatomical evaluation of the patient before and after surgery. It is unlikely that any simple anatomical explanation will explain alterations in this very complex elastohydrodynamic system.

What, then, are the basic studies required to evaluate the patient with urinary incontinence? Obviously, the patient must have a complete general medical assessment. Predisposing causes such as chronic lung disease, obesity, and intra-abdominal and pelvic abnormalities must be noted. Examination of a clean-catch urine, cystoscopy, and urethroscopy, intravenous pyelography, particularly for patients with loss of tissue integrity, and a cystometrogram are basic studies for all patients who are incontinent. Neurologic examination is necessary to rule out specific metabolic diseases and neurologic conditions such as multiple sclerosis, cord tumor, and herniated nucleus pulposis. When urethroscopy and cystoscopy are performed, it is appropriate to observe the loss of urine in the lithotomy position and also test the bulbocavernosus reflex. This is accomplished by touching the glans of the clitoris and noting the contraction of the external anal sphincter. Production of this reflex indicates integrity of the lower spinal cord and its S2, S3, and S4 segments. The examiner should also evaluate the tone of the pubococcygeal muscles by placing two fingers in the vagina and requesting the patient to elevate the fingers. With minor degrees of relaxation, exercise of these muscles may improve support and result in continence.

If the patient has obvious loss of the posterior urethrovesical angle, the vesical elevation test may indicate the degree of retropubic suspension of the urethra that will result in continence.

It is clear that the evaluation of the patient with urinary incontinence requires considerable judgment and a certain amount of appropriate instrumentation. Every practicing obstetrician and gynecologist should not own the instrumentation necessary for urodynamic assessment. True anatomical stress incontinence occurs rarely in the normal practice of obstetrics and gynecology; therefore, the observer can hardly become facile in the use of this equipment. Too many patients are operated on because of alterations in their so-called urodynamic profile. One can visualize the office of the "well-equipped" obstetrician-gynecologist with its colposcope and associated photographic equipment, ultrasound instrumentation, and a variety of urodynamic instruments, including a "potty chair" for the measurement of urine flow. If the history and physical examination suggest anatomical stress incontinence, it is probably wise to refer the patient to a well-equipped urodynamic laboratory or at least to a colleague who has special expertise in the evaluation and treatment of this disorder.

Disorders of Micturition

URGENCY INCONTINENCE

Urgency incontinence is characterized by the involuntary loss of urine associated with an intense desire to void. Sensory urgency implies local irritative symptoms unassociated with detrusor contractions until urination is initiated. Motor urgency is associated with detrusor activity that may or may not be perceived by the patient. The distinction between sensory and motor urgency is the presence or absence of local irritative factors.[13]

Sensory urgency is more often associated with disorders of the urethral meatus, urethritis, significant bacilluria, aseptic urethrotrigonitis, interstitial (autoimmune) cystitis, urethral diverticula, senile mucosal atrophy, vaginal and cervical infections, and local pelvic pathologic changes. Clearly, the symptoms of urgency and urgency incontinence must be related to the specific disorder responsible in order for treatment to be effective. In addition to an accurate history and physical examination, urine culture and appropriate investigation of vaginal secretions are helpful. Urethroscopy with the female urethroscope and cystoscopy may reveal urethral and bladder abnormalities, including senile changes and urethral diverticulae. With the exception of autoimmune interstitial cystitis, treatment is directed toward the specific cause, that is, estrogen replacement therapy for senile changes and appropriate antibacterial therapy for obvious significant bacilluria. A number of organisms have been associated with nongonoccal urethritis, including *Chlamydia trachomatis.* Yeast infection has also been reported, although this seldom causes dysuria.[14]

Motor urgency implies a detrusor contraction, which may or may not be perceived by the patient. The contraction may be provoked by skeletal muscular activity, such as moving from a sitting to standing position, coughing, sneezing, etc, or it may occur spontaneously when the patient is completely inactive. A stable detrusor does not contract between voidings, and the normal patient can inhibit detrusor activity despite rapid filling of the bladder, postural change, or coughing. However, the patient with motor urgency is unable to inhibit these contractions and complains of frequency, urgency, nocturia, occasional enuresis, and involuntary loss of urine. The most important effect of the detrusor contraction is the preceding drop in urethral pressure. Thus, the unperceived detrusor contraction may be a very common cause of involuntary loss of urine and erroneously be attributed to anatomical stress urinary incontinence.

While sensory urgency is more often related to local abnormalities, motor urgency is frequently a psychosomatic problem.[15] Treatment is directed toward the emotional health of the patient. She must have a clear insight into the nature of her bladder dysfunction and an understanding of the therapeutic measures to overcome it. Supportive therapy, including sedation and anticholinergic drugs, has been recommended. However, clinical control of detrusor dysfunction including the use of various drugs is disappointing. Many cannot be tolerated and, more significantly, patients who seem to be clinically improved show no improvement of the underlying detrusor dysfunction with urodynamic testing. Bladder training by extending the periods of voiding has been suggested, but is not entirely satisfactory.

INAPPROPRIATE DETRUSOR ACTIVITY

Inappropriate detrusor activity or, as Hodgkinson[16] has called it, "detrusor dyssynergia," is characterized by detrusor contractions that are provoked by skeletal muscle activity (type I) or are completely involuntary (type II). Patients with type I dyssynergia present with "stress urinary incontinence." If asked when they lose urine, they correctly state that it is associated with coughing or sneezing. However, with careful examination, particularly in the upright position, it will be noted that there is no *immediate* loss of urine with coughing. Leakage occurs a few seconds *following* skeletal muscle activity. Patients with type II dyssynergia complain of involuntary loss of urine while standing still or with the slightest activity.

There has been an increase in diagnosis of dyssynergia associated with the use of carbon dioxide cystometry. However, Hodgkinson, using electronic direct urethrocystometry, noted that only 10% of his patients with recurrent incontinence had detrusor dysfunction in the form of dyssynergia.[16] Drutz and associates, using gas cystometry, reported that 74% of their patients with recurrent stress incontinence had "unstable bladders."[11] It is clear that unless one uses appropriate diagnostic studies, a number of patients will be operated on for anatomical stress incontinence who in fact have some form of detrusor dysfunction. Hodgkinson has noted: "To withhold operation for over 70% of patients with recurrent stress urinary incontinence because they showed evidence of "unstable bladder" syndrome by retrograde cystometry would be a gross injustice."[16]

The true incidence lies somewhere between the 10% of Hodgkinson and the 74% reported by Drutz. In addition to medical treatment, Ingelman-Sundberg has suggested partial denervation of the bladder for inappropriate detrusor activity in the absence of neurologic disease.[17] The operative treatment is preceded by the injection of a local anesthestic agent into the parametrium. If this produces a favorable result, the hypogastric plexus is sectioned. His reports indicate that the primary results are good and the rate of recurrence low.

ANATOMICAL STRESS URINARY INCONTINENCE

Characteristics

The comments concerning anatomical stress incontinence must be tempered by the knowledge that approximately 40% of young women claim some degree of stress incontinence.[18] Since no patient dies of this condition, it is important to realize that in the following discussion we are concerned with the evaluation and treatment of the patient with *socially* disabling incontinence.

When the loss of urine occurs with an increase in intra-abdominal pressure—coughing or sneezing, jumping, etc—the pressure in the bladder must then exceed the resistance in the urethra. In the normal patient, increases in intra-abdominal pressure are distributed equally to the urethra and the bladder. If during stress there is incomplete transmission of intravesical pressure, a drop in urethral resistance occurs and incontinence results. The normal resting urethral pressure is approximately 25 to 85 H_2O. Loss of the posterior urethrovesical angle allows the proximal urethra to become functionally part of the bladder. Since the distal urethra is not affected by an increase in intra-abdominal pressure, the resting urethral pressure drops and incontinence results. If the urethral pressure is low at resting levels, even weak detrusor contractions result in the loss of urine. A low resting pressure may be due to poor perineal musculature or loss of hormonal support associated with the menopause. Urethral resistance may be increased by appropriate exercises and the administration of estrogen, or detrusor contractions may be reduced or eliminated by the use of anticholinergic drugs. Conservative therapy with sympathomimetic drugs has been suggested. Recent reports have demonstrated limited effectiveness of an oral sympathomimetic medication, phenylpropanolamine hydrochloride combined with chlorpheniramine maleate and isopropamide iodide (Ornade).[3]

When the resting urethral pressure is high, and an increase in intra-abdominal pressure results in loss of urine, the urethra has not responded to the increase of pressure because of some anatomical disadvantage. To correct this situation, the upper urethra must be replaced in its normal anatomical position. Almost all of the successful operative procedures accomplish relocation of the urethra.

Scar tissue that prevents the urethra from responding to increases in intra-abdominal pressure is an increasing cause of stress urinary incontinence. Patients referred for recurrent anatomical stress incontinence often have had an inappropriate or poorly performed retropubic suspension of the urethra, with the result that the urethra is a solid tube incapable of responding to increases in intra-abdominal pressure.

Recommended Treatment

Minor degrees of anatomical stress incontinence may be corrected with repetitive pubococcygeus exercises. These were first popularized by Kegel,[19] and various modifications have been suggested, including the contraction of the pubococcygeus during voiding.

Sympathomimetic drugs increase urethral resistance and initial reports have been encouraging.[3] The use of α- and β-adrenergic blocking agents has also been suggested. α-Adrenergic blocking agents decrease resistance of the proximal urethra, thereby decreasing residual urine. Unfortunately, to date, no randomized statistical studies have reported the effects of these agents when matched against a placebo.

Surgical correction of anatomical stress incontinence is also controversial, although many authorities are now recommending some form of retropubic suspension as the initial procedure. Interestingly, a recent article has recommended a vaginal operation for restoration of anatomical bladder neck incompetence in preference to any retropubic approach.[20]

Clearly, patients with major degrees of pelvic relaxation, including prolapse, do not have true anatomical stress incontinence. Retention is more often discovered. However, for patients with minimal loss of support, anterior colporrhaphy with plication of the vesical neck produces satisfactory results. Obviously, overcorrection of a cystocele may result in iatrogenic stress incontinence. The extent of any posterior repair will depend on the age and sexual activity of the patient. Tightening of the levator sling makes it almost impossible for the patient to void, since the first phase of voiding is voluntary relaxation of this muscle. If the vaginal approach is to be used, the anterior vaginal wall must be opened widely and the dissection carried far laterally to expose the urethra and bladder neck. The mattress sutures used to support the bladder neck, when tied, must not be under tension. This may require additional lateral dissection before the final sutures are placed. Various suture materials have been used, including chromic catgut, fine silk, and polyglycolic sutures. The last have much to recommend them, since they are completely hydrolyzed in approximately three months.

Patients with minor degrees of relaxation and demonstrable anatomical stress incontinence may be cured with a properly executed retropubic suspension of the urethra. The usual operative approach is through the space of Retzius. If abdominal surgery is to be performed, this procedure should be carried out before the retropubic suspension. It is, however, helpful to leave the peritoneum open for exposure before the suspension is performed. It is not absolutely essential to remove the uterus in order to achieve satisfactory results. A number of modifications of the original Marshall-Marchetti-Krantz procedure have been advocated, including the use of a variety of suture materials. It is recommended that the periurethral or vaginal connective tissue be sutured to the cartilage of the symphysis. In some cases, the sutures are carried to Cooper's ligament (Burch modification). The operation, to be successful, requires excellent exposure, adequate hemostasis, and accurate placement of sutures. A minimum of two sutures on either side of the urethra is recommended, although Krantz has recently indicated that he uses a single suture on either side of the bladder neck.[21] Chromic catgut, silk, and polyglycolic sutures have been used; however, because of the possibility of intravesical placement of the suture, nonabsorbable sutures should be avoided. Placement of the sutures is facilitated by elevation of the vagina and approximation of the appropriate vaginal tissues to the posterior surface of the symphysis.

Patients with recurrent stress urinary incontinence must have complete reevaluation of their bladder status. A number of these patients will be found to have inappropriate detrusor activity and should not have an additional surgical procedure. For those who have demonstrable anatomical stress incontinence, a variety of additional surgical procedures may be necessary. In many patients, incontinence is the result of scarring in the periurethral area because of a previous retropubic suspension. The scar tissue must be removed, the urethra mobilized, and an attempt made to restore the posterior urethrovesical angle and bladder base to permit response to increases in intraabdominal pressure.

A number of modifications of the retropubic approach have been suggested. Lee and Symmonds prefer to open the bladder directly and place the sutures in the bladder neck under direct vision.[22] Drukker and Miller have suggested a retropubic suspension with the creation of a suburethral sling consisting of vaginal wall at the level of the urethrovesical junction.[23] More recently, Hodgkinson has suggested a retropubic urethropexy using the round ligaments; their proximal ends are crossed beneath the urethra and joined with nonabsorbable sutures.[16]

Occasionally, some modification of the urethral sling will be required. Several of these operations have been carried out, including the use of the pyramidalis, gracilis, transverse perineal, levator ani, and bulbocavernosus muscles. More often, strips of fascia lata are used. All of these operations have the same basic principle of placement of a musculofascial sling beneath the bladder neck and urethra.

Reported results with any one or a combination of the above procedures fall far short of 100% success. Depending on the skill of the surgeon and the extent of the preoperative evaluation, the cure rate varies from less than 50% to well over 90%. Almost all of the operations are successful for a few months. However, one can ascertain success or failure only after 1 or 2 years of constant observation. A follow-up system similar to that used for the cancer patient is essential to determine the results. Many patients fail to return to the operating surgeon because of embarrassment or because they believe that the continued loss of urine is an incurable situation. Minor degrees of urgency incontinence are common and are usually controlled with appropriate antibacterial medication or anticholinergic drugs.

INCONTINENCE DUE TO LOSS OF TISSUE INTEGRITY

Incontinence After Bladder or Ureteral Injury

Incontinence following injury to the bladder or ureter may be due to a vesicovaginal or ureterovaginal fistula. Fistulas resulting from obstetric causes are exceedingly rare. Most of the injuries to the bladder or ureter are associated with radical surgery for pelvic malignancy or the result of a combination of surgery and radiotherapy. Injuries to the urinary tract after radical pelvic surgery must be expected because the principal consideration is removal of the carcinoma. On the other hand, surgery for benign disease should not be followed by serious complications involving the urinary tract. That such is not the case is obvious from a survey of the literature. Sampson, in 1902, stated that injury occurred in 1.5% of patients during 955 major gynecologic operations; Newell, in 1939, cited an incidence of 0.4% in 3,144 hysterectomies; and Rusch and Bacon, in 1940, reported an incidence of 0.05%.[24] Benson and Hinnman, in 1955, in a review of 6,211 major surgical operations performed between 1938 and 1952, cited an incidence of ureteral injury of 0.83%.[24] It seems reasonable to conclude that the incidence of urinary tract injury associated with routine surgical procedures for benign conditions should not exceed 0.5% and if this figure includes minor gynecologic operations, 0.1%.

Most of the injuries after surgery for benign disease are related to inadequate preoperative evaluation, careless mobilization and ligation of the pelvic vessels, and inadequate hemostasis. Predisposing conditions can be summarized as (1) congenital anomalies, (2) large pelvic tumors (myomas and tubo-ovarian masses), (3) cervical my-omas, (4) endometriosis, (5) pelvic inflammatory disease, (6) diverticulitis, and (7) massive ovarian cysts. The injuries include (1) crushing of the ureter, (2) division of the ureter, (3) damage to the blood supply, and (4) inadvertent cystotomy. The end result may be ureterovaginal fistula or vesicovaginal fistula.

Three factors are of paramount importance in the prevention of urologic injuries, whether they are associated with surgery for benign disease or the more radical procedures for pelvic malignancy. These are: (1) a knowledge of the anatomy of the pelvis, especially the blood supply to the pelvic viscera; (2) sharp dissection in anatomical planes with isolation of vascular bundles; and (3) adequate exposure.

The points of injury associated with total abdominal hysterectomy or removal of the adnexa are at the infundibulopelvic ligament and at the bifurcation of the uterine artery as it reaches the uterine wall. It is clear that ligation of the infundibulopelvic ligament in the region of the common iliac artery is hazardous without prior exposure of the ureter at this point. It is equally clear that careless ligation of the uterine artery may result in crushing of the ureter. Displacement of the vesicouterine fold after cesarean section or its involvement by tumor invite inadvertent cystotomy or, more serious, unrecognized damage to the bladder.

The surgical techniques associated with abdominal hysterectomy should be based on secure anatomical knowledge and clean, sharp dissection wherever possible. This is accomplished by judicious use of traction, proper exposure, appropriate assistance, and adequate lighting. For most pelvic procedures the modified Trendelenburg position presents a clear view of the pelvic structures with minimal packing. Self-retaining retractors should be used after ligation and division of the round ligaments and sharp dissection of the anterior proximal leaves of the broad ligament. This technique provides direct exposure of the infundibulopelvic ligament, and palpation of the medial leaf of this dissection will reveal the ureter, which can be followed toward the infundibulopelvic ligament and toward the cervix distally.

The vesicouterine fold should be mobilized by sharp dissection in the midline until it can be gently pushed with the index finger toward the vagina. Blunt dissection in this area is facilitated by placing a sponge in the vagina to act as countertraction. Sharp dissection will provide exposure of the uterine artery, which is easily ligated and divided by applying clamps close to the body of the uterus, avoiding constriction of the tissue adjacent to the ureter as it passes beneath the uterine artery somewhat more laterally. Perhaps the most common reason for ureteral injury is inadequate hemostasis and the frantic effort to control bleeding by blindly placing ligatures or hemostats into this area. In addition to adequate exposure and clean dissection, some type of suction is absolutely essential. For patients with endometriosis, pelvic inflammatory disease, or fibrosis after radiation therapy, it is often advisable to insert ureteral catheters prior to the surgical procedure. These can be palpated in the medial leaf of the broad ligament or near the cervix prior to the application of the clamps.

Injury to the bladder may occur after removal of the uterus as the vaginal cuff is closed. If mobilization of the vesicouterine fold is incomplete, a suture may inadvertently pass through the bladder and result in a vesicovaginal fistula.

The prevention of injury and incontinence begins with the proper preoperative evaluation of the patient. Since anatomical changes in the urinary tract are often associated with large pelvic tumors, demonstration of the course of the ureters is mandatory and is easily achieved with an intravenous pyelogram. Occasionally, a double dose of dye is required to visualize the kidneys. In some cases an infusion intravenous pyelogram will be required to outline the collecting system. Failure to demonstrate one segment of the ureter may be due to peristaltic action. However, if there is obstruction, appropriate retrograde studies may be necessary. Retrograde injection can be accomplished by placing a cone-tip catheter against the ureteral orifice and injecting contrast material. Drainage films should be taken to ascertain the degree of obstruction as well as its location. Occasionally, radioisotope renography is helpful. Although the renogram is nonspecific, being an appearance-disappearance curve for a radioactive substance entering the renal region, it embodies in its wave pattern much of the information previously obtainable only by excretory urography or by bilateral ureteral catheterization.

Preoperative cystoscopy is essential for complete evaluation of patients with significant pelvic pathology. In addition to observation of the urethra and the bladder, cytologic examination of the urine and bacteriologic evaluation should be made. Cystoscopic evaluation should be performed after the intravenous pyelogram has been reviewed.

Surgical Management of Injuries of the Bladder and Ureter

A fistula may develop in 3 or 4 days or 3 or more weeks after surgery. It is usually heralded by abnormal drainage per vaginam or a systemic reaction including pain, fever, chills, and little drainage. Management consists of immediate assessment of renal function, including blood urea nitrogen and creatinine, supplemented by an intravenous pyelogram or a radioisotope renogram. Unless bilateral injury has occurred, the blood urea nitrogen and creatinine levels will be normal. The renogram and intravenous pyelogram indicate the functional and anatomical status of the kidneys. A poorly functioning kidney, as demonstrated by the intravenous pyelogram, may be the source of abnormal drainage per vaginam. The affected kidney does not concentrate the dye; however, large amounts of dilute urine pass through the collecting system into the ureter and vagina.

Additional studies that may be of value and should immediately follow the evaluation of the upper urinary tract include cystoscopy and retrograde pyelography. Inspection of the bladder reveals the presence or absence of a vesicovaginal fistula. Confirmation may be obtained very simply by placing methylene blue or a similar solution in the bladder and noting its appearance on the vaginal sponge. The administration and recovery of intravenous indigo carmine may be helpful in confirming a ureterovaginal fistula. Most vesicovaginal fistulas are obvious at the time of cystoscopy. If a large fistula is present, a finger inserted into the vagina will tamponade the flow of fluid and permit distention of the bladder and accurate observation. If a ureterovaginal fistula is present, an attempt should be made to pass a whistle-tip catheter beyond the point of obstruction. This seldom is successful, but if the catheter can be placed in the renal pelvis for 10 to 14 days, healing usually takes place. If this maneuver fails, treatment depends on renal function as noted by serial radioisotope renograms or intravenous pyelography. If successful decompression of a stricture has been accomplished by the fistula it may not be necessary to decompress the kidney by nephrostomy. When optimal local tissue conditions are present, repair should be performed. Deteriorating renal function necessitates a temporary nephrostomy on the affected side. Closure of a ureterovaginal fistula is best accomplished by reimplantation of the ureter into the bladder. Because of poor blood supply in the lower end of the ureter, direct end-to-end anastomosis is seldom successful. In most cases, the ureter can be transplanted into the base of the bladder. The bladder is opened and the trigone visualized. The clean end of the ureter is passed directly or obliquely through the base of the bladder and a direct mucosa-to-mucosa anastomosis performed with 4-0 or 5-0 chromic catgut. The anastomosis may be splinted with a no. 6 whistle-tip catheter advanced to the renal pelvis and attached to a suprapubic catheter, or passed directly through the urethra and attached to an indwelling Foley catheter. The splint is left in place for 7 to 10 days. If it is not possible to implant the severed end of the ureter into the bladder, the kidney may be mobilized to accommodate the ureteral length. In most cases a bladder flap must be provided or the finger may be inserted into the bladder and a nipple pushed out and sutured to the appropriate psoas muscle, and the ureter is then anastomosed by direct mucosa-to-mucosa technique.

Occasionally, the definition of a vesicovaginal fistula is difficult. Additional information can be obtained by using vaginography. This procedure is carried out with sterile technique and consists of insertion of a 30-ml Foley catheter into the vagina. The bulb is filled with water or air until it fits snugly and effectively blocks the introitus. Contrast material is injected into the vagina via the catheter, under fluoroscopic control. Sequential spot films are taken as required to identify the fistula.[3]

Summary

Urinary incontinence is a sign of a disorder, not a diagnosis. Careful history and physical examination often suggest the correct diagnosis. However, complete accuracy can only be obtained by the judicious use of appropriate ancillary procedures, including careful neurologic assessment and urodynamic evaluation of the bladder and urethra. The fact that the varieties of urinary incontinence occur infrequently poses a significant medical and legal problem. Unless the facilities for complete urologic evaluation are available and unless the surgeon by training and experience has demonstrated success in the treatment of urinary incontinence, most, if not all, of these patients should be considered for referral.

REFERENCES

1. Marchant, D. J.: Urinary incontinence, in deAlvarez, R. R. (ed): *Textbook of Gynecology*. Philadelphia, Lea and Febiger, 1977, p 443.
2. Turner-Warwick, R.: Some clinical aspects of detrusor dysfunction. J. Urol. 113:539, 1975.
3. Marchant, D. J.: Urinary incontinence, in Wynn, R. M. (ed): *Obstetrics and Gynecology Annual*. New York, Appleton-Century Crofts, 1980, p 261.
4. Cryer, P. E.: Physiology and pathophysiology of the human sympathoadrenal neuroendocrine system. N. Engl. J. Med. 303:436, 1980.
5. Rohner, T. J., and Hannigan, J.: Effect of norepinephrine and isoproterenol on in vitro detrusor muscle contractility and cyclic AMP content. Invest. Urol. 17:324, 1980.
6. Cardozo, L. D., and Stanton, S. L.: A comparison between bromocriptine and indomethacin in the treatment of detrusor instability. J. Urol. 123:399, 1980.
7. Gershon, C. R., and Diokno, A. C.: Urodynamic evaluation of female stress urinary incontinence. J. Urol. 119:787, 1978.
8. Ostergard, D. R., and McCarthy, T. A.: Diagnostic procedures in female urology. Am. J. Obstet. Gynecol. 137:401, 1980.
9. Wein, A. J., et al.: The reproducibility and interpretation of carbon dioxide cystometry. J. Urol. 120:205, 1978.
10. Green, T. H.: Letter to the Editor. Am. J. Obstet. Gynecol. 132:228, 1978.
11. Drutz, H. P., Shapiro, B. J., and Mandel, F.: Do static cystourethrograms have a role in the investigation of female incontinence? Am. J. Obstet. Gynecol. 130:516, 1978.
12. Hodgkinson, C. P.: Stress urinary incontinence: diagnosis and treatment. Clin. Obstet. Gynecol. 21:649, 1978.
13. Oravisto, K. J.: Female aseptic dysuria. Ann. Chir. Gynaecol. Fenn. 61:295, 1972.
14. Holmes, K. K., et al.: Etiology of nongonococcal urethritis. N. Engl. J. Med. 292:1199, 1975.
15. Frewen, W. K.: Urgency of micturition and urge incontinence in women. Obstet. Gynecol. Digest p 19, 1975.
16. Hodgkinson, C. P.: Recurrent stress urinary incontinence. Am. J. Obstet. Gynecol. 132:844, 1978.
17. Ingelman-Sundberg, A.: Partial bladder denervation for detrusor dyssynergia. Clin. Obstet. Gynecol. 21:797, 1978.
18. Scott, J. C., Jr.: Stress incontinence in nulliparous women. J. Reprod. Med. 2:96, 1969.
19. Kegel, A. H., and Powell, T. H.: The physiologic treatment of stress urinary incontinence. J. Urol. 63:808, 1950.
20. van Rooyen, A. J. L., and Leibenberg, H. C.: A clinical approach to urinary incontinence in the female. Obstet. Gynecol. 53:1, 1979.

21. Krantz, K.: Personal communication.
22. Lee, R. A., and Symmonds, R. E.: Repeat Marshall-Marchetti procedure for recurrent stress urinary incontinence. Am. J. Obstet. Gynecol. 122:219, 1975.
23. Drukker, B. H., and Miller, D. W.: Retropubic urethropexy by the vaginal wall technique in stress urinary incontinence. Clin. Obstet. Gynecol. 21:775, 1978.
24. Higgins, C. C.: Ureteral injuries during surgery. JAMA 199:118, 1967.

Classification of Vaginal Relaxation. Precise agreement on the components of vaginal relaxation is necessary in gynecologic practice. Clayton T. Beecham[10-1] (American Assoc. of Obstetricians and Gynecologists Found., Sunbury, Pa.) presents a classification that has been found useful in describing the anatomical pathology of vaginal relaxation and which is proposed in the interests of standardization. Definitions apply when the patient is not straining and no traction is being applied to any structure. Directed muscle contractions evaluate function and have no place in an anatomical classification.

Rectocele is classified from first degree, in which a saccular protrusion of the vaginorectal wall is visible when the perineum is depressed, through third degree, in which the sacculation protrudes or extends outside the introitus. Cystocele is classed from first degree, in which the anterior vaginal wall is visible at the introitus, through third degree, in which the cystocele is part of a third-degree uterine prolapse or total prolapse of a posthysterectomy vaginal apex, and the entire urethra and bladder are outside the vagina. In first-degree uterine prolapse, the cervix is visible when the perineum is depressed; in second-degree prolapse the cervix extends through the introitus; in third-degree prolapse, the cervix and uterine corpus totally extend outside the introitus.

An enterocele may be part of a high rectocele. The peritoneal sac may or may not contain bowel. Three degrees of enterocele are recognized, in analogy with the other conditions. Prolapse of the vaginal apex after hysterectomy similarly has three degrees of severity. Urethrocele can be part of a primary cystocele. Failure of repair of a cystourethrocele can result in a distinct iatrogenic urethrocele.

▶ [There certainly is a need for a classification of vaginal relaxation in order to enhance communication and standardize reporting. This proposal by Beecham seems reasonable to us and we plan to institute its use on our service.] ◀

Diverticula of Female Urethra are discussed by Samir N. Hajj and Mark I. Evans[10-2] (Univ. of Chicago). Urethral diverticula are estimated to occur in 1.85–4.6% of women. Diverticula are symptomatic in over 80% of patients, causing recurrent urinary tract infections, postmicturition dribbling, or dyspareunia. These symptoms are not related to diverticulum size.

The diverticulum appears to originate as the result of inflammation. Once established, it can grow, serve as a reservoir of urine stagnation, and be a site of calculus formation. Rarely, carcinoma develops.

(10-1) Am. J. Obstet. Gynecol. 136:957–958, Apr. 1, 1980.
(10-2) Ibid., pp. 335–338, Feb. 1, 1980.

Surgical excision using a transvaginal approach through either a longitudinal or inverted U incision is the most common treatment. The risk of complications with various procedures ranges from 5% to 46%. Complications include urethrovaginal fistula, incontinence, and incomplete excision of the sac or sacs. A new surgical technique was developed which reduces the inadequate exposure and mobilization associated with standard techniques.

Over a $2^1/_2$-year period, 18 women were treated. Most had a preoperative voiding cystourethrogram. At operation the patients were divided into two groups based on the presence or absence of a diverticular communication to the urethral floor.

TECHNIQUE.—Adequate exposure of the urethra and diverticulum is imperative. By starting the dissection from normal, healthy planes, it is easier to prevent rupture of the sac. An inverted T incision in the vaginal mucosa is begun near the cervix and extended to the external urethral meatus. The vaginal flaps are developed to expose the entire urethra and bladder neck, as well as the intact diverticular sac. A longitudinal incision is made in the sac, exposing the neck of the diverticulum. The operator can visualize the indwelling Foley catheter that is introduced prior to the procedure. The sac is excised close to the urethral floor. The defect is then closed and a second imbricating suture applied in the periurethral tissue and tied. Repair is then complete and the vaginal mucosa is closed.

In the present series, communicating diverticula were more often associated with urinary tract infections; the data suggest an increased incidence of purulent discharge or dribbling when a communication is present. Patients with communicating diverticula were of significantly higher gravidity and parity, and their lesions tended to be more proximal on the urethra.

Complications occurred in 3 patients: 2 treated with a standard vertical incision had residual disease at 6 weeks postoperatively, and 1 patient had a Foley catheter stitched into the urethra. Fistulas, strictures, or necrosis did not develop.

▶ [W. C. Keettel of the University of Iowa reviewed this paper at our request and commented as follows:

"This is a timely review of a fairly common clinical problem which can easily be overlooked by physicians not familiar with the symptoms associated with urethral diverticula. The key to the authors' success is careful mobilization of tissue, proper removal of just the diverticular sac, and a multilayered closure without tension on the suture line, rather than the type of incision on the anterior vaginal wall. In certain patients where there is insufficient fascia for a second layer, the use of the bulbocavernous fat pad from the inner aspect of the large labia is useful. It is refreshing to note that the authors do not feel the use of a Foley catheter interferes with urethral healing."] ◀

Fascia Lata Urethrovesical Suspension for Recurrent Stress Urinary Incontinence. It is generally believed that a competent urethrovesical neck is necessary for urinary continence. This underlies the management of stress urinary incontinence by release of periurethral fascia and grafting of a supporting sling of autologous fascia beneath the restored urethrovesical junction. Roy T. Parker, W. Allen Addison, and Christopher J. Wilson[10-3] (Duke Univ.) reviewed the results of suburethral sling procedures done in 50 patients with stress

(10–3)   Am. J. Obstet. Gynecol. 135:843–852, Dec. 1, 1979.

urinary incontinence in 1958 to 1978. The age range was 27 to 70 years. Forty-seven patients had had 1 to 8 previous operations for incontinence, including 62 colpoplastic repairs and 60 retropubic suspensions. Fascia lata is preferred for use as a sling. The technique is illustrated in Figure 10–1. Where fascia lata cannot be acquired, the Aldridge technique is utilized.

Forty-two patients (84%) are cured of incontinence on follow-up for 1 to 21 years. Five of 8 patients with bladder instability were cured. Five other patients were improved, including the remaining ones with detrusor instability. Three patients with pure stress inconti-

Fig 10–1.—Abdominal and vaginal incision and retropubic placement of fascia lata strap. (Courtesy of Parker, R. T., et al.: Am. J. Obstet. Gynecol. 135:843–852, Dec. 1, 1979; from Parker, R. T.: Perspect. Surg. 1:1, 1978.)

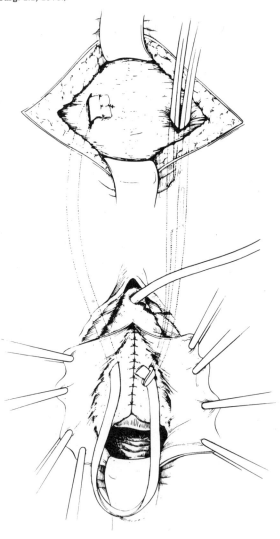

nence had a recurrence within 6 months of surgery. Two of them had previously had the Aldridge sling procedure without colpoplastic repair. An average of 12 days was needed for reestablishment of a satisfactory voiding pattern; in 4 exceptions, 2 to 6 months were necessary. One patient had pulmonary embolism, and 1 required repair of a urethrovaginal fistula. The average hospitalization was 18.5 days.

Anterior colporrhaphy combined with a fascia lata urethrovesical junction suspension offers the best chance of permanent relief in properly selected patients who have previously had unsuccessful surgery for stress urinary incontinence.

▶ [This is an excellent description of an anatomically sound procedure for the troublesome patient with recurrent stress incontinence in whom scarring from previous attempts at repair have fixed and shortened the urethra. We have had some experience with a similar technique employing heterologous fascia lata; the use of the patient's own fascia lata is more appealing.] ◀

Medical Management of the Unstable Bladder. R. Hal Younglove, Robert L. Newman, and Leonard A. Wall[10-4] (St. Luke's Hosp., Kansas City, Mo.) reviewed the treatment of 70 incontinent females with unstable bladder seen from 1976 to 1978. The patients lost urine during a variety of activities such as laughing, lifting, and exercising. A trial-and-error approach with various drugs was used. Initially flavoxate hydrochloride was used in a daily dosage of 800 mg. Another approach combined chlorpheniramine maleate and phenylpropanolamine hydrochloride used twice daily. Second-line drugs included oxybutynin chloride and propantheline bromide. Phenytoin sodium was used as well. Diazepam, hyoscyamine, and chlordiazepoxide were also used in combination with the other agents.

Unstable bladder was diagnosed from symptoms on increased intraabdominal pressure, a midurethral pressure of 60 to 80 cm water, a bladder filling resistance of 15 to 30 cm water, severe urgency before closure of the urethrovesical sphincter, and a bladder capacity of about 200 ml. The patients usually exhibited well-supported urethrovesical angles on performance of the Valsalva maneuver. Forty patients considered themselves to be cured, 11 showed marked improvement on treatment, 6 failed to improve, 12 were lost to follow-

UNSTABLE BLADDER CURES	
Drug	**No. of patients**
Urispas	21
Ornade	12
Ditropan	3
Pro Banthine	1
Dilantin	1
Ornade plus Valium	1
Ornade plus Urispas	1
Total	40

(10–4) J. Reprod. Med. 24:215–218, May 1980.

up, and 1 is still trying different drugs. The success of various medications is indicated in the table.

Medical management cured or improved over two thirds of patients with unstable bladder in this series. Perseverance is necessary until each patient finds the drug that will improve her condition. Not all patients respond to the same medication. Pharmacotherapy alone helps most women with unstable bladder, but there will always be treatment failures. The operation described by Ingleman-Sundberg to resect the inferior hypogastric plexus has been reported to be helpful in a few selected patients.

▶ [These authors use the term "unstable bladder" to describe a type of incontinence other than pure stress incontinence. Other terms include detrusor dysfunction or dyssynergia and urgency incontinence. It is important to note that these patients may give a history of urine loss with coughing and sneezing but they are also incontinent under other conditions (eg, when in bed or on hearing running water). Approximately three fourths of the patients were either cured or improved with drug therapy. The list of drugs used is a long one and they were apparently used in a trial-and-error fashion until success was achieved.] ◀

Simple Transvesical Repair of Vesicovaginal Fistula was used by Ralph R. Landes[10-5] (Univ. of North Carolina) in the management of 40 consecutive patients with vesicovaginal fistulas due to surgical mishap. All but 5 fistulas occurred following total abdominal hysterectomy. Although more extensive procedures using combined intraperitoneal-transvesical approaches, with extensive dissection and omental flaps, probably are needed to repair large, complicated, or irradiated fistulas, these are not often encountered in urologic practice. Repairs have been delayed for 2 to 3 months. Use of the vaginal diaphragm catheter is helpful during this time.

Fig 10–2.—Placement of sponge rubber ball in vagina. Traction on wire suture helps in the dissection and separation of layers. (Courtesy of Landes, R. R.: J. Urol. 122:604–606, November 1979.)

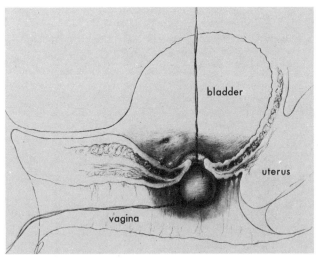

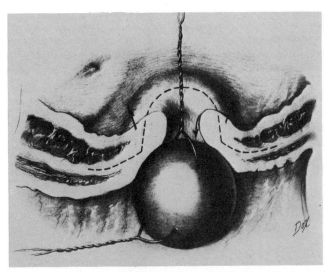

Fig 10–3.—Dotted line indicates dissection of layers. Fibrotic ring of fistula is allowed to remain with vaginal layer. (Courtesy of Landes, R. R.: J. Urol. 122:604–606, November 1979.)

TECHNIQUE.—A ball tractor is used in repair of the fistula. Sponge rubber is more satisfactory to use than a Foley catheter balloon because it cannot be inadvertently punctured. Wire is preferable to sutures for attachment to the ball for the same reason. A Foley catheter bag is passed into the bladder with the patient in a frog-leg position; the bladder is then exposed and opened. A ureteral catheter is passed through the fistula into the vagina and tied to one wire of the ball tractor (Fig 10–2). The bladder mucosa is incised just outside the fibrous ring of the fistula leaving the unyielding ring intact (Fig 10–3). After the bladder layer is separated from the vagina for 1–2 cm around the fistula, the vaginal edges are joined with horizontal mattress sutures inverting the scarred edges into the vagina (Fig 10–4). A middle layer of bladder

Fig 10–4.—Closure done in three layers with 4-0 chromic catgut. Vaginal layer is inverted into vagina. Crossed suture line of muscularis. Bladder mucosa inverted into bladder. (Courtesy of Landes, R. R.: J. Urol. 122:604–606, November 1979.)

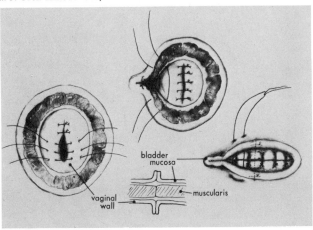

muscle then is brought together with interrupted sutures, with inversion of
the bladder mucosal layer into the bladder. The repair is done with 4–0
chromic gut sutures. A large suprapubic catheter is placed with its head distant from the suture line, and a Foley catheter is also inserted. Drainage
tubes are fixed to opposite sides. The urethral catheter is removed in one
week, and the suprapubic catheter in 2 weeks.

No failures occurred in this series. Simple, benign, small vesicovaginal fistulas can be closed by this direct method. The important principles are to allow sufficient time for maturation of the fistula, to
bring broad raw surfaces together without tension, and to maintain
free postoperative drainage.

▶ [What gynecologists do from below, urologists do from above. This description of a
transvesical repair of a small vesicovaginal fistula is similar to that which would be
done transvaginally, except that the reinforcing layers in this operation come from the
bladder side rather than the vaginal side. The ultimate results are probably similar with
either approach. The author's sponge rubber ball tractor seems like a good idea.] ◀

Vesicovaginal Fistula Repair—Revisited. Troublesome vesicovaginal and rectovaginal fistulas occasionally develop during treatment of gynecologic malignancies. Effective repair of these defects in
the presence of irradiated and scarred tissues is difficult and often
fails. W. Gary Smith and Gary H. Johnson[10-6] (Univ. of Utah) evaluated the method described in 1928 by Martius, involving introduction
of a pedicled blood supply from the labial fat pad to cover the suture
lines with tissue having a good blood supply. Experimentals indicated
that small arteriolar vessels migrate from these autografts into the
surrounding compromised and ischemic tissues.

TECHNIQUE.—A large Foley catheter is placed in the bladder suprapubi-
cally for postoperative decompression of the bladder. Every effort is made to
mobilize the involved tissues to close the fistula primarily without tension. A
combined vaginal-abdominal approach may be necessary. After excision of
the scarred fistula tract, the bladder defect is closed in two layers with interrupted gut and Dexon sutures designed to invert the bladder mucosa and
placed so the fistula is closed in a horizontal direction. The pubovesical-cer-
vical fascia is dissected from the vaginal flaps and mobilized to cover the
repair site. A pedicled flap is taken by an incision lateral to the labium majus
and brought medially to the repair site through a separate vaginal incision

Fig 10–5.—Transfer of fat pad to fistula
repair site. (Courtesy of Smith, W. G., and
Johnson, G. H.: Gynecol. Oncol. 9:303–309,
June 1980.)

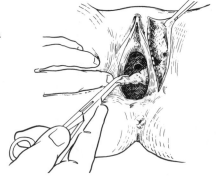

(10–6) Gynecol. Oncol. 9:303—309, June 1980.

(Fig 10–5), where it is fixed in place with interrupted sutures. The skin incision is closed over a drain, and the vaginal wall is replaced and sutured vertically.

Eight patients with vesicovaginal fistulas have undergone closure with a bulbocavernosus fat pad after treatment for invasive cervical carcinoma in the past four years. Seven repairs were successful. The other patient is still incontinent after two attempts at fistula closure.

Use of the bulbocavernosus fat pad as a pedicled blood supply is a safe and easy way to revascularize radiation-induced ischemic and fibrosed tissues. Vaginal closure should be considered in every case. Many patients can obtain successful closure through use of conventional methods that prevent suture line tension and mobilization of a pedicled blood supply to the closure site.

▶ [Vesicovaginal fistulas developing as a result of radiation are notoriously difficult to repair successfully. Because of the scarring and fibrosis, the irradiated tissues are poorly vascularized and the degree of mobility that can be achieved is limited. The technique described here of using the bulbocavernosus fat pad as a pedicle graft is essentially the same as that described by Martius 40 years ago. By covering the repair site with a vascularized pedicle, successful closure was achieved in 7 of 8 patients, including 4 of 5 previously irradiated for cancer of the cervix.] ◀

▶ ↓ For a nonoperative approach to urinary fistulas, read on. ◀

Vesicouterine Fistula Treated by Amenorrhea Induced With Contraceptive Steroids: Two Case Reports. Vesicouterine fistulas are becoming more frequent with the increasing use of cesarean section. The accepted treatment is surgical. S. M. Rubino[10-7] (Univ. of Palermo) describes 2 women with vesicouterine fistulas who were successfully managed by inducing amenorrhea with continuous administration of an estrogen-progestogen combination for 6 months.

CASE 1.—Woman, 26, with amenorrhea and 6 episodes of hematuria at monthly intervals, was seen 7 months after lower segment cesarean section. A fistula and a 3-cm opening in the posterior bladder wall were observed. The patient used Ortho-Novum 1/50 daily for 6 months. Normal menses ensued, with no hematuria, and the patient conceived and underwent an elective cesarean section without recurrence of the fistula.

CASE 2.—Woman, 24, with a postsection fistula, was treated in the same way, and also did well. She is now pregnant again.

Fistulas seldom close spontaneously because the flow of fluid through them inhibits healing. In these 2 patients, prevention of menstrual flow through the vesicouterine fistulas permitted the fistulas to close. This approach should be tried in women with vesicouterine fistulas but no urine leakage before resorting to operation.

▶ [This suggested therapy for patients with vesicouterine fistulas causing amenorrhea and cyclic hematuria is certainly simple and, at least in the two reported cases, effective.] ◀

New Technique for Vulvar Skin Grafting. The cosmetic results of vulvar skin grafting are important to young patients to avoid both deformity and sexual dysfunction. Handling of the free graft may be difficult when the graft edges curl, and suturing often is made more difficult by slippage or tearing of the graft. Don J. Hall, Dean R. Go-

(10–7) Br. J. Obstet. Gynecol. 87:343–344, April 1980.

plerud, and Leo J. Dunn[10-8] (Med. College of Virginia, Richmond) describe an easy, rapid method of handling and applying split-thickness skin grafts to the vulva. The method has been used in 3 cases of intraepithelial squamous cell carcinoma.

TECHNIQUE.—Grafts are taken from the lateral portion of the buttock at a thickness of 0.018 in. and applied to petrolatum gauze with the epidermal surface in contact with the gauze. The graft is smoothed out with a finger moistened in saline, and excess gauze then is trimmed off, using the graft as a template. Fine bleeding points are controlled by electrocoagulation. After the graft bed is prepared, the graft is applied with its dermal surface in contact with the wound bed and the edges are secured to the wound margins using a skin stapler, avoiding tension on the graft. Scattered staples may be used to secure central parts of the graft. Petrolatum gauze then is applied in several layers and, after insertion of a urethral catheter, a pressure dressing is applied. The patient is placed on a low-residue diet and Lomotil, and subcutaneous heparin is used to prevent venous thrombosis. The layers of petrolatum gauze are removed starting at 48 hours, and all dressings are removed by day 5. Staples are removed by day 7, when the graft backing is easily removed and areas of dead tissue may be debrided. The total area of loss was less than 10% in each case.

Use of this method has made handling of vulvar grafts easier and reduced anesthesia time. The only disadvantage is the occasional need to remove a buried staple from a deep position in the interstitial tissue.

▶ [These technical suggestions concerning the handling and application of vulvar skin grafts are helpful.] ◀

Incidence of Pain Among Women Undergoing Laparoscopic Sterilization by Electrocoagulation, Spring-Loaded Clip, and Tubal Ring. I-Cheng Chi and Lynda Painter Cole[10-9] analyzed data from five comparative studies conducted at three centers in Thailand, El Salvador, and Costa Rica. In each study two techniques of laparoscopic sterilization were randomly assigned to 300 women requesting sterilization for family planning purpose. None had been pregnant for at least 42 days. In the two studies at Center A, Bangkok, Thailand, 100 mg of meperidine and 2.5 mg of droperidol were injected intravenously about 10 minutes before surgery; 10 to 20 cc of 1% lidocaine was injected into the subumbilical abdominal wall after the patient was prepared for surgery. In the three studies conducted at Center B, San Salvador, El Salvador, and Center C, San José, Costa Rica, anesthetic and operative procedures were similar to those used at Center A except that 2 cc of thalamonal (0.05 mg fentanyl citrate and 2.5 mg droperidol per cc) was injected intravenously before the patient entered the operating room. Tubal topical anesthetics were not used. All laparoscopies were performed with a single incision. Nearly all patients were discharged 2 to 5 hours after the procedure.

Sociodemographic characteristics, surgical complications, and mean surgical times were similar for all groups. During the sterilization procedures, tubal rings were associated with greater pain than electrocoagulation and spring-loaded clips, and electrocoagulation was as-

(10–8)   Obstet. Gynecol. 54:343–345, September 1979.
(10–9)   Am. J. Obstet. Gynecol. 135:397–401, Oct. 1, 1979.

INCIDENCE OF ABDOMINAL OR PELVIC PAIN DURING LAPAROSCOPY, RECOVERY PERIOD AND AT EARLY FOLLOW-UP VISIT

Center	Tubal occlusion technique	Total patients	Moderate or severe pain during procedure (%)	Pain during recovery period (%)	Pain at early follow-up visit (%)
A	Electrocoagulation	136	15.4	14.0*	14.7*
	Spring-loaded clips	115	11.3	24.1	27.6
B	Electrocoagulation	132	22.7*	18.3*	2.3
	Spring-loaded clips	122	3.3	29.2	4.5
A	Electrocoagulation	139	19.4*	15.8*	25.9
	Tubal rings	143	39.9	51.7	29.4
C	Electrocoagulation	143	11.2	16.1*	1.4
	Tubal rings	137	8.7	29.2	2.9
B	Spring-loaded clips	139	5.1*	44.6	36.7
	Tubal ring	141	14.2	46.8	26.4

*$P < 0.05$.

sociated with greater pain than clips (table). After the procedure and before discharge from the center, both mechanical tubal occlusion techniques (clips and rings) were associated with higher rates of abdominal or pelvic pain than electrocoagulation. These differences in pain did not persist to the early follow-up visit (usually 7 to 21 days after the procedure), which was made by more than 90% of the patients in each study.

▶ [The random patient assignment, pain evaluation by someone other than the operator, and multinational nature of this study are commendable. The difference in prevalence of pain postoperatively between the spring-loaded clip groups at Center B is hard to understand. On balance, the study suggests that intraoperative pain is most likely with rings and least likely with clips and that postoperative pain is less likely with electrocoagulation than with either mechanical occlusion technique.] ◀

Cul-de-sac Insufflation: Easy Alternative Route for Safely Inducing Pneumoperitoneum. Since 1977, Dirk A. F. van Lith, Kees J. van Schie, Willem Beekhuizen, and Marijke du Plessis[10-10] (Leiden, The Netherlands) used cul-de-sac insufflation to induce pneumoperitoneum for outpatient pelvic laparoscopy in 350 consecutive patients undergoing elective sterilization. Either a three-barreled insufflation trocar or a double-barreled Steptoe-type pneumoperitoneum needle was used. A van Schie-van Lith intrauterine tenaculum provides maximum uterine anteflexion, necessary for secure atraumatic culdocentesis. No preoperative preparation is necessary. Local anesthesia is achieved by paracervical block and 1% lidocaine-adrenaline. The insufflation needle is introduced between the sacrouterine ligaments in the midline of the posterior vaginal fornix, 0.5 cm dorsal to the cervix. Gas is insufflated with the patient in a moderate Trendelenburg position.

The procedure was successful in 341 patients. Most failures occurred early in the series. The second attempt at insufflation always was made via an infraumbilical puncture. These findings, as well as reported data and anatomical considerations, appear to justify cul-de-sac insufflation via culdocentesis as the method of choice for the creation of pneumoperitoneum. The abdominal route may be considered

(10–10) Int. J. Gynaecol. Obstet. 17:375–378, Jan.–Feb. 1980.

when the cul-de-sac method is contraindicated or when it fails. Contraindications include a fixed retroverted uterus, cul-de-sac adhesions or masses, second-trimester pregnancy, and amputation of the uterine cervix.

▶ [Although we do not necessarily agree with these authors that the cul-de-sac is the preferential route for inducing pneumoperitoneum prior to laparoscopy, it is a technique that can occasionally be put to good use. We have found it especially helpful in obese patients.] ◀

Noninvasive Measurement of Cardiac Output During Laparoscopy. Ray McKenzie, Rajindar K. Wadhwa, and Richard C. Bedger[10-11] (Univ. of Pittsburgh) used noninvasive transthoracic impedance cardiography to evaluate cardiac function in 18 healthy patients undergoing laparoscopy. Stroke volume and cardiac output were determined with the chest in the resting expiratory position at 5-minute intervals before, during, and after pneumoperitoneum or before and during laparotomy. Fourteen patients had laparoscopy and 4 had hysterectomy or abdominal tubal ligation without insufflation of the peritoneum.

Both cardiac output and stroke volume fell significantly during insufflation of the peritoneum. Cardiac output was depressed to 60% of baseline in the patients undergoing laparoscopy. The effects were reversed on release of the pneumoperitoneum. No differences were found between nitrous oxide and oxygen insufflation. The variables did not change significantly during laparotomy. The fall in cardiac output during laparoscopy was due to a decline in stroke volume, with no significant change in heart rate. Intra-abdominal pressures did not exceed 20 torr during laparoscopy.

Some unexplained cardiac arrests that occur during laparoscopy in healthy females may be due to impaired venous return caused by the increased intra-abdominal pressure of pneumoperitoneum. Lethal cardiac output values can result. Routine transthoracic impedance cardiography could alert the anesthesiologist to this danger, and by leading to immediate release of pneumoperitoneum, prevent a catastrophic situation.

▶ [This is important information. A substantial decrease in cardiac output occurred during laparoscopy, presumably secondary to impaired venous return caused by the pressure of the pneumoperitoneum. If we are informed from the head of the table of cardiovascular disturbances during the course of a laparoscopic procedure, the authors' recommendation to immediately release the pneumoperitoneum makes good sense.] ◀

New Technique for Minilaparotomy is described by B. Palaniappan[10-12] (Madras, India). Minilaparotomy appears to be superior to other methods as a simple means of voluntary female sterilization that can be used with local anesthesia. It results in relatively little morbidity and a reduced recovery time. The safety record of this procedure makes it ideally suited for use in a well-equipped office with a recovery room. It is also suitable for puerperal and postabortion patients. Paramedical personnel can easily be trained in the technique.

A short transverse suprapubic incision is made. Local or short

(10-11) J. Reprod. Med. 24:247–250, June 1980.
(10-12) Int. J. Gynaecol. Obstet. 17:260–262, Nov.–Dec. 1979.

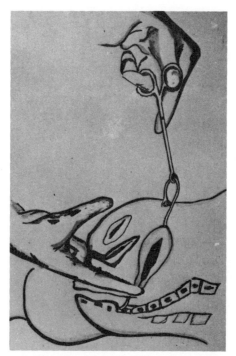

Fig 10–6.—Elevation of uterus toward surface by gloved fingers inserted into vagina. (Courtesy of Palaniappan, B.: Int. J. Gynaecol. Obstet. 17:260–262, Nov.–Dec. 1979.)

spinal anesthesia is used. An elevator is used to raise the uterus toward the skin surface. A gloved hand suffices for this maneuver (Fig 10–6). A retroverted uterus is moved by insertion of the left index finger behind the uterus and its elevation with the vaginal fingers. The technique has been used in 500 patients, without difficulty. It is applicable to obese women. The tubes are easily ligated by the Pomeroy technique or by applying Bleier plastic clips. Movements should be made in a gentle, calculated manner.

Minilaparotomy has achieved high patient acceptance in developing countries because of the short convalescence. Use of the fingers rather than a metal uterine elevator precludes the need for cervical dilation and local anesthesia and avoids the risks of uterine perforation and contamination, cervical trauma, and endometritis. Minilaparotomy performed by well-trained personnel is a safe and effective method of female sterilization that can be offered to large numbers of women throughout the world.

▶ [Many devices have been described for elevating the uterus at minilaparotomy. Palaniappan suggests the gloved hand. His description of "handy" uterine elevators and his contention that minilaparotomy in the "hands" of well-trained personnel is especially applicable in developing countries merit applause.] ◀

Contact Hysteroscopy: New Technique to Explore the Uterine Cavity was evaluated by Michael S. Baggish[10-13] (Hartford, Conn.).

(10–13) Obstet. Gynecol. 54:350–354, September 1979.

Direct visualization of the uterine cavity by hysteroscopy has many potential advantages, including localization of pathology, determination of the adequacy of dilation and curettage or biopsy, an exact diagnosis of anomalies and synechiae, the detection of ectopic pregnancy, and localization of a "missing" intrauterine contraceptive device. In addition, hysteroscopy may be satisfactorily performed under local anesthesia. The contact hysteroscope consists of a transparent rod of optical glass, terminating as a nonreflective mirror and encased in a steel jacket. An adjustable focusing magnifier is attached directly to the lens. A paracervical block can be used for the procedure.

Sixty-five women were examined with the contact hysteroscope at the time of dilation and curettage, suction curettage, or laparotomy. Fifteen others were examined in an office setting. Forty patients were examined under paracervical block anesthesia, and 25 under general inhalational anesthesia. Endometrial abnormalities were distinguished from normal secretory or proliferative phase epithelium. Early embryos sometimes were evaluated without disrupting the amnion. No complications resulted from contact hysteroscopy.

Initial evaluation of the contact hysteroscope has given satisfactory results. Use of this instrument should provide substantial advantages to the physician who wishes to view the interior of the uterus. So long as contact with the endometrium is established, bleeding will not obscure vision. The principal disadvantage of contact hysteroscopy is the lack of a panoramic view. The contact hysteroscope is useful for examining the vagina and cervix in virginal girls. Perhaps the most important use of this method is in the diagnosis of endometrial carcinoma and its precursors. The observations may be helpful in planning treatment. Directed endometrial biopsy will permit outpatient diagnosis and eliminate a general anesthetic, and disease staging should be improved. Frequent observations of the effects of progestin therapy on hyperplastic endometrium should increase confidence in conservative management.

▶ [This preliminary report of a new type of hysteroscope is intriguing. Since the uterine cavity is not distended, no delivery system is required; in addition, the device is thinner than conventional scopes. Ambient room light is all that is required for illumination. The chief disadvantage is the lack of a panoramic view of the uterine cavity.] ◀

Corpus Luteum Surgery. Hemorrhage within a corpus luteum can produce a tender adnexal mass, and the presence of an unruptured corpus luteum cyst can lead to diagnostic confusion. Lester T. Hibbard[10-14] (Univ. of Southern California) reviewed 200 consecutive emergency laparotomies done in the past 6 years. There were 140 cases of ruptured corpus luteum, 26 of ruptured corpus luteum in pregnancy, 23 of corpus luteum cyst of pregnancy, and 11 of corpus luteum cyst.

Most patients presented with pain (table). More than half the women had delayed menstruation, but only 13 had irregular vaginal bleeding at admission, and none had excessive bleeding. The general physical findings were unremarkable. An ovarian cyst was palpated

(10–14) Am. J. Obstet. Gynecol. 135:666–670, Nov. 1, 1979.

CORPUS LUTEUM: DIAGNOSTIC FEATURES

	Ruptured corpus luteum	Ruptured corpus luteum of pregnancy	Corpus luteum cyst of pregnancy	Corpus luteum cyst
Pain	139/140	21/26	14/23	11/11
Delayed menstruation	69/125	26/26	23/23	6/10
Vaginal bleeding	9/132	2/26	1/23	1/10
False pregnancy test	5/126	2/22	0/22	1/8
False culdocentesis	2/140	1/25	3/16	1/7
Palpable mass	33/140	15/26	22/23	7/11

in 29 of 34 cases of unruptured cyst but in only 48 cases of ruptured cyst. Ruptured corpus luteum was more frequent on the right side.

Only 73 cases of ruptured corpus luteum in this series were correctly diagnosed preoperatively. No case of corpus luteum cyst was correctly diagnosed. All but 7 of the 49 patients with a corpus luteum of pregnancy had a primary preoperative diagnosis of ectopic pregnancy. Laparotomy was necessary in 13 cases, usually to control bleeding. Laparoscopy sufficed in most cases of both ruptured corpus luteum and corpus luteum cyst. Seven patients had a corpus luteum of pregnancy removed. Three of these pregnancies went to term. Six of 18 patients with a ruptured corpus luteum of pregnancy who were managed by observation or hemostatic measures went to term. No major operative complications occurred, and morbidity was minimal. The average hospital stay after laparoscopy was 1.2 days.

Routine culdocentesis and pregnancy testing will identify most patients with corpus luteum cyst or ruptured corpus luteum who can safely be managed by expectant observation or should have a diagnostic operative procedure such as laparoscopy before exploratory laparotomy is performed. When a laparotomy is done, the ovary should be conserved if possible.

▶ [This is a typical Hibbard paper—a concise, thoughtful, and practical approach to a clinical problem. It contains a number of suggestions for differentiating the ruptured corpus luteum from the ectopic pregnancy. One of these is entirely new to us—in ectopic pregnancy, the hematocrit on the cul-de-sac aspirate is nearly always more than 12%.] ◀

Ectopic Pregnancy: Current Clinical Trends. The diagnosis and management of ectopic pregnancy continue to be major problems. James D. Kitchin III, Robert M. Wein, Wallace C. Nunley, Jr., Siva Thiagarajah, and W. Norman Thornton, Jr.[10-15] (Univ. of Virginia) reviewed experience with 191 cases of ectopic pregnancy seen in the 16-year period ending in 1978. The overall incidence was 1 in 126 deliveries, but in the last 3 years of the study the incidence was 1 in 60 deliveries. An intrauterine device (IUD) was in place at the time of ectopic implantation in 10.5% of cases. Pregnancy had occurred at least twice previously in 56% of patients. Adequate follow-up was possible in 152 cases.

There was no history of a missed period in 20.4% of women, including 30% of those wearing an IUD. No vaginal bleeding or spotting had occurred since the last period in 31.4% of patients. Pain had been

(10–15)   Am. J. Obstet. Gynecol. 134:870–876, Aug. 15, 1979.

present for over a week in about one fourth of patients. Adnexal tenderness was a feature of 94.2% of cases and was often bilateral. An adnexal mass was palpated in 43% of patients, sometimes on the side opposite that of the gestation. The preoperative hematocrit correlated poorly with clinical shock. There were 3 ovarian pregnancies in the series. The corpus luteum was on the same side as the ectopic implantation in 57 of 84 evaluable cases. Salpingectomy was done in all but 1 of the patients with tubal implantations. There was 1 postoperative death. Blood transfusions were unnecessary in 38.2% of cases. Subsequent conception has occurred in 36.8% of the women followed, but only 36 of these 56 women have carried pregnancies to term. Ectopic pregnancy recurred in 13 women.

Current trends in ectopic pregnancy are discouragingly similar to those in earlier reports. Serious consideration should be given to methods of management that may offer better potential for future reproduction. Aggressive extirpative surgery may not be necessary in all cases. Improved tubal reconstructive procedures may improve the outlook for fertility in selected instances.

▶ [This review of the experience of the University of Virginia with ectopic pregnancy over a 16-year period underscores several important features of the condition. (1) The frequency seems to be increasing, related perhaps to increased gonorrhea prevalence or partially effective antibiotic therapy, or both, with the role of the IUD problematic. (2) The textbook clinical picture of a missed period, pain, bleeding, and a tender adnexal mass is far from invariable; with respect to all aspects except pain, 20% of patients had not missed a period, 30% gave no history of bleeding since the last menstrual period, 57% had no palpable mass, and 37% had either bilateral or no adnexal tenderness. (3) The prognosis for future reproduction is poor; scarcely more than a third of followed patients conceived and only two thirds of these carried their pregnancies to term. The standard operative treatment in this series was salpingectomy, and some would argue that the conception rate might be higher with conservative surgery.] ◀

Female Sterilization and Subsequent Ectopic Pregnancy. Ectopic pregnancy is one of the few true surgical emergencies facing the gynecologist on a relatively frequent basis. Its etiology remains controversial. Gordon C. Wolf and Nicholas J. Thompson[10-16] (Wright State Univ. School of Medicine, Dayton, Ohio) conducted an 8-year retrospective study in the Dayton, Ohio, area from 1970 to 1977, during which time there were 86,809 births and 721 tubal pregnancies. Thirty-three ectopic pregnancies were preceded by tubal sterilization. A total of 23,739 tubal sterilizations had been performed.

The median age of the 33 patients was 30.8 years. The average gravidity/parity was 3.2/2.7. Two thirds of the patients presented within 2½ years of their surgery. All had abdominal or pelvic pain, and only 2 patients reported normal menses. Twenty-nine patients had positive pregnancy tests; 3 negative tests were done before 1974. Eighteen patients had had a Pomeroy procedure and 15, laparoscopic sterilization. Both the "three-burn" and "burn and divide" techniques were used.

In only 15 patients was a correct diagnosis made at admission, although in 26 a correct preoperative diagnosis was made. The average

(10–16) Obstet. Gynecol. 55:17–19, January 1980.

time between admission and surgery was 28 hours. Fifteen patients had bilateral, and 12 unilateral, salpingectomy; 12 of these also had unilateral oophorectomy. Three patients had hysterectomy and bilateral salpingo-oophorectomy, 1 had hysterectomy only, and 2 had cornual resection. In 25 patients, ectopic pregnancy was in the distal segment or fimbria. Only 2 pregnancies were in the proximal segment. Distorted tubal anatomy secondary to the sterilization procedure was noted in 26 case reports.

The 7.4% rate of tubal sterilization preceding ectopic pregnancy in the past 4 years indicates the increasing importance of this factor as an etiologic agent in ectopic gestation. Candidates for sterilization should be counseled as to both the possibility and risk of extrauterine as well as intrauterine gestation subsequent to all methods of sterilization.

▶ [The number of tubal pregnancies appears to be increasing in Dayton, Ohio, as does the ratio of tubal to intrauterine gestations. This has been noted elsewhere and is thought to be due in part to an increased incidence of tubal infection, the use of intrauterine contraceptive devices, and perhaps, as suggested by this report, an increased prevalence of tubal sterilizations. Because we do not know the denominator (ie, the number of women who have had tubal sterilizations), we cannot estimate the risk of tubal pregnancy in sterilized women in this population. The point, of course, is to remember to consider the diagnosis of ectopic pregnancy in a patient with a suggestive history even though her tubes have been "tied"; 7.4% of patients with tubal pregnancies in 1974–1977 described here had had previous tubal sterilizations.] ◀

Incidental Appendectomy at the Time of Surgery for Ectopic Pregnancy. Although incidental appendectomy at the time of elective pelvic surgery is safe, it is not clear whether such an incidental procedure is prudent in nonelective and emergency cases. A. Dena Cromartie, Jr., and Paul J. Kovalcik[10-17] (Naval Regional Med. Center, Portsmouth, Va.) undertook a retrospective study to determine whether incidental appendectomy could be done safely in patients having surgery for ectopic pregnancy. Of 560 patients having surgically documented ectopic pregnancies in 1956–1976, 67 underwent incidental appendectomy at the time of primary surgery. Complication rate was 16.4% in the study group and 21.3% for the control group. Rate of specific complications possibly attributable to gastrointestinal surgery per se was 6.0% in the study group and 6.5% in the control group. Comparable numbers of patients in the two groups were operated on under emergency conditions. Significantly fewer study patients were admitted in hypovolemic shock.

It is concluded that incidental appendectomy can be done safely in selected patients at the time of surgery for ectopic pregnancy. The operative risk is not increased, and the patient is spared the possible subsequent development of acute appendicitis.

▶ [A number of studies have indicated that incidental appendectomy can be done safely in conjunction with various obstetric and gynecologic operations. Yet we suspect that most obstetrician-gynecologists would express some reluctance about the operation in a patient with ectopic pregnancy, citing such factors as the emergency nature of the surgery, the presence of blood in the peritoneal cavity, etc. This retrospective review seems to indicate that incidental appendectomy is safe at the time of operation for ectopic pregnancy. However, only 12% of ectopic patients had appen-

(10–17)   Am. J. Surg. 139:244–246, February 1980.

dectomy, so there was undoubtedly considerable selection exercised. This is borne out by the lower incidence of the incidental surgery in patients in shock. A definitive answer requires a prospective study with random assignment.] ◄

Analysis of Macrosurgical and Microsurgical Techniques in Management of Tuboperitoneal Factor in Infertility. Alvin M. Siegler and Vasilios Kontopoulos[10-18] (SUNY, Downstate Med. Center) analyzed 160 tubal reconstructions, half done just before and half after the adoption of microsurgical principles that included optimal magnification, gentle handling and constant irrigation of tissues, lysis of adhesions and tubal incisions with a unipolar microelectrode, and the use of fine sutures and microsurgical instruments. The average patient age was 28 years. In the more recent cases, the occluded tubal ends were removed serially with microscissors until patency was ascertained with indigo carmine dye. Corticosteroids were used with prophylactic antibiotics perioperatively in almost all patients until the most recent 40 operations. When antibiotics were used alone in alternate women, there was no difference in postoperative infectious morbidity between the two groups. Hydrotubation was not routinely carried out in cases of distal tubal obstruction.

No term pregnancies occurred in 20 patients who had ampullary or isthmic segments implanted. The outcome was not improved by varying the site of implantation from the cornu to the posterior uterine wall or by using microsurgical techniques for preparing the implanted tubal segment. Two patients had tubal pregnancies. Five of 20 patients who had anastomoses done without magnification conceived; 3 had tubal gestations. Six of the 16 patients who had anastomoses with microsurgical methods had term pregnancies; 2 are currently pregnant, and 1 had a tubal pregnancy. Fifteen salpingoneostomies done before the advent of microsurgery resulted in 2 term pregnancies and 3 tubal pregnancies. Twenty-three microsurgical procedures resulted in 5 term pregnancies and 3 tubal gestations, and 1 patient currently has an intrauterine pregnancy. Two of 11 patients who had conventional fimbrioplasties were delivered at term, and 2 had tubal gestations. Five of 9 patients who had microsurgical fimbrioplasties were delivered at term, and 1 tubal pregnancy occurred. In all, 12.5% of women conventionally operated on were delivered at term and 17% had tubal gestations. The respective figures for microsurgery were 28% and 11%. Three women with current intrauterine pregnancies could improve the microsurgical success rate to 31%.

Microsurgical tubal reconstruction does appear to improve postoperative pregnancy rates and to reduce tubal pregnancies.

► [Dr. Anthony A. Luciano of the University of Iowa reviewed this paper at our request and commented as follows:
"In this study, the authors report that the use of microsurgical techniques in the management of infertility associated with tuboperitoneal factors significantly improved the outcome. The overall success rate, determined by term pregnancy, more than doubled in the microsurgical series. As the authors point out and I wish to emphasize, microsurgery does not simply imply the use of magnification; the whole concept of fine surgery included embodies gentle handling and constant irrigation of tissues, meticulous hemostasis, the use of microsurgical instruments and fine sutures, careful

(10–18) Fertil. Steril. 32:377–383, October 1979.

dissection and precise tissue approximation. The principles, though recognized for many years, have been greatly refined and reemphasized with the advent of microsurgery. To what extent magnification alone contributes to the improved results cannot be ascertained either from this study or from any other yet published, since the patients in the microsurgical series benefited not only from the magnification of the microscope but also from the fine surgical techniques and the greater experience acquired by the surgeon in these procedures. Each of these factors might have contributed significantly toward a better outcome. However, whether or not the microscope is used by the infertility surgeon, the adoption of fine surgical techniques, as described above, is strongly recommended."

In a related study, Diamond (Fertil. Steril. 32:370, 1979) reported a 4.7 times improvement in term pregnancy rate with microsurgical techniques over gross approaches in cases of cornual occlusion.] ◄

Microsurgical Reversal of Female Sterilization: A Reappraisal. Reversal of female sterilization has been requested increasingly in the past decade. Earlier reports have claimed better results from microsurgical than from conventional reversal methods, but relatively few cases have been included in these studies. Victor Gomel[10-19] (Univ. of British Columbia) reviewed the results of microsurgical reversal of sterilization in 118 women, aged 21 to 39 years, treated in a 10-year period. All were cases of tubotubal anastomosis with the intramural segment forming part of the oviduct. The procedure was unilateral in 22 cases. The length of reconstructed tubes ranged from 2.5 to 8.5 cm. The interval from sterilization to request for reversal ranged from 1 week to 16 years. The proximal tubal lumen was enlarged where necessary because of significant discrepancy between the segments and unfreed stumps.

Seventy-six patients (64.4%) had achieved intrauterine pregnancy at follow-up. Many pregnancies occurred 18 months or more after operation, the mean interval being 10.2 months. One ectopic pregnancy occurred in an early case. The spontaneous abortion rate was 9.4%. Most patients who aborted achieved a viable pregnancy before or after this event. Of 36 patients in whom the only or the longest reconstructed oviduct measured 4 cm or less, 61.1% achieved pregnancy, a mean of 19.1 months after surgery. No significant complications occurred.

The satisfactory results of microsurgical reversal of tubal sterilization and the very low ectopic gestation rate are made possible by magnification and microsurgical technique, which permit total excision of the diseased segment, proper alignment, and accurate approximation of tissue planes with fine, inert sutures.

Microsurgical Reversal of Female Sterilization: Role of Tubal Length. Sherman J. Silber and Robert Cohen[10-20] (St. Louis) performed microsurgical reanastomosis of the fallopian tubes in 25 women who had undergone tubal sterilization by a variety of techniques. The only selection criterion was the presence of fimbriae on at least one side. Anatomical patency was achieved in all patients. Two patients had less than 2 cm of extrauterine tubal length, whereas 7 had more than 5 cm. Eleven patients required ampullary-isthmic anastomosis, 13 ampullary-cornual anastomosis, and 1 an

(10–19) Fertil. Steril. 33:587–597, June 1980.
(10–20) Ibid., pp. 598–601.

RELATION OF TOTAL TUBAL LENGTH TO PREGNANCY

Tubal length

	0–2 cm	2–3 cm	3–4 cm	4–5 cm	>5 cm
Total no. of patients	2	5	7	4	7
Pregnant	0	0	4	4	7
Not pregnant	2	5	3	0	0
Normal intrauterine pregnancy rate	0%	0%	43%	100%	100%

isthmic-cornual anastomosis. All patients have been followed for over 1 year.

Fifteen patients had achieved pregnancy at follow-up. One pregnancy was ectopic. The chance of a normal pregnancy was directly related to the length of the tube remnant (table). About half the patients with 3 to 4 cm of tube on the longer side remaining achieved a normal intrauterine pregnancy, as did all 11 with more than 4 cm of tube remnant. None of 7 patients with less than 3 cm of tube remaining achieved pregnancy despite accurate anastomosis. Ampullary length had no substantial effect on outcome so long as at least 1 cm of ampulla remained. Most patients had undergone laparoscopic cauterization. The only type of sterilization that reliably left a long segment of tube was the Falope-Ring procedure.

The findings support the view that tubal length is a critical factor in tubal reanastomosis, but the length of residual ampulla is less important than was previously thought. Insurance of the least amount of tissue damage is important in making sterilization as reversible as possible. The chance of reversibility is considerably reduced if more than half the tube is destroyed on both sides. If tubal destruction is extensive, an autotransplant to the opposite side, using microvascular anastomoses, may usefully create one long tube rather than two short ones.

▶ [Both this article and the preceding one emphasize the importance of tubal length to successful reversal of female sterilizations. As long as the frimbriae and 1 cm of the ampulla were present, the site of the anastomosis was not the critical factor. The results of these two microsurgical series are certainly excellent.] ◀

Prevention of Postoperative Tubal Adhesions: Comparative Study of Commonly Used Agents. Development of adhesions after pelvic surgery is a major cause of bowel obstruction and failure of reconstructive tubal surgery. Gere S. diZerega and Gary D. Hodgen[10-21] (Natl. Inst. of Health) compared the efficacy of several commonly used regimens in preventing adhesions following trauma to the fimbriated end of the fallopian tubes in rhesus monkeys. None of the animals had preexisting tubal adhesions. Tubal patency was assessed immediately prior to operation and 2 weeks postoperatively.

Five monkeys had only tubal abrasion without prior assessment of tubal patency. Five had tubal abrasion with assessment of tubal pa-

(10–21) Am. J. Obstet. Gynecol. 136:173–178, Jan. 15, 1980.

tency before and after traumatization. Five had identical studies performed, but were treated with intramuscular dexamethasone (0.5 mg), promethazine (5 mg), and ampicillin (125 mg) twice daily, beginning 2 days preoperatively and continuing for 5 days postoperatively. Another five monkeys underwent identical surgical procedures, but received 20 ml of 10% dextran 40 in normal saline intraperitoneally before the abdomen was closed. Another group received 20 ml of 32% dextran 70 in dextrose intraperitoneally after tubal abrasion. Two additional monkeys also received the 32% dextran 70 protocol; biopsies of the fimbriae were performed before the abrasion and 2, 5 and 7 days later, at which times the presence or absence of 32% dextran 70 was noted.

Following tubal abrasion, extensive bilateral adhesions developed in all of the untreated animals and in those treated with dexamethasone-promethazine-ampicillin and 10% dextran 40. The adhesions involved fimbria, omentum, ovary, uterus, bowel, and bladder. However, only 1 monkey treated with 32% dextran 70 had a slight unilateral adhesion.

Of the 10 tubes evaluated in the 32% dextran 70 group, 9 were patent prior to abrasion. All 9 were patent 2 weeks after trauma. In the other groups in which patency was evaluated, 27 tubes were patent before tubal abrasion, but only 1 remained so 2 weeks later. This difference is highly significant.

Microscopic changes including epithelial swelling and vacuolization, stromal edema, hemorrhage, and neutrophil infiltration were observed in the fimbriae within 15 minutes after tubal abrasion. By 2 days later, frank epithelial sloughing and massive stromal changes were seen. Significant healing with reepithelialization was seen by 5 days postoperatively. Restoration of normal tubal epithelium had taken place by day 7. The 32% dextran 70 was evident in the pelvic cavity on day 5, but not on day 7 after administration. These observations support the idea that 32% dextran 70 is efficacious because it prevents tissue apposition during the period of epithelial repair.

▶ [The results of this experimental animal study seem quite clear—systemic drugs alleged to prevent adhesion formation were ineffective against tubal adhesions in the monkey, as was 10% dextran 40, but striking protection was afforded by 32% dextran 70. Presumably, the higher concentration and higher molecular weight dextran remains as some type of coating long enough to prevent coapting of abraded tissues. In a limited experience with this approach in patients, we have been impressed with an increased incidence of postoperative ileus.] ◀

Prevention of Postoperative Thromboembolism by Dextran 70 or Low-Dose Heparin was assessed by Michael K. Hohl, Klaus P. Lüscher, Jan Tichý, Marianne Stiner, Raimund Fridrich, Ulrich F. Gruber, and Otto Käser[10-22] (Univ. of Basel).

The 232 women over 40 years of age admitted for major gynecologic surgery were randomly assigned to two treatment groups. One group (117 patients) received intravenous dextran 70 during and after the procedure. The second group (115 patients) received subcutaneous low-dose heparin before and for 7 days following operation. During

(10–22) Obstet. Gynecol. 55:497–500, April 1980.

the first study, all patients had ^{125}I fibrinogen uptake tests in the perioperative period. Positive leg scans were confirmed by venogram. During the second phase of the study, fibrinogen uptake studies were not done, but when deep vein thrombosis was suspected clinically, it was confirmed by venogram.

Positive leg scans were seen in 14.5% of the patients treated with dextran, but only in 1.7% of the heparinized patients. Of the deep vein thromboses, 26% were bilateral; 57% occurred within 3 days postoperatively. Deep vein thromboses developed more often in patients with malignant disease rather than benign conditions. These patients were also older than those without deep vein thrombosis.

The type of operation influenced the incidence of deep vein thrombosis in the dextran-treated group. Significantly more deep vein thromboses occurred after vaginal hysterectomy with colporrhaphy than after abdominal hysterectomy.

Nonfatal pulmonary embolism was confirmed in 2 patients treated with dextran, and venous thromboembolic disease was a contributing factor in the death of another dextran 70-treated patient within a month after operation.

These data indicate that heparin was more effective than low-dose dextran in the prevention of deep vein thrombosis postoperatively. The benefit to hazard ratio appears to favor the use of heparin rather than dextran 70 for the prophylaxis of deep vein thrombosis following major gynecologic surgery.

▶ [Just which gynecologic surgical patients should receive prophylactic anticoagulation remains a matter of dispute. Obesity and malignancy are frequent indications on our service for low-dose heparin anticoagulation of patients undergoing major gynecologic procedures. Heparin did a better job than dextran 70 when administered according to this study's protocol.] ◀

Posttransfusion Purpura as Gynecologic Complication. Posttransfusion purpura is a recently separated category of thrombocytopenic purpura occurring mainly in women. Brian H. Rank, Charles Gay, Lillian Burke, Keith Wright, Donald J. Nollet, and David J. Blomberg[10-23] review this condition and report an illustrative case.

Woman, 54, was admitted for anemia and menometrorrhagia of five weeks' duration. She received a transfusion of 2 units of blood, and on the fifth day of hospitalization total abdominal hysterectomy, salpingectomy, and oophorectomy were performed; another unit of blood was given postoperatively. Recovery was uneventful until the fourth postoperative day when a fresh clot in the incision, purpura, multiple petechiae in the groin, copious vaginal bleeding, and epistaxis were noted. Platelet count was 29,000 mm³. Clotting studies were normal. Bone marrow biopsy showed decreased basophils and increased megakaryocytes and megakaryocyte precursors. All medications were discontinued and prednisone therapy initiated. A platelet isoantibody in the serum was identified by clot retraction inhibition, complement fixation, and ^{51}Cr release methods. Following exchange transfusion, the patient's condition improved and she has had no further complications.

The differential diagnosis in this case included immune-drug purpura, bone marrow suppression secondary to medication, disseminated intravascular coagulation, posttransfusion purpura, and idio-

(10–23) Obstet. Gynecol. 55(Suppl.):72S–75S, March 1980.

pathic thrombocytopenic purpura. The diagnosis of posttransfusion purpura depends on the demonstration of antiplatelet antibodies. Several laboratory techniques are available to detect these antibodies and more than one method should be used when posttransfusion purpura is suspected.

Posttransfusion purpura is rare, but may be life-threatening and may considerably lengthen a hospitalization. Adequate methods are available for treatment, however, preferably exchange transfusion or plasmapheresis unless contraindicated. A high index of suspicion and knowledge of this entity are necessary to avoid unnecessary morbidity and mortality.

► [This report was abstracted to call attention to an entity that we had not heard of, posttransfusion purpura. Severe thrombocytopenia presenting 5 to 12 days after blood transfusion should suggest the possibility of this rare condition. Just as one seems likely to soon see or hear a word that has been recently added to his or her vocabulary, we anticipate that we will soon see such a patient. Our hematologists recommend plasmaphoresis as therapy for this problem.] ◄

Psychiatric Status After Hysterectomy: One-Year Prospective Follow-up. Adverse psychiatric sequelae have traditionally been ascribed to hysterectomy, but prospective studies have not supported a posthysterectomy syndrome. Ronald L. Martin, William V. Roberts, and Paula J. Clayton[10-24] (Washington Univ.) evaluated 44 randomly selected women, who underwent hysterectomy for indications other than cancer, before and 1 year after operation. The Zung Self-Rating Depression Scale was administered. Mean follow-up interval was 11.7 months. There had been 1 surgical and 5 medical hospitalizations at the time of follow-up.

All but 2 of the 17 patients who received anxiolytic drugs after operation and all 4 given antidepressants or stimulants had also received them before hysterectomy. Two patients received outpatient psychiatric care, 1 for the first time. One patient was psychiatrically hospitalized with signs of psychosis, but they rapidly remitted. Hysteria was diagnosed in 13 women and primary affective disorder, depression, in 9. Secondary depression was diagnosed in 6. All but 3 depressed patients had an index psychiatric illness. The group as a whole showed a nonsignificant decrease in depression ratings at follow-up. Posthysterectomy syndome was diagnosed in 11 women (25%). Ten of these patients were hysterical. Sexual dysfunction was not significantly more frequent after operation. Presenting complaints were relieved or improved in 89% of the patients. Fatigue and headaches were related to less than total oophorectomy.

Hysterectomy was not associated with adverse psychiatric sequelae in this series. Women with psychiatric symptoms at follow-up generally had had similar problems before operation. Many symptoms were associated with a preoperative diagnosis of hysteria. When hysteria is diagnosed, surgical decisions should be based on objective findings rather than on the patient's subjective complaints.

► [This is a follow-up report of a study abstracted in the 1979 YEAR BOOK (p. 254). Hysterectomy was not followed by an excess of psychiatric symptoms in these patients.

(10–24) JAMA 244:350–353, July 25, 1980.

The initial prevalence of hysteria was high (27%), and 38% of the hysterics (vs none of the nonhysterics) reported unsatisfactory relief of their presenting complaints. Hysterectomy clearly is not appropriate therapy for hysteria! The authors point out that hysterics are often inconsistent and unreliable historians. Several office visits may be required to decide whether a particular patient will truly be benefited by hysterectomy.] ◀

11. Tumors

Vulvar Neoplasia in the Young. Vulvar carcinoma in situ occurs most frequently in the fifth and sixth decades of life, but a trend toward development of this lesion in younger patients has been noted recently. George D. Hilliard, Fred M. Massey, and Robert V. O'Toole, Jr.[11-1] (Lackland AFB) encountered 6 patients under age 30 with intraepithelial neoplasms and 1 with microinvasive cancer in 1972–1977. The age range at diagnosis was 20–28 years. Tissue diagnosis was significantly delayed in 4 patients. Three were asymptomatic, but 1 of these patients noted an enlarging lesion. Three patients had abnormal Papanicolaou smears, 1 of which was categorized as class II. All 3 of these patients had concurrent cervical disease. Five patients were thought clinically not to have neoplasia.

Four patients had carcinoma in situ, 2 had severe dysplasia, and 1 had microinvasive carcinoma of the vulva. Five had significant intraepithelial neoplasia in the cervix or vagina. Most of the lesions, which had a wide anatomical distribution, had the gross appearance of condyloma acuminatum. Most were multicentric. Chronic dermal inflammation was usually present. Dysplasia was regularly observed adjacent to lesions interpreted as carcinoma in situ. Treatment included simple vulvectomy, wide local excision, and application of 5-fluorouracil (5-FU) cream. In 3 of 4 patients treated with 5% 5-FU ointment, response was complete, and there have been no recurrences on short-term follow-up.

Serious vulvar lesions, which may be mistaken for more benign growths, can develop in young women. These lesions respond poorly to various creams and solutions in common use. The entire genital tract must be evaluated when early neoplasia is found in the cervix, vagina, or vulva, and early biopsy must be considered, even in the young patient. Close follow-up is necessary after treatment of these vulvar lesions.

▶ [This report illustrates that vulvar dysplastic changes are not limited to middle-aged or elderly patients. The coexistence of vaginal or cervical intraepithelial neoplasia is again shown to be common (5 of the 7 patients described). Although 5-FU is mentioned in this report, it has not been an effective therapy of vulvar neoplasia on our service.] ◀

Carcinoma In Situ of the Vulva: Continuing Challenge. Eduard G. Friedrich, Jr., Edward J. Wilkinson, and Yao Shi Fu[11-2] reviewed the epidemiologic, clinical, and histologic findings in 50 cases of carcinoma in situ of the vulva. The mean patient age was 38.9; 76% of patients were premenopausal. Parity was highly variable; nearly a third of patients were nulligravid. Condyloma acuminatum, herpes simplex, gonorrhea, syphilis, *Hemophilus vaginalis* and tri-

(11–1) Am. J. Obstet. Gynecol. 135:185–188, Sept. 15, 1979.
(11–2) Ibid., 136:830–843, Apr. 1, 1980.

chomonas were present alone or in combination in 60% of patients. Condyloma acuminatum was or had been present in 13 patients. Fifteen patients had a total of 21 tumors, the most common associated neoplasm being cervical carcinoma. Most lesions were not deep. Eleven patients had anal involvement. Twenty-four patients (48%) were completely asymptomatic.

Ten patients were managed primarily by shallow or deep total vulvectomy. One died postoperatively of pulmonary embolism. One patient with positive urethral margins had a recurrence after 4 years. Partial vulvectomy was done as a primary procedure in 10 patients. One of 7 patients with disease-free margins had a recurrence, but 2 of 3 with involved surgical margins have been free of disease for 2 and 4 years, respectively. Wide local excision was done as primary therapy in 17 patients. All but 2 of 15 patients with tumor-free margins have been free of disease for 2 to 9 years. Three women failed to respond to topical 5-fluorouracil therapy. In only 1 patient did an in situ lesion progress to invasive carcinoma. Five patients had spontaneous regression of disease. All these had aneuploid lesions at the time of diagnosis. Multiple clones were observed in 2 of these.

Nearly one third of these patients had antecedent or concomitant evidence of DNA viral infection of the vulva. Treatment should be individualized. Reliable patients may safely be observed for 1 or 2 years for spontaneous regression, especially if the diagnosis is made during pregnancy. Prompt therapy is indicated for immunosuppressed patients and those in later life. The extent of excision is dictated by the extent and location of the lesions.

Carcinoma In Situ of the Vulva. Joseph Buscema, J. Donald Woodruff, T. H. Parmley, and R. Genadry[11-3] (Johns Hopkins Hosp.) reviewed 106 cases of carcinoma in situ of the vulva occurring over the past 15 years in order to identify the pathology and evaluate the results of various therapeutic methods. Clinical data and follow-up were available for 102 patients.

Average age of the 102 patients was 47 years; however, 40% were under age 41. Associated cervical malignancies were found in 28 of the 106 patients (27%). A slightly higher than expected incidence of multicentric disease in the lower genital canal was noted. Because about 20% of the patients were asymptomatic, discovery of the lesions was the result of the high index of suspicion based on the known frequency of multicentric disease.

Pathologic studies revealed various grossly observable patterns with more than one clinical feature frequently noted in the same patient. "Warty" tumors were seen by the physician or noted by the patient in about 20% of the cases. Due to the multiplicity of patterns, a biopsy of all unusual lesions is imperative.

Microscopic examination also showed the lesions to vary greatly. The lesion with little, if any, abnormality of the surface epithelium but demonstrating atypical maturation at the base of the rete pegs is of major significance and most difficult to assess. Tissue sections from

(11–3) Obstet. Gynecol. 55:225–230, February 1980.

the initial lesion in a patient who eventually developed invasive cancer showed such an atypicality with intraepithelial keratin pearls dropping off at the base into the underlying tissue. This finding is histopathologically classic for squamous cell carcinoma and reemphasizes the histologic classification of carcinoma of the vulva as a squamous cell, not epidermoid, lesion.

Patients treated by wide local excision had an incidence of recurrence comparable to that of patients treated by vulvectomy. Specimens taken during vulvectomy often showed little or no evidence of histologic abnormality, and it was assumed that vulvectomy was not necessary in many of these patients. It is suggested that carcinoma in situ of the vulva be treated only by local excision.

Invasive cancer developed in only 4 of the 102 patients, 2 whose disease appeared after age 70 and 2 who had been treated with immunosuppressive agents for systemic disease.

▶ [This article and the preceding one together present the largest series of vulvar carcinoma in situ published. They confirm numerous associations found in earlier studies, notably those with sexually transmitted diseases and malignancies elsewhere in the genital tract. This disease differs greatly from cervical carcinoma. In the first place, the vulvar condition is often associated with symptoms (itching in approximately half) or a gross lesion, or both. Moreover, the histologic picture is highly variable and lesions that appear relatively innocent by standards for cervical pathology may be quite aggressive; an example is illustrated in Figure 5 in the original article, which would probably be diagnosed as something like "basal cell hyperplasia" in the cervix and would not be considered especially dangerous. Spontaneous regression does occur, so there may be a place for observation without surgical excision for a year or two in carefully selected instances. Treatment should be individualized since, in the words of Friedrich and colleagues, "The probability of recurrent in situ disease depends more upon the presence or absence of tumor at the surgical margins than upon the magnitude of the operative procedure." Although histologic examination of the surgical margins is important, it is not completely accurate; three of Friedrich's 37 patients with tumor-free margins developed recurrences.] ◀

Alternate Approach to Early Cancer of Vulva. The traditional management of vulvar carcinoma has been radical vulvectomy with inguinal and pelvic lymphadenectomy. Improved patient survival has resulted from this approach and morbidity has been reduced in recent years; however, the procedure has serious adverse effects on body image and sexual function. Philip J. DiSaia, William T. Creasman, and William M. Rich[11-4] used a modified approach in 18 patients, median age 46, with early invasive carcinoma of the vulva, the goal being to preserve vulvar tissue and sexual function without sacrificing curability. The patients had primary lesions 1 cm or less in diameter confined to the vulva or perineum; focal invasion was limited to 5 mm in depth. Only squamous carcinomas were included. Six patients had a history of intraepithelial neoplasia of the cervix or vagina.

The superficial inguinal nodes are used as sentinel nodes in treatment planning. Wide local excision of the vulvar skin is carried out with removal of adequate subcutaneous tissue, leaving a 3-cm margin of normal skin on all sides of the primary lesion. Skin grafts, if needed, are generally taken from the medial thigh. The mean length of follow-up after wide local excision was 32 months. No recurrences

(11–4) Am. J. Obstet. Gynecol. 133:825–832, Apr. 1, 1979.

developed in this series. Two other patients had metastatic disease in the superficial inguinal nodes and underwent radical vulvectomy and node dissection. Adequate sexual function was preserved in the 18 patients having wide local excision. The mons veneris and clitoris, as well as most of the superior aspect of the vulva, were preserved in these women.

Dissection of the superficial inguinal nodes through small groin incisions permits adequate assessment of vulvar carcinoma. Early invasive but nonaggressive lesions can be managed by wide local excision, with careful follow-up of the remaining vulvar skin. Many of the most erogenous zones of the female anatomy may be preserved using the described modified approach, and sexual function is minimally altered.

▶ [Microinvasive carcinoma of the vulva can be associated with positive lymph nodes. In a previous edition (1979 YEAR BOOK, p. 267–268), we agreed with the view that radical vulvectomy with bilateral inguinal lymphadenectomy was the procedure of choice in this condition. The authors of the present report suggest that tumor emboli from a primary lesion are rapidly deposited in the draining lymph nodes and that disease between the early primary (<1 cm diameter; ≤5 mm of focal invasion) and the regional nodes is unusual. Therefore, they performed wide local excision and bilateral superficial inguinal lymphadenectomy. If the nodes were positive (2 of 20 patients), radical vulvectomy and bilateral inguinal lymphadenectomy and an ipsilateral pelvic node dissection were carried out. If the nodes were negative, radical vulvectomy was not performed. More experience is required to know whether or not this lesser procedure is as effective in these early cases as is radical vulvectomy. The authors' point that this less mutilating procedure is more acceptable to patients in terms of body image and sexual function is well taken.] ◀

Malignant Melanoma of the Vagina: Report of 19 Cases is presented by Arthur F. Chung, Murray J. Casey, J. T. Flannery, James M. Woodruff, and John L. Lewis, Jr.[11-5] Average age of the 19 patients, seen from 1934 to 1976, was 60 years. Seven patients were nulligravidas. No patient had a family history of melanoma. Thirteen women had vaginal bleeding; 11 were postmenopausal. The lesions were most commonly in the lower third of the vagina, on the anterior wall. About half the lesions showed a mixture of nevoid, spindle, and epithelioid cells. Many showed cellular pleomorphism. Vascular invasion was seen in only 1 specimen. No lesion was confined to the vaginal epithelium.

Seven women initially underwent radical surgery, 8 had primary radiotherapy, and 3 had wide local excision. One was untreated because of widespread metastases at diagnosis. Primary radical surgery provided local control in 5 of the 7 cases. All patients who underwent wide local excision had recurrent disease and died with metastatic melanoma. Primary radiotherapy produced local control in only 1 patient. Fourteen patients had recurrent or metastatic disease, or both, after primary treatment. Median time to recurrence was 9 months. One of 9 patients was cured of recurrence by radical surgery. Median survival time after recurrence was 1 year. Only 1 patient has lived more than 5 years after treatment of recurrence. Overall 5-year survival was 21%.

(11–5) Obstet. Gynecol. 55:720–727, June 1980.

Patients with primary vaginal melanoma should be treated by removal of the entire vaginal mucosa, adjacent tissues, and regional lymphatic drainage. Pelvic node dissections should be done when the upper two thirds of the vagina is involved. In lower-third cases, vulvectomy should be included. Radiotherapy and cytotoxic chemotherapy may be useful adjuncts. Immunotherapy may also have a role after surgical excision, especially in patients with microscopic node disease.

▶ [Malignant melanoma of the vagina is a rare tumor with a poor prognosis (related in part to a tendency for deep invasion, according to the authors of this article). Based on this series, radical surgery appears to be the therapy of choice.] ◀

Evaluation of Smears Obtained by Cervical Scraping and an Endocervical Swab in Diagnosis of Neoplastic Disease of the Uterine Cervix. Preben Johansen, Erik Arffmann, and Gorm Pallesen[11-6] (Aalborg, Denmark) examined the diagnostic value of endocervical swab specimens as an adjunct to the usual cervical scraping method in the diagnosis of neoplastic disease of the uterine cervix. Studies were done in 312 women seen consecutively in a 9-month period because of abnormal cervical smears or known intraepithelial neoplasia of the cervix. A scraping from the squamocolumnar junction was followed by an endocervical swab procedure. Both samples were satisfactory in 168 cases and were obtained within 3 months of tissue sampling. These patients had a mean age of 33 years. Cone biopsy or hysterectomy was performed on 57 patients.

Correlation between cytologic and histologic findings was exact in 65% of 182 cases when cervical scrapings were used and in 63% when the endocervical swab method was used. These methods correctly anticipated the histologic diagnosis of mild to moderate dysplasia in 45% and 66% of cases, respectively, and that of severe dysplasia or carcinoma in situ in 66% and 46%. Invasive squamous carcinoma was diagnosed by cervical scraping in 6 of 8 cases, whereas abnormal findings were underestimated in the endocervical swab specimen in 4 cases. The combination of cytologic methods resulted in exact correlation with the histologic findings in 69% of cases. False negative rates are given in Tables 1 and 2. There were no false positive cytologic diagnoses of neoplasia among the 57 patients in whom cone biopsy or hysterectomy was done, and the combination of cytologic methods had an accuracy of 70% in these patients.

TABLE 1.—FALSE NEGATIVE RATES FOR SMEARS OBTAINED BY CERVICAL SCRAPING, ENDOCERVICAL SWAB, AND COMBINATION OF THE TWO TECHNIQUES IN MILD-MODERATE DYSPLASIA GROUP

Cell collection technique	False negative rate %
Cervical scraping	36
Endocervical swab	25
Cervical scraping and endocervical swab	13

(11–6) Acta Obstet. Gynecol. Scand. 58:265–270, 1979.

TABLE 2.—FALSE NEGATIVE RATES FOR SMEARS OBTAINED BY
CERVICAL SCRAPING, ENDOCERVICAL SWAB, AND COMBINATION
OF THE TWO TECHNIQUES IN SEVERE DYSPLASIA-CARCINOMA IN
SITU GROUP

Cell collection technique	False negative rate %
Cervical scraping	10
Endocervical swab	14
Cervical scraping and endocervical swab	6

The endocervical swab smear contributes to the detection of mild and moderate cervical dysplasia, but cervical scrapings reveal more severe dysplasias and carcinomas in situ. A combination of the two methods is optimal for detecting both mild to moderate dysplasia and severe dysplasia-carcinoma through reducing the false negative rate. The endocervical swab method should not be used alone because unsatisfactory smears are more frequent, and the severity of epithelial lesions may be underestimated.

▶ [Articles over the past several years have come down on both sides of the issue of whether an endocervical cytologic sample should be obtained in addition to the cervical scraping. In the present report, a moistened cotton swab was used to sample the endocervix after the exocervical scraping had been taken. This second sample reduced the false negative rates, especially in cases of mild to moderate dysplasia. One patient with invasive cancer had an abnormal endocervical smear but a negative cervical scraping. Whether the beneficial effects of sampling the endocervix were due to the location of small dysplastic lesions in the cervical canal or simply to the provision of more cells for analysis is unclear. Stated differently, would a second exocervical scraping have decreased the false negative rate to a similar degree (see Luthy, et al.: Obstet. Gynecol. 51:713, 1978)?] ◀

An Etiologic Survey of Clinical Factors in Cervical Intraepithelial Neoplasia: Transverse Retrospective Study. Cervical intraepithelial neoplasia has been steadily increasing since 1970. Bernard Lambert, Richard Morisset, and Pierre Bielmann[11-7] (Montreal, Que.) examined the factors possibly associated with intraepithelial neoplasia in a retrospective survey of 123 patients and 112 control patients. Fourteen epidemiologic variables were assessed by stepwise logistic multiple regression analysis. Double-blind questionnaires were administered to all patients.

The neoplasia patients were slightly younger than the controls and appeared to have a lower educational level. More neoplasia patients were from lower socioeconomic families. The variable most related to development of neoplasia was the first sexual contact, patients with the earliest sexual exposure tending to have a higher incidence of cervical intraepithelial neoplasia. This factor remained of prime importance when nulliparas were excluded from analysis. Socioeconomic status, as reflected by the husband's or father's occupation, was the next most important factor.

These findings appear to deny a role to a number of epidemiologic factors in appearance of cervical dysplasia and carcinoma in situ.

(11–7) J. Reprod. Med. 24:26–31, January 1980.

Promiscuity and contraception did not appear to be significant factors in the incidence of cervical intraepithelial neoplasia. The most significant factors were age at first sexual contact and socioeconomic status. Future studies should examine variations in food intake, personal hygiene, and immunoresistance and its possible variations with socioeconomic status. Other factors such as vitamin A will also have to be correlated with carcinogenesis of the cervix. A target population should be females aged 19 to 20 years.

▶ [As medical students, we learned of several demographic and behavioral variables that are associated with the development of carcinoma of the cervix and presumably with cervical intraepithelial neoplasia as well. Many of these variables are interrelated, and therefore the connection between a particular variable and the development of cervical dysplasia or cancer is problematic. The statistical tool of stepwise multiple regression analysis should be useful in establishing which factors are independently important. The present study suggests that age at first intercourse is the most important variable. This view is consistent with that found in a report concerning abnormal cervical cytology in Taiwanese prostitutes (1979 YEAR BOOK, p. 271). Apparently the cervical transformation zone in the young is especially susceptible to carcinogenic influences.] ◀

Cervical Crypt Involvement by Intraepithelial Neoplasia. Local treatments for cervical intraepithelial neoplasia (CIN) destroy only a superficial layer of tissue, but CIN may involve the cervical crypts, and abnormal epithelium may be present several millimeters beneath the cervical surface, even without invasion. Subsequent colposcopy and cytologic study may yield normal findings, but theoretically the buried islands of CIN could become invasive. M. C. Anderson and R. B. Hartley[11-8] (London) examined the involvement of cervical crypts by CIN grade 3 (severe dysplasia and carcinoma in situ) to define the depth of destruction needed for adequate treatment. Review was made of 343 conization specimens obtained between 1970 and 1978. Mean patient age was 32 years. An average of 15 sections per cone was examined.

The mean depth of uninvolved crypts was 3.4 mm; the deepest uninvolved crypt extended 7.8 mm beneath the surface. No crypt involvement was demonstrated in 11.4% of women with CIN grade 3. The mean depth of involved crypts was 1.2 mm; the deepest involved crypt was 5.2 mm from the surface. Crypt involvement did not exceed 2.9 mm in 95% of cases and did not exceed 3.8 mm in 99.7%. Deeper sectioning of the specimens did not alter the findings significantly. The depth of crypt involvement increased gradually with age, but not significantly.

If nonsurgical techniques such as diathermy or cryocautery are used to treat patients with grade 3 CIN, consistent and effective destruction of tissue to depths of 3 and 4 mm should eradicate the disease in 95% and 99.7%, respectively. Destruction should extend at least 4 mm throughout the transformation zone when conservative methods are used to treat patients with grade 3 CIN.

▶ [This study has important implications regarding nonextirpative treatment (ie, cryotherapy, electrocautery, laser) of cervical intraepithelial neoplasia. The mean depth of crypt involvement was 1.24 mm; thus, assuming normal distribution, 95% of

(11–8) Obstet. Gynecol. 55:546–550, May 1980.

involved tissue would be included in a depth of 2.92 mm and 99.7% in a depth of 3.8 mm. Destructive therapy to depths less than this is presumably responsible for CIN recurrence after local treatment.] ◄

Study of Cryosurgery for Dysplasia and Carcinoma In Situ of the Uterine Cervix. There has been increasing interest in cryosurgery for benign and premalignant lesions of the uterine cervix. B. Elmfors and N. Stormby,[11-9] in a study at two hospitals in Sweden, examined the effects of cryosurgery in women under age 40 with abnormal cervical smears in whom dysplasia or carcinoma in situ had been diagnosed by punch biopsy.

A total of 89 patients with carcinoma in situ and 22 with dysplasia were studied during 2 years. The age range was 18 to 39 years. Mean parity was 1.8; 13 patients were nulliparous. Cryosurgery was done with the use of liquid nitrous oxide as refrigerant and a 25-mm cone-shaped cervical probe with a 20-mm endocervical extension.

Of the 91 patients treated by cryosurgery, 16 had severe dysplasia and 75 had carcinoma in situ. Normal smears were obtained from 86% of the patients after one cryosurgical treatment. Of the other 17 patients, 11 had further cryosurgery, with normal smears developing in 8 of them, and 6 had a conization. Among 33 pregnancies that followed cryosurgery were 2 low birth weight infants, 1 with meningomyelocele. Two patients with previous secondary infertility conceived after cryosurgery.

Seven of 62 biopsies obtained 1 year after cryosurgery showed slight atypia, and 2 showed residual carcinoma in situ. All subsequent smears were negative without further measures.

These results support reports that cryosurgery is an effective means of treating preinvasive cervical carcinoma and allied conditions. Expertise in colposcopy is necessary for adequate cryosurgical treatment. Conization may be indicated in the few patients in whom cryosurgery fails. Further prolonged follow-up of treated patients is needed to prove that cryosurgery is a definitive treatment for precancerous lesions of the cervix.

► [The "cure rate" of 90% for cryotherapy of cervical intraepithelial neoplasia grade 3 (ie, carcinoma in situ and severe dysplasia) noted here is almost exactly that found with previous studies with shorter durations of follow-up. To temper the enthusiasm evident in this and earlier articles, we would point out the obvious—a 90% cure rate means a 10% failure rate. In our opinion, cryotherapy of cervical intraepithelial grade 3 lesions should be used only in very carefully selected instances in which compelling reasons exist to avoid other approaches (hysterectomy or conization) and careful follow-up is assured.] ◄

High-Power Density Carbon Dioxide Laser Therapy for Early Cervical Neoplasia is discussed by Michael S. Baggish[11-10] (Mount Sinai Hosp., Hartford, Conn.). The carbon dioxide (CO_2) laser has recently become available as a treatment modality for early cervical neoplasia. Aggressive, high-power density CO_2 laser beam therapy was used to treat 115 women with various grades of cervical intraepithelial neoplasia.

The laser functions surgically by vaporizing tissue. A helium neon

(11–9) Br. J. Obstet. Gynaecol. 86:917–921, December 1979.
(11–10) Am. J. Obstet. Gynecol. 136:117–125, Jan. 1, 1980.

laser with a visible red aiming beam operates coincidentally to provide a visual target at the treatment site. Safety for both the patient and operator must be insured by careful precautions.

Patients ranged from 18 to 82 years of age. The first 50 women were followed every other day for 4 weeks after laser treatment to observe healing. The other patients were examined at 3 and 6 weeks posttreatment, then at 6-month intervals. If persistent atypia were found, retreatment was initiated. Follow-up ranged from 8 months to 2 years.

Laser power densities of approximately 1000 watts/cm^2 second and continuous time modes provided better depth of destruction in affected tissues.

The healing process involved 48 hours of maximum sloughing of necrotic tissue. Spotty bleeding was present in 10% of the patients, but none had substantial blood loss. Moderate leukorrhea peaked by 96 hours. Margins surrounding the treated area remained pink. By 7 days, the discharge ceased; by 14 days the depression was fully covered by squamous cells. Healing was substantially complete in 3 weeks, and by 4 weeks the treatment site could not be identified if not previously marked.

Initially, only small areas were treated at each session, but experience showed that laser treatment did not cause scarring, adhesions, or stenosis, so that extensive lesions could be treated at a single sitting. If heat buildup in the tissues was allowed to dissipate, there was little discomfort.

The failure rate was 4.34%. Of 25 patients with mild dysplasia, none required more than two treatments. In the 43 patients with moderate dysplasia, 9 required two sessions and 2 patients required a third treatment. Of 47 patients with more advanced lesions, 12 required more than one treatment. Most of the persistent lesions occurred early in the study when the peripheral extent of treatment and depth of destruction were more limited.

Advantages of laser therapy include the precision with which it destroys tissue; accessibility to small, difficult-to-treat foci of disease; a bloodless field; destruction of bacteria in infected areas; and minimal or no pain after the procedure.

▶ [Laser, the newest wrinkle therapeutically in intraepithelial neoplasia, has considerable theoretical appeal because it permits precise treatment of small areas of abnormality without destroying large amounts of adjacent normal tissue, as occurs with electrocautery or cryocautery. This study outlines the histologic and clinical effects of CO_2 laser treatment of cervical neoplasia lesions in 115 patients. The results seem moderately encouraging, with a residual recurrence rate of 4.34%, but follow-up periods were relatively short (8 months to 2 years). More study is needed.] ◀

Cell-Mediated Cytotoxicity in Preinvasive and Invasive Squamous Cell Carcinoma of the Cervix. Cell-mediated immune responses have been observed in patients with invasive cervical carcinoma, and circulating antibodies to cervical tumor antigens have been detected in patients with invasive cancer and carcinoma in situ. Morteza M. Dini, Kianoosh Jafari, and Isidoro Faiferman[11-11] (Chi-

(11–11) Obstet. Gynecol. 55:728–731, June 1980.

cago) determined whether blood leukocytes from patients with pre-cancerous lesions are sensitized to cervical tumor antigens, as determined by cytotoxic reactivity to a tissue culture cell line of cervical cancer origin. Coincubation of the target cell line of human squamous carcinoma and blood leukocytes was performed in 22 patients with squamous cell cancer of the cervix and 9 with other tumors, and in 9 normal females.

The degrees of cell reduction were 90.1% in mild dysplasia, 91.1% in moderate dysplasia, 91.6% in severe dysplasia, 85.0% in carcinoma in situ, and 85.0% in invasive squamous cell carcinoma of the cervix. Blood leukocytes of patients with squamous neoplasia showed no significant cytotoxicity against a cell line from ovarian adenocarcinoma. Lymphocytes from patients with other tumors showed no significant cytotoxicity against the cell line derived from squamous cell carcinoma. Cells from normal subjects appeared to enhance the growth of cells from both test tumors.

Strong cytotoxic reactions can be found between patient blood leukocytes and an appropriate target cell line even at early stages of cervical dysplasia. The findings suggest that dysplasia is an early stage of a neoplastic process, which if unchecked may progress to an invasive stage. Patients with such lesions should be treated definitively whenever discovered, and close follow-up should be part of management.

▶ [Lymphocytes from patients with cervical dysplasia demonstrated cytotoxicity against an established line of human cervical squamous cell carcinoma cells. This not only suggests that cervical dysplasia and carcinoma represent different degrees of the same process (which is, after all, quite generally considered to be the case), but also that the apparently localized, basement membrane-bound, intraepithelial phenomenon has had a systemic influence on the organism as reflected by this leukocytic hypersensitivity.] ◀

Factors Influencing Treatment of Patients With Stage IA Carcinoma of the Cervix. Recommended treatments for stage IA, or microinvasive cervical carcinoma, range from conization to radical surgery and radiotherapy. T. Iversen, V. Abeler, and K. E. Kjorstad[11-12] (Oslo) followed 122 patients with stage IA cervical carcinoma for 5–25 years. Primary surgery had led to apparently complete tumor removal. Microinvasion was defined as tumor infiltration to a depth no greater than 5 mm. Mean age of patients was 44. Diagnosis was made on conization specimens in 53 patients, on hysterectomy specimens in 65 and on large wedge biopsies in 4. Treatment was by conization in 2 patients; hysterectomy in 19; extended hysterectomy in 53; conization plus radium in 34; and hysterectomy plus radium in 14. Three patients had adenocarcinoma, 2 had adenosquamous lesions, and 116 had squamous cell carcinomas.

Forty-two patients were classified as having carcinoma in situ with minimal stromal invasion. Tumor cells were seen in vascular channels in 8. One patient had tumor at the resection margin and 7 others had in situ lesions. Five of the 8 recurrences were observed after 5 years. One patient had a pelvic node metastasis detected 13 years

(11–12) Br. J. Obstet. Gynaecol. 86:593–597, August 1979.

after primary treatment. The 5-year crude survival rate was 99%. Four central recurrences and four pelvic wall recurrences developed. Four patients with recurrences had tumor cells in blood or lymph vessels. Only 1 patient without blood vessel or lymphatic invasion, who had an adenocarcinoma, developed a pelvic wall metastasis.

Accurate assessment of microinvasive carcinoma of the cervix requires systematic histologic examination of an adequate specimen, at least a cone biopsy containing the entire lesion. If minimal stromal invasion is found without carcinoma in situ or tumor at the margin, no further treatment is necessary. If there is stromal invasion for less than 5 mm with free margins and no tumor in vessels, total hysterectomy with conservation of the ovaries is recommended for younger patients. Older patients may undergo hysterectomy with salpingo-oophorectomy or may be treated with intracavitary radium. If atypical epithelium is present at the resection margins, extended hysterectomy without node dissection is recommended unless such surgery is contraindicated, in which case radiotherapy may be preferable. Wertheim hysterectomy or radiotherapy is indicated when vascular spaces are involved.

▶ [The management of stage 1A ("microinvasive") carcinoma of the cervix is controversial. Whereas the overwhelming majority of patients do well with simple surgical removal (ie, simple hysterectomy and perhaps even conization), a few develop recurrence. This study underscores the significance of two factors—stromal invasion of 5 mm or more and presence of tumor in vascular and lymphatic channels—in identifying patients at high risk in whom more radical therapy is needed. It also documents the long latent period between primary therapy and recurrence; in 5 of 8 recurrences more than 5 years had elapsed.] ◀

Invasive Cervical Carcinoma in Young Women. Ross S. Berkowitz, Robert L. Ehrmann, Risa Lavizzo-Mourey, and Robert C. Knapp[11-13] (Harvard Med. School) have frequently diagnosed cervical carcinoma in patients under age 35 in recent years. Review was made of 110 newly diagnosed cases of invasive cervical cancer seen from 1975 to 1978. Twenty-seven patients (24.5%) were aged 35 years or less (average, 29.6). Only 1 of these patients had never been pregnant.

Stage I disease was present in 93% of the younger and in 52% of the older patients. Two younger patients had stage II disease at initial diagnosis. Seven younger and only 8 older patients had cervical adenocarcinoma. All but 1 of the younger patients were treated surgically. Four had metastatic cancer in pelvic nodes at radical hysterectomy. All young stage I patients are presently free from disease clinically. Three of those with pelvic node metastasis received postoperative radiotherapy. The other patient developed a pelvic side wall recurrence and is doing well 2 years after external beam radiotherapy. Both young patients with stage IIb disease developed pulmonary metastases after primary radiotherapy. One died and the other is receiving chemotherapy. Fifteen of 25 younger patients had normal cervical cytologic reports within 2 years of the detection of invasive cancer. Review of the smears in 10 cases showed missed cervical neopla-

(11–13) Gynecol. Oncol. 8:311–316, December 1979.

sia in 5 and unsatisfactory technique for adequate interpretation in 2.

The findings do not indicate that cervical cancer in young women has a poor prognosis. Cervical cancer is a potential problem in any sexually active female, and all suspected and symptomatic cervical lesions should be promptly biopsied, regardless of a prior normal cervical cytologic report.

Vaginal Smear History in Patients With Invasive Cervical Carcinoma. Although a decrease in incidence of cervical cancer has been claimed since the institution of mass screening programs, cases of invasive cervical cancer have appeared in screened groups. H. Grundsell, J.-E. Johnsson, L.-G. Lindberg, H. Ström, E. Tekavec, C. Tropé and Z. Bekassy[11-14] (Univ. of Lund) reviewed the findings in 53 consecutive patients with a mean age of 55 years seen during 1977–1978 with invasive cervical cancer. Cytologic study had never been done in 30 patients (about 57%), who had a mean age of 68 years. Three patients had ignored invitations to participate in a mass screening program. Eleven of the 23 screened patients had had a benign smear within four years (mean, $2^1/_2$) before diagnosis. Five smears had been less than adequately evaluated, but two of these showed only minimal abnormalities. Four of 12 patients with dysplasia did not respond to repeated calls for follow-up procedures. Five other patients had not had further studies other than repeat smears.

All atypical cervical cytologic smears must be evaluated clinically and treated to make an early diagnosis in the approx 10%–15% of cancer patients who lack frankly malignant cells in their cytologic cell samples. The results of therapy may then be controlled by repeat cytologic studies until normal samples are obtained over a considerable period of time.

▶ [This article and the preceding one, from Sweden and Boston, respectively, highlight similar problems in cervical cancer screening. Both describe series in which about half of the patients with invasive cervical cancer had had negative cytologic screening a year or two prior to diagnosis. Of those with smears originally read as benign, some had suspicious or malignant cells on rereview that had been overlooked or misinterpreted. Others had varying degrees of dysplasia reported, but either refused follow-up or were followed with repeat smears *without* histologic evaluation.

Potential sources of failure to diagnose cervical cancer by cytologic screening can be attributed to the physician (failure to obtain a proper smear and failure to evaluate reported dysplasia histologically), to the laboratory (failure to recognize abnormal cells on the slide), and to the patient (failure to participate in cytologic screening or in the indicated follow-up of abnormal smears).

Finally, the point needs constant emphasis that a Papanicolaou smear is a screening test. It is not a substitute for cervical biopsy when a patient presents with abnormal vaginal bleeding or has an abnormal cervix on physical examination.] ◀

Accuracy of Lymphangiography in Diagnosis of Para-aortic Lymph Node Metastases from Carcinoma of the Cervix was investigated by R. C. Brown, H. J. Buchsbaum, H. H. Tewfik, and C. E. Platz[11-15] (Univ. of Iowa). Lymphangiography, celiotomy, para-aortic lymph node excision, and postoperative abdominal radiography were performed in 25 patients with carcinoma of the cervix, most of whom

(11–14) Ann. Chir. Gynaecol. 68:127–129, 1979.
(11–15) Obstet. Gynecol. 54:571–575, November 1979.

TABLE 1.—CORRELATION OF RADIOGRAPHIC AND
PATHOLOGIC FINDINGS

Radiographic/pathologic	+/+	−/−	−/+	+/−
No. of cases	13/5	8/7	8/1	13/8

+: Positive; −: negative.

TABLE 2.—CORRELATION OF RADIOGRAPHIC AND
PATHOLOGIC FINDINGS

Radiologic/pathologic	+/+	+/−
Filling defect	9/3	9/6
Obstruction	2/1	2/1
Stasis	3/1	3/2
Lack of no.	6/5	6/1
Collateral circulation	0/0	0/0

+: Positive; −: negative.

had stage IIIb disease. Four patients were deleted from evaluation because the postoperative film revealed suspicious lymph nodes.

Of the 21 lymphograms evaluated, 13 were positive and 8 were negative. Five of the 13 positive and 1 of the 8 negative lymphograms were found to be positive by pathologic examination (Table 1). The most reliable lymphographic signs of lymph node metastasis were decrease in number of nodes and filling defects in the nodes (Table 2). Stasis, collateral circulation, and obstruction were of no value as radiographic signs.

Of the 6 histologically positive cases, 5 were radiologically positive and 1 was radiologically negative. This gives a sensitivity (true positive cases among the pathologically proved positive cases) of 0.833 and a specificity (true negative cases among pathologically proved negative cases) of 0.467. Although the sensitivity seems to favor use of lymphangiography in screening patients with far-advanced carcinoma of the cervix, the specificity of the test is so low that each patient having a positive result would have to have a surgical biopsy before radiation therapy. Lymphangiography can be of assistance in locating suspicious lymph nodes, but it can not be used as the sole method of treatment planning.

▶ [Although this report indicates a relationship between the radiographic appearance of the paraaortic lymph nodes and the presence or absence of metastases, this relationship is not precise enough to make lymphangiography useful in the therapeutic management of patients with cervical cancer.

In a related study, Lee and associates (Radiology 135:771, 1980) described 21 patients irradiated for periaortic lymph node metastases from cervical or endometrial cancer and concluded that cure was possible. However, the numbers are too small and the follow-up too short for us to concur.] ◀

Lung Metastases in Cervical and Endometrial Carcinoma.
Lung metastasis is not uncommon in patients with cervical or endometrial carcinoma, and the lung is involved in more than one third of patients with distant metastases. Carl J. D'Orsi, James Bruckman,

Peter Mauch, and Edward H. Smith[11-16] (Boston) reviewed the records of 352 patients with cervical carcinoma and 669 with endometrial carcinoma seen in 1968–1977. Forty-four developed lung metastases, and radiographs were available for study in 42 cases.

Incidence of pulmonary metastases was 5.1% in patients with cervical carcinoma and 3.6% in those with endometrial carcinoma. Respective median ages were 55 and 66 years. Median time from presentation to the detection of lung metastases in both groups was one year. Median time to death was 5 months; 80% of these patients died within 1 year of the discovery of the metastases. Fifteen patients died from pulmonary causes. Eleven had a solitary lung metastasis at relapse. Median time to death in these cases was 5 months after discovery of the metastasis, compared to 9 months for those with more than one lesion. The size of the metastases found at radiographic examination of the chest varied greatly. Three patients had mediastinal or hilar adenopathy, 5 had pleural effusions or thickening in addition to the parenchymal lesions, and 1 had only a pleural effusion.

One quarter of the patients in this series had a solitary pulmonary metastasis. Four fifths of affected patients died within 1 year of developing pulmonary metastases. The lesions were smooth, noncavitating masses, but were not characteristic enough to be distinguished from other tumors.

▶ [Lung metastases are generally considered to be unusual with cervical and endometrial cancer though, as indicated by this study, (5.1% and 3.6%, respectively), they are by no means rare. Of patients who developed pulmonary spread, 80% did so within 30 months of initial presentation and 80% died within a year of diagnosis of lung metastases. The metastatic lesions were generally well-circumscribed and noncavitary but had no features to distinguish them from other tumors of other origins.] ◀

Factors Influencing the Occurrence of Advanced Cervical Carcinoma. Many patients still are being seen with invasive squamous cell carcinoma of the cervix, although mortality rates have declined in some populations. Leslie A. Walton, Wallace Kernodle, Jr., and Barbara Hulka[11-17] (Univ. of North Carolina) reviewed the records of 170 patients seen in 1975–1977. Patients had a tissue diagnosis of invasive squamous cell carcinoma or adenocarcinoma of the cervix and stage II–IV disease by conventional staging procedures. There were 83 cases of stage II, 79 of stage III, and 8 of stage IV disease in the series. The number of nonwhites included was disproportionate to area population. Most patients were aged 50–69 at diagnosis.

Only 12% of cases were diagnosed by screening examinations or Papanicolaou smears before the onset of symptoms (table). Vaginal bleeding was the presenting feature in 84%. Sixty-two patients who had diagnosis after the onset of symptoms were being followed by the health care system for some nonpelvic medical problem, often hypertension, heart disease, or diabetes. More screened than unscreened patients had stage II disease. This was especially true for blacks,

(11–16) AJR 133:719–722, October 1979.
(11–17) South. Med. J. 72:808–811, July 1979.

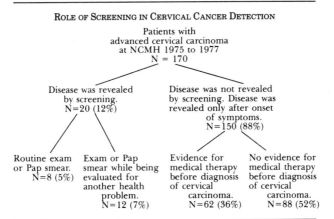

ROLE OF SCREENING IN CERVICAL CANCER DETECTION

Patients with
advanced cervical carcinoma
at NCMH 1975 to 1977
N = 170

Disease was revealed
by screening.
N=20 (12%)

Disease was not revealed
by screening. Disease was
revealed only after onset
of symptoms.
N=150 (88%)

Routine exam
or Pap smear.
N=8 (5%)

Exam or Pap
smear while being
evaluated for
another health
problem.
N=12 (7%)

Evidence for
medical therapy
before diagnosis
of cervical
carcinoma.
N=62 (36%)

No evidence for
medical therapy
before diagnosis
of cervical
carcinoma.
N=88 (52%)

among whom 58% of screened patients and 34% of unscreened patients had stage II disease.

Of patients with advanced cervical carcinoma, 73% were from the lower socioeconomic group and from agricultural regions. It remains to be seen whether local, regional, or community efforts will lead to a system whereby poor, educationally deprived, lower-socioeconomic, parous women can be screened and rescreened so that the incidence of cervical carcinoma will decline.

▶ [Only 12% of these patients with advanced (stage II–IV) cervical cancer had their cancers detected by screening examinations. It is distressing that 36% of the patients in the entire series were receiving medical attention for some nonpelvic problem. These patients apparently did not have the benefit of a routine pelvic examination and Papanicolaou smear as part of their medical care. Death from cervical cancer is preventable, but only if both patients and physicians insist on regular cytologic screening.] ◀

Death from Cervix Uteri Carcinoma: The Changing Pattern. Patients with cervical carcinoma traditionally have died of hemorrhage, local infection, and renal failure, but the mortality pattern appears to be changing. Henry J. Katz and J. N. P. Davies[11-18] (Albany Med. College) reviewed autopsy records of 133 patients who died before 1965 and 30 who died afterward of cervical carcinoma. A remarkable reduction in the degree of ureteral involvement resulting in uremia is apparent since 1965, despite an increase in the average age at death. Only 1 of 29 treated patients with ureteral blockage producing uremia died. The proportions of cervical adenocarcinoma and squamous carcinoma remained virtually unchanged. Mortality from uremia was 27.7% during 1935–1964 and only 6.7% during 1965–1979. Ureteral blockage was substantially less frequent after 1965. The overall pattern of spread and organ involvement has not changed appreciably, but the extent of local spread has been limited by better treatment of the local lesion.

(11–18) Gynecol. Oncol. 9:86–89, February 1980.

For practical purposes, the classic pattern of mortality from cervical carcinoma has disappeared and been replaced by pulmonary embolism, myocardial infarction, bronchopneumonia, and cachexia and septicemia. The change is related to treatment methods that have much improved the control of disease with respect to the ureters. More efficient radiotherapy is chiefly responsible.

▶ [As medical students, we learned that uremia was an important cause of death in patients with cervical cancer. According to the authors of this report, this is no longer true. Although ureteric involvement is still common, blockage and uremia are less frequent. Better control of pelvic disease has resulted in a wider distribution of extrapelvic metastases and a changing pattern of terminal illnesses in these patients.] ◀

Evaluation of Office Endometrial Biopsy in Detection of Endometrial Carcinoma and Atypical Hyperplasia. Outpatient endometrial biopsy has several important advantages over conventional dilatation and curettage for obtaining a tissue diagnosis of intrauterine lesions. Steven M. Greenwood and D. John Wright[11-19] (Danville, Pa.) reviewed 1 year's experience with endometrial biopsy in 891 women whose first endometrial sample in 1974 was obtained by the biopsy method. The results were compared with those for subsequent samples obtained over 3 years by biopsy, dilatation and curettage, or hysterectomy. The Novak suction curet was used without anesthesia in most cases.

Hysterectomy, done in 26% of the patients, showed endometrial carcinoma in 21 and atypical hyperplasia in 25. The rate of each of these conditions among all first biopsy specimens was 2%. The first endometrial biopsy was positive in 76% of the women with proved endometrial carcinoma. All four patients who had second diagnostic procedures had their lesions detected. In 1 patient who had only one biopsy that was inadequate, the lesion was not diagnosed preoperatively. The first biopsy detected atypical hyperplasia in 48% of these cases. Eleven women had a second diagnostic procedure, and in 36% the lesion was diagnosed. Two of 4 women with two negative biopsy specimens had the lesion diagnosed by a third procedure, 1 by a third biopsy. Nearly 10% of initial biopsies yielded inadequate material. No patient is known to have died with or of endometrial carcinoma during the 3-year study period.

Endometrial biopsy is a useful means of detecting endometrial carcinoma. It is highly accurate, with no false positive results, and it obviates the need for hospitalization for dilatation and curettage. If an inadequate or nondiagnostic biopsy specimen is obtained in a subject with nonmenstrual bleeding, another attempt should be made to obtain diagnostic material, preferably by dilatation and curettage. The endometrial biopsy also is of definite value in the diagnosis of precancerous hyperplasia. An inadequate biopsy specimen should never be considered negative.

▶ [This study reaffirms the value of the office endometrial biopsy in the detection of endometrial carcinoma, but, more importantly, it illustrates that this technique is not without a few false negative results. A patient with postmenopausal bleeding and a negative office endometrial sampling should have dilatation and curettage.] ◀

(11-19) Cancer 43:1474–1478, April 1979.

Precursors of Endometrial Carcinoma. Various abnormal endometrial lesions have been linked to endometrial cancer over the years, and the histologic classification of endometrial lesions is now starting to exhibit greater uniformity among pathologists. Alfred I. Sherman and Saul Brown[11-20] (Detroit) evaluated 235 patients aged 60 and over with a diagnosis of endometrial adenocarcinoma in whom at least one curettage specimen had been obtained within 10 years before the diagnosis of cancer. In another group of 216 patients, endometrial hyperplasia had been diagnosed at age 50 or over; these patients were untreated for at least 2 years after the diagnosis.

Seventy-two percent of all patients who developed invasive endometrial carcinoma had a previous diagnosis of a precursor lesion. Only 3% had cystic hyperplasia, and only 17% showed proliferative endometrium. In the precursor group, 7 of 12 patients who were not operated on and who had a diagnosis of carcinoma in situ developed endometrial cancer. Lesions in 4 of 5 patients treated with progestins reverted to a more benign state; the other progressed to cancer. Cancer developed in 38% of patients with adenomatous or atypical adenomatous changes. In only 18% of these patients did the endometrium revert to a benign state.

The designation of adenomatous and atypical adenomatous hyperplasia of the endometrium as precursor lesions appears to be warranted. Cystic hyperplasia should not be considered to be a precursor lesion. It is suggested that adenomatous and atypical adenomatous lesions and carcinoma in situ be referred to as intraepithelial carcinomas of the endometrium (ICE) and graded 1 to 3 according to severity. Total excision by complete hysterectomy should offer a chance for complete cure in these patients. Curettage is also a possibility, but it is a less controllable procedure. Endocrinopathy may be managed by cyclic progestin or progesterone therapy, ovarian resection, or clomiphene administration.

▶ [This paper confirms how prescient Gusberg was 30 years ago in recognizing the relationship between adenomatous hyperplasia, particularly when atypical, of the endometrium and later endometrial cancer. Of 235 women with endometrial cancer who had had endometrial sampling 1 to 10 years prior to diagnosis, nearly 45% exhibited atypical adenomatous hyperplasia and 25% exhibited adenomatous hyperplasia at the earlier study. Of patients with the precursor lesions followed 2 to 18 years, 57% with atypical adenomatous hyperplasia and 22% with adenomatous hyperplasia developed endometrial cancer.] ◀

Serum Androgens and Estrogens in Postmenopausal Women With and Without Endometrial Cancer. The exact role of endogenous estrogen production in the genesis of endometrial adenocarcinoma has not been clearly defined. Howard L. Judd, Bert J. Davidson, Anthony M. Frumar, Issa M. Shamonki, Leo D. Lagasse, and Samuel C. Ballon[11-21] (Univ. of California, Los Angeles) report a prospective study of 35 consecutive patients with endometrial adenocarcinoma and control subjects matched for age and percentage of ideal body weight. The diagnosis had been made by fractional curettage in each case. The cancer patients had at least 6 months of amenorrhea before

(11–20) Am. J. Obstet. Gynecol. 135:947–956, Dec. 1, 1979.
(11–21) Ibid., 136:859–871, Apr. 1, 1980.

bleeding and all but 2 of the controls had at least 6 months of amenorrhea before study.

Mean concentrations of serum androstenedione, testosterone, estrone and estradiol were similar in the cancer patients and control subjects. Estrogens but not androgens correlated closely with body weight and percentage of ideal weight, with higher estrogen levels in the heavier patients. None of the hormone levels correlated with age or time since the menopause. Cancer patients with diabetes tended to be more obese and to have higher estrogen levels than those without diabetes. Those who had used estrogens in the past were more slender and had lower endogenous estrogen levels than nonusers. Two thirds of cancer patients exhibited excess body weight, high endogenous estrogen levels or a history of previous estrogen use. Hypertension was comparable in the two groups.

These findings strongly suggest that androgen and estrogen metabolism is similar in postmenopausal women with and those without endometrial cancer when the groups are matched for age and weight. Two thirds of cancer patients in this series had presumed risk factors for acquiring endometrial cancer. Conditions associated with persistent, unopposed estrogen stimulation of the endometrium appear to increase the likelihood of malignant transformation occurring.

▶ [In this study, androgen and estrogen levels were no different in patients with endometrial cancer and age- and weight-matched controls. In both cancer and control subjects, estrone and estradiol levels correlated well (r approximately 0.6) with body weight expressed as a percent of ideal, reflecting the by now well-known phenomenon of conversion of androstenedione to estrogens in fat tissue. As we may have commented before, the fat's the thing, it seems.] ◀

Endometrial Disease After Treatment With Estrogens and Progestogens in the Climacteric. The possible role of exogenous estrogens in endometrial carcinoma remains controversial. M. E. L. Paterson, T. Wade-Evans, D. W. Sturdee, Margaret H. Thom, and J. W. W. Studd[11-22] report a prospective study of 745 women receiving different hormonal regimens for the climacteric. Overall, the study covered 21,736 months. The women received cyclic low- or high-dose estrogen therapy for 3 of every 4 weeks in the form of piperazine estrone sulfate, estradiol valerate, conjugated equine estrogens, or estriol hemisuccinate; or as sequential oral estrogens with added progestogen (norgestrel or norethisterone); or as subcutaneous estradiol implants, with or without testosterone, and oral norethisterone. Endometrial biopsies were obtained by vacuum aspiration curettage.

Of the 1,002 biopsies attempted, 827 yielded satisfactory specimens. Cystic hyperplasia occurred in 7% of the women taking low-dose cyclic estrogen therapy and in 14.8% of those in the high-dose group. When progestogens and estrogens were taken, the rate of hyperplasia was 1.2%. The rate in patients receiving an estradiol implant was 14.8%, but it was 55.8% for those not taking any progestogen. No hyperplasia occurred when norethisterone was given for over 10 days. The rate of adenomatous and atypical hyperplasia was increased in patients given only estrogens. Also, the rate of hyperplasia increased

(11–22) Br. Med. J. 1:822–824, Mar. 22, 1980.

with the duration of Premarin administration. Evidence of an adeno-carcinoma was found in 1 pretreatment biopsy specimen.

These findings confirm the value of giving a progestogen for at least ten days in each cycle to prevent both cystic and adenomatous hyper-plasia in estrogen-treated postmenopausal women. Regular endome-trial curettage is also advisable, especially in women receiving only estrogens. The bleeding response during treatment does not provide a useful guide to the status of the endometrium.

▶ [Theoretically, the addition of terminal progestational therapy to cyclic estrogens should lessen the risk of endometrial hyperplasia, a theory that seems to be borne out in this study. The overall incidence of endometrial abnormalities was 14.8% with high-dose oral estrogen, 7% with low-dose oral estrogen, and 1.2% with oral estrogen and added progestin. Among patients with estradiol implants, hyperplasia occurred in 14.8%, but this frequency fell progressively with longer periods of progestin use, and no hyperplasias were found if progestin was taken for more than 10 days each month. The implication seems clear that added progestin is a good idea in the patient treated with estrogen during the climacteric.] ◀

Endometrial Carcinoma: Clinical-Pathologic Comparison of Cases in Postmenopausal Women Receiving and Not Receiving Exogenous Estrogens. Many case-control studies of estrogen ther-apy in endometrial cancer have lacked histopathologic review of slides, and another criticism is that postmenopausal women receiving estrogen are also likely to be receiving good medical care. Steven G. Silverberg, Dennis Mullen, Jack A. Faraci, Edgar L. Makowski, Al-exander Miller, Jack L. Finch, and Jeffrey V. Sutherland[11-23] com-pared the clinical and pathologic findings in 43 postmenopausal pa-tients with endometrial carcinoma who had received exogenous estro-gens before diagnosis and 79 similar patients not exposed to estro-gens. Most of the former had received oral preparations only. Respective mean ages were 61.3 and 63.7 years.

Constitutional risk factors for endometrial cancer were less fre-quent in the estrogen users (table). Average durations of symptoms were 4.6 months in the estrogen users and 7.8 months in the controls. More hysterectomy specimens from estrogen nonusers showed myo-metrial invasion, but no major difference in extent of disease was seen in cases in which preoperative radiotherapy had not been used. Mixed adenosquamous carcinoma was twice as frequent in estrogen nonusers than in users (28% vs 14%). Stromal lipid histiocytosis and

---

PREVALENCE OF DIABETES, HYPERTENSION, AND OBESITY IN
POSTMENOPAUSAL ENDOMETRIAL CARCINOMA PATIENTS WITH AND
WITHOUT PRIOR ESTROGEN EXPOSURE

	Estrogen	No estrogen
Diabetic	4/43 ($\chi^2 = 7.67, P < 0.01$)	25/79
Hypertensive	12/43	33/78*
Obese	12/32† ($\chi^2 = 8.99, P < 0.005$)	47/68†

*Hypertension status unknown for 1 patient in no-estrogen group.
†Status unknown for 11 in estrogen group and 11 in no-estrogen group.

(11–23) Cancer 45:3018–3026, June 15, 1980.

vascular invasion were observed more often in specimens from estrogen nonusers. Only 5 of 20 recurrences in estrogen nonusers occurred among the 19 such patients who did not have surgical treatment.

The reasons for the better survival of estrogen-using patients with endometrial cancer is unclear. These tumors appear to be highly sensitive to estrogen stimulation or deprivation. If the excellent prognosis in estrogen-related cases is confirmed, the risk-benefit ratio for estrogen administration may well balance out on the side of benefit.

▶ [This article suggests, as others have previously, that endometrial cancers associated with estrogen use may be generally less aggressive, as indicated by grade and myometrial invasion, than those unassociated with estrogen exposure. More experience is needed to speak definitively concerning prognosis. It is interesting that the constitutional factors considered to predispose to endometrial cancer were less common in the estrogen group. Perhaps those factors act through a mechanism which is "provided" by exogenous estrogens in the absence of the predisposing factor.] ◀

Risk of Exogenous Estrogen Therapy and Endometrial Cancer. Most studies relating the use of exogenous estrogens to endometrial cancer risk have been retrospective case-control investigations. Frederick R. Jelovsek, Charles B. Hammond, Brett H. Woodard, Richard Draffin, Kerry L. Lee, William T. Creasman, and Roy T. Parker[11-24] (Duke Univ.) carried out a retrospective study of 431 patients with endometrial cancer and 431 controls matched for age, race, and parity, seen from 1940 to 1975. All the former had a pathologic diagnosis of invasive adenocarcinoma of the endometrium. They were more often obese, hypertensive, and diabetic than were the controls.

The overall risk that endometrial carcinoma might develop was 2.38. Increased risk was associated with estrogen therapy for over 5 years in white patients. The risk was confined to stage I, grade 1 lesions and more superficial myometrial invasion. No risk relation to dosage of estrogens could be clearly established. The 5-year survival of estrogen users with stage I, grade 1 lesions was 94.7%. Survival of patients with similar lesions who did not use estrogen was 93.3%. The 5-year survivals for all stages of disease were 86.5% for estrogen users and 73.4% for estrogen nonusers. Estrogen use in the study group ranged from 4.4% to 6.9% between 1940 and 1970, and it was 33% from 1970 to 1975.

The authors believe that a real risk that endometrial cancer may develop is associated with long-term estrogen replacement therapy. Therapy for individual patients must be carefully considered. Any abnormal uterine bleeding must be promptly and thoroughly evaluated. Annual endometrial sampling and added progestin therapy are recommended at the authors' institution. The benefit-risk ratio is reassessed at each patient visit.

Estrogen and Endometrial Cancer: Cases and Two Control Groups From North Carolina. Barbara S. Hulka, Wesley C. Fowler, Jr., David G. Kaufman, Roger C. Grimson, Bernard G. Greenberg, Carol J. R. Hogue, Gary S. Berger, and Charles C. Pulliam[11-25] evaluated the endometrial cancer risk associated with exposure to ex-

---

(11–24) Am. J. Obstet. Gynecol. 137:85–91, May 1, 1980.
(11–25) Ibid., pp. 92–101.

ogenous estrogen for 256 cases, 224 gynecology controls, and 321 community controls. Carcinomas in situ were excluded. The cases included 170 adenocarcinomas, 49 adenoacanthomas, 13 adenosquamous carcinomas, 14 clear cell lesions, and 10 undifferentiated carcinomas. Both control groups were matched with the study cases for age and race.

Among black women there were no differences in estrogen use between cases and either set of controls. White women showed risk values of 3.6 and 4.1 after $3^{1}/_{2}$ years or more of estrogen use. No increase in risk was found for shorter periods of use, regardless of dosage, type of estrogen, or mode of administration. Obese women exhibited no increase in risk with exogenous estrogen use. The highest risks, 5 to 8, were in nonobese, nonhypertensive women after $3^{1}/_{2}$ years or more of estrogen use. The minimum latency period after the first administration of estrogen was 3 to 6 years. An estrogen-free interval of 2 years reduced elevated risks to nonuser levels. With prolonged estrogen use, the risks of cancer were high for stage IA and grade 1 lesions, and either small or not significant for more advanced disease. This may be attributable to increased medical surveillance resulting in earlier diagnosis or to less aggressive lesions.

The findings are consistent with carcinogenic promotion rather than an initiator action for estrogen use. The target cells of obese women are already exposed to estrogen, and if a predisposition toward endometrial cancer exists, more exogenous estrogen may have no appreciable incremental effect.

▶ [The two studies presented in this article and the preceding one, from different North Carolina institutions, reached a number of similar conclusions regarding exogenous estrogen and endometrial cancer. (1) Cancer risk appears to be increased threefold to fourfold by estrogen usage. (2) The increased risk applies to white women only. (3) A positive correlation exists between duration of estrogen use and risk. (4) Obesity, another risk factor for endometrial cancer, seems to lessen the increased risk with estrogen. We agree that the preponderance of evidence indicates an association between perimenopausal and postmenopausal estrogen treatment and subsequent endometrial cancer development which must be taken into account in developing an individualized approach to therapy of the menopause.] ◀

Incidence of Endometrial Cancer in Relation to Use of Oral Contraceptives. Several studies have shown that among young women with endometrial cancer who had used oral contraceptives, a greater proportion had taken sequential preparations, particularly Oracon (0.1 mg ethinyl estradiol and 25 mg dimethisterone). Noel S. Weiss and Tom A. Sayvetz[11-26] (Seattle) evaluate the hypotheses that users of sequential preparations are at increased risk of endometrial cancer, or, conversely, that there is a decreased risk among users of combined preparations.

All white female residents aged 35–49 years living in two counties in Washington and who had newly diagnosed endometrial cancer were interviewed approximately 1 year after diagnosis. They were asked about menstrual and reproductive history, contraceptive and noncontraceptive use of estrogens, and other matters relevant to the development of endometrial cancer. White women, aged 36–55, were used as controls.

(11–26) N. Engl. J. Med. 302:551–554, Mar. 6, 1980.

USE OF COMBINED ORAL CONTRACEPTIVES* AMONG WOMEN WITH
ENDOMETRIAL CANCER AND AMONG CONTROLS

USE OF COMBINED ORAL CONTRACEPTIVES	PATIENTS WITH CANCER	CONTROLS	RELATIVE RISK †	95 PER CENT CONFIDENCE LIMITS
Yes‡	17	76	0.5	0.1–1.0
No	93	173	1.0	—

*Subjects who had used sequential oral contraceptives for one or more years
are excluded.
†Standardized for age and use of menopausal estrogens.
‡Use for one or more years.

A higher proportion of women with endometrial cancer had used
sequential oral contraceptives than had controls. The risk factor for
users was more than twice that of nonusers. There was a very strong
relationship between Oracon use and the development of endometrial
cancer. The relative risk to Oracon users was 7.3; the use of other
sequential preparations was actually less common among patients
with this type of cancer than among controls.

The small number of patients limited the ability of the study to
determine whether particular patterns of Oracon use were especially
hazardous.

The table illustrates that patients with endometrial cancer had not
used combined oral contraceptives as often as control women had. The
risk of endometrial cancer among users of combined preparations was
estimated to be 50% that of nonusers.

The effect of combined oral contraceptives on the development rate
of endometrial cancer seemed to be influenced by subsequent use of
menopausal estrogens. The relative protection afforded by combined
preparations was present only in patients who either had not used
estrogens or who had used them for less than 2 years. However, these
estimates of risk have very wide confidence limits. The protective effect of combined oral contraceptives was not evident among women
who used estrogen for 3 or more years.

These data suggest that the development of endometrial neoplasia
can be extremely sensitive to hormonal factors. Oral contraceptives
which emphasize the estrogen component may promote cancer,
whereas preparations which emphasize the progestational component
may provide a protective effect.

▶ [These results are interpreted as indicating that Oracon, a high-estrogen sequential
oral contraceptive, predisposes to endometrial cancer whereas combination agents
apparently partially protect against its development. It should be noted, however, that
the patients were at the younger end of the age group for endometrial cancer (mostly
less than age 50) and interpretation of endometrial neoplasia in premenopausal
women is notoriously difficult. In any event, the point is really moot, because Oracon
is no longer available.] ◀

**Stage III Adenocarcinoma of Endometrium: Two Prognostic
Groups.** James E. Bruckman, William D. Bloomer, Abraham Marck,
Robert L. Ehrmann, and Robert C. Knapp[11-27] (Harvard Med. School)

(11–27) Gynecol. Oncol. 9:12–17, February 1980.

STAGE III ENDOMETRIAL CANCER: PROGNOSIS AND DISTRIBUTION OF DISEASE

Extrauterine sites of tumor

Authors	Ovary and/or tube	Other pelvic structures
Milton and Metters	14/17* (82%)	0/12 (0%)
Frick *et al.*	12/22* (55%)	3/12 (25%)
Antoniades *et al.*	4/6† (67%)	10/31 (32%)
Bruckman *et al.*	12/15† (80%)	3/11 (27%)

*Five-year survivors.
†Relapse-free survivors at time of analysis.

analyzed diagnoses of 26 patients with stage III endometrial cancer. In 15 patients (group A), extrauterine disease was confined to the ovary or fallopian tube, or both. In 11 patients (group B), disease extended beyond these organs to the vagina or other pelvic structures. Treatment included a combination of radiation and surgery in all but 1 patient, who was given radiation therapy alone.

The median follow-up was 65 months and the median time to relapse was 9 months. Group A patients had a significantly better relapse-free survival rate than did group B patients. The actuarial relapse-free 5-year survival rate for all stage III patients was 54%; it was significantly different for group A (80%) and group B (15%). This prognostic difference could not be predicted with the current classification system for carcinoma of the corpus uteri, although it is common practice to use surgical-pathologic staging in reporting results when extrauterine tumor is found during surgery.

Other authors have previously reported that patients with solitary ovarian metastases from endometrial cancer had a better prognosis than those in whom disease had extended to pelvic nodes or peritoneum (table). Analysis of their data supports the findings of the present study that patients with endometrial cancer involving only the ovary and tube have a good prognosis. Patients with endometrial cancer involving structures other than ovary and tube are clearly candidates for adjuvant hormonal or drug therapy because of their poor prognosis.

▶ [This sort of division of patients with stage III endometrial cancer has been previously suggested by others. It makes good sense, as the prognosis is clearly related to which pelvic structures are involved with metastatic disease.] ◀

Medroxyprogesterone Acetate (Depo-Provera) Versus Hydroxyprogesterone Caproate (Delalutin) in Women with Metastatic Endometrial Adenocarcinoma. Progesterone therapy remains the treatment of choice for metastatic endometrial adenocarcinoma that is not amenable to surgery or radiation therapy. In a prospective study, M. Steven Piver, Joseph J. Barlow, John R. Lurain, and Leslie E. Blumenson[11-28] (Roswell Park Meml. Inst.) evaluated whether the use of Depo-Provera significantly improves the objective

(11–28) Cancer 45:268–272, Jan. 15, 1980.

response and survival rate of patients with metastatic endometrial adenocarcinoma over results previously obtained in patients treated with a similar dose of Delalutin.

Of the 114 patients with metastatic or recurrent disease, 44 received Depo-Provera over a 5^{1}/$_2$-year period; 70 controls received Delalutin over 11^{1}/$_2$ years. Follow-up ranged from 2 to 17 years. A complete response to progesterone therapy included complete regression of all x-ray and clinical evidence of tumor for at least 3 months. A decrease of 50% or more in the product of the perpendicular diameters of the tumor masses for 3 or more months was considered a partial response. Stable disease was defined as no change, or less than a 50% decrease in size of the measurable lesion. Progression was defined as increased tumor size.

The results indicate that there was no significant increase in objective response to Depo-Provera (18.9%) as compared to Delalutin (13.7%). The addition of localized radiation therapy to pelvic recurrences did not increase the response rate to Depo-Provera (14.3%) compared to Delalutin plus radiation therapy (15.8%). Of the 114 patients who received progesterone therapy, 15.8% achieved an objective response, with 7.0% having a complete response. The mean duration of response was not significantly different between the two groups.

There was a significant correlation between response to progesterone and the time interval from original treatment to recurrence. Patients having recurrences 3 or more years after initial therapy had a significantly better rate of response (33.3%) compared to those having recurrences in less than 3 years (8.3%). There was no significant increase in objective response with respect to size of the tumor masses, number of metastases, histologic grade of the lesions, site of metastases, or prior radiation therapy.

Although there was only a 15.8% overall objective response, those patients who had such a response lived significantly longer than those with stable disease or progression. The median survival for patients responding to Delalutin was 59.8 months, compared to 12 months for patients with stable disease and 2.8 months for patients with progression. For women who responded to Depo-Provera, the median length of survival was 28.8 months, compared to 11 months for those with stable disease and 3.8 months for those with progression.

Although only 1 in 6 women responded to progesterone therapy, these patients had a significant prolongation of life. Therefore, progesterone therapy should remain a part of the management of metastatic endometrial adenocarcinoma, but should be combined with other active cytotoxic agents.

▶ [The groups of patients receiving Depo-Provera and Delalutin were treated at different times and are not strictly comparable. Given this caveat, the treatment results were similar with the two drugs. The objective response rate was 16% and was independent of most variables analyzed. A well-differentiated metastasis was perhaps more likely to respond (the differences relating response to grade of tumor were not statistically significant, however). Patients with late recurrences (≥3 years) did better with progestin therapy than did those with early recurrences. Because of the modest overall response rate, the authors suggest combining progestin treatment with other chemotherapeutic agents (see 1979 YEAR BOOK, p. 292).] ◀

▶ ↓ For a possible explanation of differential response to progestins, read on. ◀

Clinical Correlates of Estrogen- and Progesterone-Binding Proteins in Human Endometrial Adenocarcinoma. Adenocarcinoma of the uterus is the most common female pelvic malignancy. Progestins have been the preferred treatment for metastases, although only one third of the tumors respond to hormonal therapy alone. Techniques which permit identification of tumors with a high potential for response to hormonal therapy are needed. W. T. Creasman, K. S. McCarty, Sr., T. K. Barton, and K. S. McCarty, Jr.[11-29] (Duke Univ.) evaluated 78 endometrial carcinoma specimens from 74 patients for estrogen and progesterone receptors by multiconcentration saturation and sucrose density gradient analyses. The clinical stage and histologic grade of the tumors, as well as the patient's clinical course, were compared to the receptor levels.

Of the primary tumors, 67.2% were estrogen-receptor positive and 67.2% were progesterone-receptor positive. Both receptors were present in 60.9%. Among the 14 recurrent tumors, 36% contained estrogen receptors, 43% contained progesterone receptors, and 36% contained both receptors.

Several relationships between receptor content and morphological differentiation were noted. Higher levels of both receptors were seen more often in grade I tumors, and grade I tumors tended to include a higher proportion of estrogen- and progesterone-positive lesions. Also, there was a relationship between the quantitative levels of both receptors for grade I and grade II lesions, but not for grade III lesions.

No correlation was seen between clinical stage or uterine cavity size and the estrogen or progesterone receptor content.

Myometrial invasion or extrauterine disease did not appear to correlate with the presence or absence of receptors at the time of diagnosis. Receptor-positive lesions tended to be less aggressive than those with neither receptor.

When malignant peritoneal cytology demonstrated extrauterine disease, response to progestins appeared to correlate with the presence or absence of receptors. Those with significant levels of receptors responded better to therapy.

Receptor analysis of a recurrent tumor was performed in 14 patients, 13 of whom were treated with progestins only. Of 8 patients with negative receptor assays, 7 did not respond to hormonal therapy.

The overall correlation of response of recurrent endometrial adenocarcinomas to progestin therapy alone and receptor analysis was 92%.

▶ [Estrogen and progesterone receptor assays may help decide which patients with recurrent endometrial cancer will respond to treatment with progestins. Twelve of 13 patients in this study responded, as would be predicted by the receptor status of their tumors (7 of 8 with negative assays failed to respond, 5 of 5 with significant receptor levels had stable disease or objective responses to hormonal treatment).] ◀

(11–29) Obstet. Gynecol. 55:363–370, March 1980.

Estradiol and Progesterone Binding in Uterine Leiomyomas and in Normal Uterine Tissues. Uterine leiomyomas are particularly sensitive to estrogen stimulation, suggesting that they have estrogen receptors similar to those in normal tissues. Emery A. Wilson, Frank Yang, and E. Douglas Rees[11-30] (Univ. of Kentucky) undertook to determine whether cells of uterine leiomyomas contain receptor proteins for estradiol-17β and progesterone. Tissues were obtained from 6 patients, aged 40 to 71 years, undergoing hysterectomy for uterine leiomyomas. Two patients were postmenopausal, and 4 were in the proliferative phase of the endometrial cycle. Estrogen receptor was assessed by the dextran-coated charcoal assay and by the sucrose density gradient technique. Progesterone receptor was measured by a glycerol density gradient method.

The concentration of cytoplasmic estrogen receptors in leiomyomas was significantly greater than that in myometrium and significantly less than that in endometrium (table). The concentration of cytoplasmic progesterone receptors in leiomyomas also was greater than that in myometrium and less than that in endometrium, but the differences were not significant because of individual variation. No significant correlation was found between the concentrations of estrogen or progesterone receptors and patient age or weight.

The finding of cytoplasmic receptor proteins in leiomyomatous tissue explains the sensitivity of leiomyomas to endogenous or exogenous steroids. If exogenous hormone is indicated for replacement therapy, estrogens with relatively low binding affinity or with short-duration receptor binding may be preferable. Progesterone administration might reduce both estrogen and progesterone receptor concentrations, leading to decreased sensitivity of leiomyomas to endogenous estrogens and possibly to a decrease in their size.

▶ [The finding of increased estrogen receptor activity in leiomyoma cytosol is consistent with what one might predict given the estrogen sensitivity of these tumors.] ◀

CONCENTRATION OF ESTROGEN RECEPTORS IN CYTOSOL FROM
MYOMETRIUM, LEIOMYOMA, AND ENDOMETRIUM
(FM/MG CYTOSOL PROTEIN)

Patient	Myometrium	Leiomyoma	Endometrium*
EC	21	60	174
LR	20	68	—
MH	13	32	130
MJ	18	30	112
NW	12	25	—
WS	15	28	108
Mean	16.5	40.5	131.0
SEM	1.5	7.6	15.1
P†		<0.05	<0.01

*—: Insufficient amount of tissue.
†Based on difference of paired samples.

(11–30) Obstet. Gynecol. 55:20–24, January 1980.

Review of Ovarian Cancer at the University of Texas Systems Cancer Center, M. D. Anderson Hospital and Tumor Institute.

Julian P. Smith and Thomas G. Day, Jr.[11-31] reviewed the records of 2,115 patients with ovarian cancer, who were treated from 1944 to 1973. Ninety percent had one of the common epithelial cancers of the ovary; the other 10% had germ cell tumors, stromal tumors, or other uncommon ovarian neoplasms. Younger patients with epithelial cancers had earlier and lower-grade lesions and a better survival rate. The best survival rates were associated with hysterectomy and bilateral salpingo-oophorectomy. Addition of omentectomy did not improve the 5-year survival rate.

Important prognostic factors included the stage and grade of tumor and the presence or absence of ascites, but probably the most important was the size of the largest tumor mass remaining after initial operation. Spillage of the contents of cystic lesions did not appreciably alter survival. Most patients had advanced disease when first evaluated and received some form of adjunctive postoperative therapy. Survival of patients given postoperative irradiation was better than that of those given chemotherapy, when compared by stage and the size of the largest residual tumor mass (Tables 1 and 2).

Postoperative radiotherapy appeared to be a better adjunct than chemotherapy in this study, but it is hoped that postoperative treatment with new multiple-drug combinations will significantly improve survival of patients with ovarian cancer.

▶ [This reported experience of the M. D. Anderson Hospital in Houston—2,115 ovarian cancer patients over a 30-year period—must be one of the largest series published. It

TABLE 1.—PERCENT SURVIVAL BY STAGE AND POSTOPERATIVE TREATMENT

Stage	*Irradiation*		*Chemotherapy*	
	2 yr.	*5 yr.*	*2 yr.*	*5 yr.*
I	90	84	83	76
II	69	48	66	37
III	49	30	28	7
IV	33	13	10	3

TABLE 2.—PERCENT SURVIVAL BY TUMOR SIZE AND POSTOPERATIVE TREATMENT AT FIVE YEARS

Residual tumor (cm)	*Irradiation*	*Chemotherapy*
None	70	67
0-1	52	32
1-2	15	16
3-6	12	4
7-9	0	0
10+	4	5

(11–31) Am. J. Obstet. Gynecol. 135:984–993, Dec. 1, 1979.

contains much valuable information about this disease. The prognostic importance of both stage and histologic grade is confirmed; in addition, the authors state that the most important prognostic factor was the diameter of the largest tumor mass remaining after initial surgery. Few conclusions about therapy can be drawn from a retrospective analysis. Although the data do seem to suggest somewhat better outcome with radiation therapy than with chemotherapy postoperatively (table), the nonrandom nature of assignment to treatment groups precludes any firm generalization. Most surprisingly, in his response to the discussion of this paper, Doctor Smith stated, "I feel very strongly that there is no place in the postoperative treatment of epithelial cancer of the ovary for irradiation therapy."] ◄

Ovarian Carcinoma: Improved Survival Following Abdominopelvic Irradiation in Patients with Completed Pelvic Operation. Ovarian carcinoma accounts for nearly half the deaths from female genital tract malignancies in North America, with no trend toward decreasing incidence or mortality being evident. About 2 of 3 patients die of the disease. Alon J. Dembo, Raymond S. Bush, Francis A. Beale, Helen A. Bean, John F. Pringle, Jeremy Sturgeon, and Joan G. Reid[11-32] (Ontario Cancer Inst., Toronto) carried out a prospective study of 190 postoperative ovarian cancer patients with stage IB, II, and III presentations. The median follow-up was 52 months.

All patients were seen within 3 months of bilateral salpingo-oophorectomy and hysterectomy (BSOH). Pelvic irradiation was given in a dose of 4,500 rad to the midplane in 20 fractions by means of supervoltage technique. Abdominopelvic irradiation consisted of 2,250 rad to the pelvic midplane, followed by the same dose to the whole abdomen and pelvis. Chlorambucil was given in a basic dose of 6 mg daily for 2 years or until relapse occurred.

Patients in whom BSOH could not be completed had a poor prognosis regardless of subsequent therapy. When BSOH was completed, pelvic plus abdominopelvic irradiation with no diaphragmatic shielding significantly improved survival, and it gave long-term control of occult upper abdominal disease in about 25% more patients than pelvic irradiation alone or with adjuvant chlorambucil therapy. The efficacy of combined radiotherapy was independent of stage or tumor grade. Addition of chlorambucil to pelvic irradiation delayed the time to treatment failure but did not reduce the number of treatment failures. Serious gastrointestinal toxicity did not occur in BSOH-completed patients. Three patients had major sepsis from chlorambucil therapy. Four patients had second neoplasms.

Pelvic radiation alone is inadequate postoperative treatment for stage II ovarian carcinoma, and adjuvant chlorambucil therapy does not improve long-term survival. Pelvic plus abdominopelvic radiation is appropriate treatment for patients with small amounts of abdominal disease and has curative potential.

▶ [This prospective study addresses the issue of the choice of postoperative adjunctive therapy in patients with stage Ib, II, and III ("asymptomatic") carcinoma of the ovary. Pelvic irradiation alone was not effective. This has been demonstrated previously and is not unexpected, given the tendency for occult intra-abdominal metastases and positive peritoneal fluid cytology in these patients. Better results were obtained here with the addition of abdominal strip irradiation than with chlorambucil. The liver was not shielded, ensuring that the diaphragms were treated. As others have reported,

(11–32) Am. J. Obstet. Gynecol. 134:793–800, Aug. 1, 1979.

the prognosis was improved if complete surgery could be performed and if there was no or little apparent residual tumor.] ◄

Advanced Ovarian Cancer: Correlation of Histologic Grade with Response to Therapy and Survival. Robert F. Ozols, A. Julian Garvin, Jose Costa, Richard M. Simon, and Robert C. Young[11-33] (Natl. Inst. of Health) reviewed the pathologic specimens of 82 patients with stage III-IV ovarian cancer, as defined by FIGO, to determine the prognostic and therapeutic importance of histologic grade. Histologic types and grades were determined in a blind manner by two pathologists. A cytologic grade was assigned based on a modification of Broder's system, which emphasizes the degree of differentiation and the number of mitotic figures present. The degree of anaplasia and the percentage of undifferentiated cells were also taken into account. A pattern grade was assigned based on the degree to which the tumor formed papillary structures or glands versus solid tumor areas. Borderline malignancy was assessed by a lack of stromal invasion and slightly atypical epithelium two to three layers thick.

The modified Broder's system was found to be particularly useful, identifying four groups with differing survival and apparent differential responses to chemotherapy. Overall improvement of survival in stage III-IV cases, observed in a prospective study of combination chemotherapy, was related primarily to an increased survival of patients with grade 2 and 3 lesions, representing intermediate degrees of cytologic differentiation. Survival in grade 1 cases, with minimal cytologic features of malignancy and very few mitoses, was markedly better than in grade 4 cases, with a high degree of cytologic anaplasia and numerous mitotic figures. In neither case did survival appear to be influenced by the choice of chemotherapy.

Clinical trials of chemotherapy for ovarian cancer should use cytologic grade as a separate stratification factor. Chemotherapy for advanced disease may have to be tailored in part to the histologic grade of disease. Both cytologic and pattern methods should be used.

► [Dr. S. G. Lifshitz of the University of Iowa reviewed this paper at our request and commented as follows:

"The results of this study in 82 patients with stage III and IV ovarian carcinoma clearly demonstrate that the cytologic grading of these tumors based on the degree of anaplasia and number of undifferentiated cells (modified Broder's grade I-IV) is useful in identifying four groups of patients with different survival as well as what seems to be an apparent differential response to chemotherapy. This work indicates that the overall improvement of survival in patients with stage III and IV ovarian carcinoma observed in a prospective study of single vs combination chemotherapy (N. Engl. J. Med. 299:1261–1266, 1978; and 1980 YEAR BOOK, p. 321) was related to improved survival of patients with grade II and III lesions. In grade I and IV lesions, survival did not appear to be influenced by the choice of chemotherapy. The authors have clearly pointed out the need to employ cytologic grading as a separate stratification factor in prospective clinical trials assessing the efficacy of chemotherapy for ovarian cancer."

Perhaps this differential response with histologic grading is the reason Park and associates, in a report from the Gynecologic Oncology Group (Cancer 45:2529, 1980), were unable to identify an improved response in advanced or recurrent ovarian epithelial carcinomas with combination chemotherapy. The complete or partial response rate

(11–33) Cancer 45:572–581, Feb. 1, 1980.

with melphalan was 29.2% and was not apparently enhanced by the addition of 5-fluorouracil, dactinomycin, and Cytoxan.] ◄

Clinicopathologic Review of 118 Granulosa and 82 Theca Cell Tumors. Granulosa cell tumors and theca cell tumors are functional ovarian tumors comprising about 3% of ovarian neoplasia and as much as 10% of ovarian malignancies. Arthur T. Evans, III, Thomas A. Gaffey, George D. Malkasian, Jr., and John F. Annengers[11-34] (Mayo Clinic and Found.) review the patients' clinical course and histologic features of 200 such tumors.

The peak incidence occurred in the fifth, sixth, and seventh decades of life. The overall mean age at initial diagnosis was 51 years. Theca cell tumors predominated in the older patients.

The two tumor types were equally distributed between the right and left ovaries. Bilateral involvement by granulosa cell tumors occurred in 3 patients. Lesions, staged retrospectively using the 1976 FIGO classification for ovarian cancer, were classified Iai in 83.1% of the patients. Of theca cell tumors, 97% were stage Ia, all but 1 being Iai. The granulosa cell tumors were less uniform, with 79% being stage Iai and 10% being stage III at diagnosis.

Various histologic patterns were seen in granulosa cell tumors, including all the recognized subtypes. The microfollicular type was the most common pattern. The thecomas featured lipid-laden stromal cells associated with spindle-shaped stromal fibroblasts. All theca cell tumors were unilateral.

Total abdominal hysterectomy with bilateral salpingo-oophorectomy was performed in 56% of the women. A more conservative procedure was often performed in younger women.

None of the patients with theca cell tumors had recurrence, but recurrence developed in 18.6% of the patients with granulosa cell tumors. The average interval between initial diagnosis and recurrence was 6 years. Average survival after recurrence of granulosa cell tumors was 5.6 years.

The initial histologic stage of a granulosa cell tumor was related to incidence of recurrence. Stage Iai tumors recurred at a rate of 8.9%; more extensive disease was associated with recurrence rates of 30% or more. The only exception occurred in 4 patients with stage Ic lesions, none of whom had recurrence.

The extent of the initial surgical procedure also affected recurrence risks. Only 6% of patients had recurrence after total abdominal hysterectomy and bilateral salpingo-oophorectomy. In contrast, those who underwent less extensive procedures had a recurrence rate of 25%.

Mortality from the primary tumor was, for the entire study, 12.5%, excluding patients whose cause of death was unknown. The benign behavior of thecomas requires that survival data be evaluated independently for granulosa cell and theca cell tumors. There was 1 death from theca cell tumor and 20 (17.9%) from granulosa cell tumors.

(11–34) Obstet. Gynecol. 55:231–238, February 1980.

Once recurrence had developed in patients with granulosa cell tumors, 72.7% died from their disease.

▶ [This paper contains no new information but it represents a large series and an excellent review of granulosa and theca cell tumors.] ◀

Distinguishing Lymph Node Metastases From Benign Glandular Inclusions in Low-Grade Ovarian Carcinoma can be extremely difficult. Early stage I undifferentiated and embryonal ovarian carcinomas are associated with a poor prognosis when microscopic aortic lymph node metastases are present. R. L. Ehrmann, J. M. Federschneider, and R. C. Knapp[11-35] (Brookline, Mass.) describe four patients in whom low-grade or borderline ovarian carcinoma was associated with glandular structures in aortic lymph nodes. Benign glandular inclusions within pelvic and aortic lymph nodes are well known. However, in three of these patients the ovarian tumors were so well differentiated that interpretation of the epithelial structures in the nodes as metastases or benign inclusions was problematic. Determining whether metastases are present may dictate further treatment and may affect long-term survival.

Glandular inclusions in lymph nodes are found exclusively in women. They are often cystically dilated and are usually lined with simple, benign-appearing, cuboidal epithelium which is often ciliated. The lining epithelium may also be simple columnar or pseudostratified columnar, and may form papillary infoldings into the lumens. Cytoplasmic or intraluminal secretion may be present as well as calcifications resembling psammoma bodies which distort the glandular shape. Mitoses are rare. The following cases illustrate some difficulties encountered in interpretation of glandular inclusions.

CASE 1.—Woman, 34, at operation had bilateral papillary cystic ovarian tumors diagnosed as papillary serous cystadenocarcinoma, grade 1, stage Ib. Figure 11–1 demonstrates the benign appearance of the aortic lymph node inclusions, which were lined by low columnar epithelium of a tubal type with ciliated and nonciliated cells.

CASE 2.—Woman, 37, had bilateral multicystic ovarian tumors with external papillary growth and extension to the right broad ligament. The diagnosis was papillary serous cystadenocarcinoma, grade 1, stage III. The glandular inclusions appeared relatively benign, as did the crypt epithelium and small gland spaces in the ovarian tumor. The lymph node structures could be either benign inclusions or metastases. The glandular structures were numerous in the nodes without destruction of nodal architecture. No papillae were found in the nodes, in contrast to the tumor. The conclusion was that the nodal inclusions were benign rather than metastatic carcinoma as originally diagnosed.

CASE 3.—Woman, 25, had bilateral nodular cystic ovarian tumors with external excrescenses and peritoneal seedings, including the diaphragm. The tumor diagnosis was papillary serous cystadenofibroma of borderline malignancy, stage III. The aortic node inclusions had epithelial papillae and psammoma bodies, features seen in the ovarian tumor. However, these features have also been seen in inclusions without carcinoma. It was concluded that the inclusions were benign.

(11–35) Am. J. Obstet. Gynecol. 136:737–746, Mar. 15, 1980.

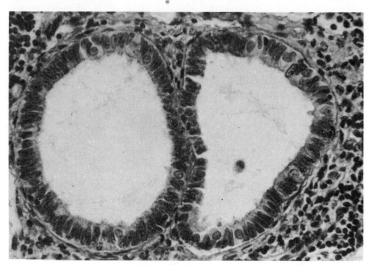

Fig 11–1.—Case 1. Aortic lymph node showing benign glandular inclusions. Hematoxylineosin; reduced from ×319. (Courtesy of Ehrmann, R. L., et al.: Am. J. Obstet. Gynecol. 136:737–746, Mar. 15, 1980.)

CASE 4.—Woman, 29, had bilateral papillary cystic ovarian tumors with widespread peritoneal implants, including the omentum, and invasion of the uterus. The diagnosis was papillary serous cystadenoma of borderline malignancy, stage III. The possibility of metastasis to the aortic lymph nodes was plausible clinically. Papillary glands and psammoma bodies in the nodes resembled the metastases. Loose rosettes and sheets of cells among the lymphocytes also suggested metastatic tumor rather than benign inclusion.

▶ [This collection of four cases calls attention to a dilemma. When lymph nodes removed for staging of low-grade ovarian carcinoma contain glandular structures, is it "benign glandular inclusions" or metastatic disease? So much—radiation, chemotherapy, etc—depends on the answer, and there do not seem to be any firm criteria on which to base judgment.] ◀

Unusual Cystadenofibromas: Endometrioid, Mucinous, and Clear Cell Types. Grace F. Kao and Henry J. Norris[11-36] (Armed Forces Inst. of Pathology, Washington, D.C.) reviewed the findings in 16 cases of cystadenofibroma with unusual epithelial components, encountered from 1957 to 1974, during which 126 cystadenofibromas of various types were collected. Ten other lesions had epithelial atypia as the unusual feature. The study cases included 12 endometrioid cystadenofibromas, 3 clear cell (mesonephroid) cystadenofibromas, and 1 cystadenofibroma with mucinous epithelium lining the cystic spaces.

The clinical and gross pathologic features of these lesions are essentially similar (table). The median age of the 12 patients with endometrioid lesions was 57 years. Eight of 10 patients were parous. Six were postmenopausal. Four of the 16 women had bilateral tumors. No patient had ascites. Six endometrioid neoplasms showed an admixture of endometrioid epithelium with a minor component of cells resembling those of the fallopian tube mucosa. Mitotic activity was seen

(11–36) Obstet. Gynecol. 54:729–736, December 1979.

CLINICAL AND PATHOLOGIC FEATURES OF ENDOMETRIOID, CLEAR CELL, AND MUCINOUS
CYSTADENOFIBROMAS COMPARED WITH ORDINARY CYSTADENOFIBROMAS

	Endometrioid	Clear cell	Mucinous	Ordinary
No. of patients	12	3	1	100
Age range (years)	30–75	54–62	49	17–86
Median age (years)	57	59	—	40.5
Race (non-white)	18%	33%	0%	6%
Size range (cm)	4–15	4.5–26	3–10.5	2–23
Median diameter (cm)	10	12	7	9
Bilateral	17%	33%	Yes	23%

in only 1 case of endometrioid cystadenofibroma. Fifteen patients were followed, 12 for 5 years or longer. One endometrioid lesion recurred, but the patient has lived for $6^{1}/_{2}$ years since initial operation without undergoing complete excision. Hysterectomy was performed in 13 patients. Leiomyomas were seen in 5 uteri, adenomyosis in 3, and endometrial polyps in 1.

The endometrioid cystadenofibroma is a benign counterpart of endometrioid adenocarcinoma of the ovary. Most ovarian clear cell tumors are carcinomas; borderline lesions are rare. Patients with clear cell cystadenofibromas with epithelial atypia should be followed closely. Mucinous cystadenofibroma is not expected to recur. The various epithelial patterns found in these unusual cystadenofibromas reflect the pluripotentiality of the cells from which they and other epithelial neoplasms of the ovary are derived.

▶ [Since the epithelial component of cystadenofibromas is thought to arise from the multipotential ovarian surface epithelium, it is not surprising that different histologic patterns are seen. Cystadenofibromas occur in middle-aged women, and these semisolid tumors are not infrequently bilateral. These features mean that the surgeon may suspect cancer in the operating room until the report of the pathologist's findings.] ◀

Second-Look Laparoscopy Prior to Proposed Second-Look Laparotomy. There has recently been an increase in women undergoing second-look laparotomy after treatment for ovarian adenocarcinoma, done so that alkylating agent therapy, which may lead to acute leukemia, can be discontinued if residual malignancy is absent. M. Steven Piver, Shashikant B. Lele, Joseph J. Barlow, and Marie Gamarra[11-37] (Roswell Park Meml. Inst.) evaluated second-look laparoscopy in patients in complete clinical remission after prolonged chemotherapy for advanced ovarian adenocarcinoma. Twenty-two patients with lesions of FIGO (International Federation of Gynecology and Obstetrics) stages IIB, III, and IV underwent second-look laparoscopy after a median of 23 months of therapy. Most patients had serous adenocarcinoma. Treatment was most often with melphalan or melphalan and 5-fluorouracil. Five patients received pelvic irradiation besides chemotherapy.

Four women with biopsy-proved persistent tumor at laparoscopy had stage III disease. Seven women had abnormal cytologic washings, and in 4 of these, all with stage II disease, this was the only laparo-

(11–37)   Obstet. Gynecol. 55:571–573, May 1980.

scopic evidence of persistent ovarian malignancy. Persistent cancer was documented in 8 patients in all (36.3%), and they were spared second-look laparotomy. Eight of 10 women undergoing second-look laparotomy after normal laparoscopic studies had no evidence of persistent disease. Two second-look laparoscopies were falsely negative. In 1 case cancer was not found on frozen-section biopsy. The other patient had a small periureteral nodule that was not biopsied.

The absence of visible tumor and malignant cells in cytologic washings at second-look laparoscopy permits laparotomy, if indicated, with the same anesthesia. The finding of tumor spares the patient second-look laparotomy. Patients with no evidence of persistent malignancy at second-look laparoscopy require a second-look laparotomy before discontinuance of effective chemotherapy is considered.

▶ [In this study, laparoscopy was done in 23 patients with complete clinical remission after chemotherapy for advanced ovarian cancer. In 4 there was gross evidence of residual tumor and in 4 more, peritoneal cytologic washings were positive; these 8 patients (36% of the total) were spared laparotomy. To utilize this approach with maximal benefit, it is necessary to have the capability for peritoneal cytologic examination while the patient is under anesthesia, so that a laparotomy can be done immediately if the results are negative.] ◄

Reexploration After Treatment for Ovarian Carcinoma. Benny P. Phillips, Herbert J. Buchsbaum, and Samuel Lifshitz[11-38] (Univ. of Iowa) reviewed information on 65 patients with documented ovarian carcinoma who underwent a second exploratory celiotomy from 1969 to 1978. Nearly 90% of the patients had epithelial tumors of the ovary. The 33 patients with stage III or stage IV disease generally received systemic chemotherapy, but a few received pelvic irradiation with an abdominal boost. The 12 patients with stage II disease were managed by pelvic irradiation followed by systemic chemotherapy. The 16 patients with stage I disease were managed variously. Median interval between celiotomies was 22 months. Chemotherapy was continued for 3 months after a second-look procedure that yielded normal findings. There were no operative deaths or major surgical complications.

In 50 patients the second operation followed appropriate staging, reduction surgery, and appropriate therapy. Twenty-four of these patients had no clinical or radiologic evidence of residual disease, and 21 of them had no evidence of tumor at operation. Only 1 patient with a second-look operation that yielded normal findings had a recurrence, and this was the only death from disease in the group. Among 26 patients who underwent exploration after regression of disease, but who had suspected or known residual carcinoma, only 27% of those found to have residual disease are alive. Twelve patients had more extensive disease at reexploration, and their average survival was 6 months. The 14 patients with less extensive disease at reexploration had an average survival of 31 months. All 8 patients who underwent exploration on surgical indications had residual disease. All died within 2 years; median survival was only 2 months. Of 6 patients who underwent reexploration before adjuvant therapy in

(11–38) Gynecol. Oncol. 8:339–345, December 1979.

whom the initial operation was inadequate for staging, reduction, or both, 4 had a higher stage of disease than was appreciated at the first operation. Two are without disease.

Second-look surgery should be part of the treatment plan for patients with ovarian carcinoma. The indications are discontinuance of therapy, resection of residual disease, and mapping of residual disease requiring a change of therapy. Morbidity is low even in irradiated patients, and the benefits far outweigh the risks.

▶ [Twenty-one of 24 patients without clinical evidence of disease had negative findings at second-look procedures. Chemotherapy could then be discontinued in these patients. Another patient had nonresectable tumor nodules. She was treated with irradiation and a different chemotherapy regimen and subsequently had a negative "third-look" laparotomy. Reexploration after the initial treatment for ovarian cancer is clearly of value in certain patients.] ◀

Conservative Management of the Zollinger-Ellison Syndrome: Ectopic Gastrin Production by an Ovarian Cystadenoma.

Sites of gastrin production other than tumors of the pancreas or duodenum found in patients with Zollinger Ellison syndrome include the parathyroid and a mucinous cystadenocarcinoma of the ovary. Thomas T. Long III, Thomas K. Barton, Richard Draffin, William J. Reeves and Kenneth S. McCarty, Jr.[11-39] describe a patient with a unilateral benign mucinous cystadenoma of the ovary in which gastrin was localized immunohistologically and from which high levels of immunoreactive gastrin were extracted. The ulcer diathesis resolved after oophorectomy without gastrectomy.

Woman, 49, had had an asymptomatic pelvic mass and epigastric pain for several months with a single episode of melena. Antacids had been given. A 10×12-cm cystic mass was found on the right side of the pelvis. Upper gastrointestinal tract roentgenographic studies showed numerous gastric ulcers, confirmed by endoscopy. Fasting serum gastrin levels were 200 to 530 pg/ml. Cimetidine was given in a dose of 300 mg every 6 hours. Laparotomy showed a cystic tumor of the right ovary, and hysterectomy and bilateral salpingo-oophorectomy were performed. Fasting serum gastrin levels were normal postoperatively, and cimetidine therapy was stopped. Gastric ulcers were absent 5 months after operation. The fasting serum gastrin level at 18 months was 45 pg/ml.

The tumor was a mucinous cystadenoma. Immunoperoxidase staining showed cytoplasmic gastrin at 1:10 and 1:100 dilutions of anti-human-gastrin I antibody. The tumor tissue contained 737 ng of extractable gastrin per gm of tumor.

Zollinger-Ellison syndrome was a likely diagnosis in this case from the preoperative test findings. The ulcer diathesis remitted after removal of the ovarian mucinous cystadenoma. Gastric acid secretion was controlled with cimetidine, permitting resection of the ovarian lesion without removal of the stomach. The Zollinger-Ellison syndrome may resolve after extirpation of a unifocal benign lesion that is producing gastrin, obviating the need for gastrectomy in selected cases.

▶ [Read on.] ◀

(11–39) JAMA 243:1837–1839, May 9, 1980.

Pheochromocytoma of the Broad Ligament: Localization by Computerized Tomography and Ultrasonography.

David C. Aron, William M. Marks, Philip R. Alper, and John H. Karam[11-40] (Univ. of California, San Francisco) report a case in which a pelvic pheochromocytoma that eluded extensive angiographic attempts at detection was successfully localized by computerized tomography (CT) and ultrasonography.

Woman, 51, with intermittent headaches and labile hypertension since childhood, had severe pain in the right posterior part of the neck and was found to have a blood pressure of 230/110 mm Hg supine, falling to 100/75 mm Hg on standing. Glucose intolerance was demonstrated. Urinary vanillylmandelic acid (VMA) and norepinephrine values were elevated. Subarachniod hemorrhage was substantiated by lumbar puncture. Extensive angiography failed to show a pheochromocytoma. Repeated urine studies showed normal catecholamine and VMA values, but elevated metanephrine levels. Phenoxybenzamine was given by mouth in a dose of 10 mg 3 times daily. Seven months later, urinary catecholamine, metanephrine, and VMA levels again were elevated. A CT scan showed a 3×4-cm mass contiguous with the left aspect of the uterus; the adrenal glands were normal. A pelvic sonogram confirmed the presence of the mass. Norepinephrine estimates on vena caval samples showed a step-up at the L5–S1 level, the region corresponding to the pelvic mass. At laparotomy, a 22.5-gm pheochromocytoma was found in the left broad ligament and was removed. The patient was normotensive off medication after surgery. Urinary catecholamine levels have returned to normal.

Computerized tomography and ultrasonography are noninvasive methods of localizing pelvic and adrenal masses, particularly pheochromocytomas. Sonography may show an echogenic or relatively echo-free mass. Low-density areas on CT studies may represent necrotic tissue. Either or both of these techniques can be recommended as the initial radiographic procedure when a pheochromocytoma is diagnosed biochemically.

► [Our residents would call both this case and the one presented in the preceding article "GRM" (Grand Rounds material). The first patient had the Zollinger-Ellison syndrome. The neoplastic source of gastrin was not pancreatic, but was an ovarian mucinous cystadenoma (a gastrin-secreting mucinous cystadenocarcinoma of the ovary has previously been described). An immunohistochemical technique demonstrated gastrin in both the stroma and the mucinous epithelium of the ovarian tumor.

The second patient had an extra-adrenal pheochromocytoma located within the leaves of the left broad ligament. This tumor was discovered on a CT scan and apparently could not be palpated in this "obese" women. We have seen the other side of this coin, ie, the putative mass on the CT scan which cannot be felt and indeed is not present at operation.] ◄

Natural History of Recurrent Molar Pregnancy.

The incidence of molar pregnancy in the United States is approximately 1:1,500 live births, and the risk of subsequent proliferative trophoblastic sequelae developing is about 1:6. Jerome M. Federschneider, Donald P. Goldstein, Ross S. Berkowitz, Ann R. Marean, and Marilyn R. Bernstein[11-41] (Boston) studied the natural history of recurrent molar pregnancy and assessed its implications in the woman's future reproductive potential.

(11–40) Arch. Intern. Med. 140:550–552, April 1980.
(11–41) Obstet. Gynecol. 55:457–459, April 1980.

Over 13½ years, 7 patients with recurrent hydatidiform mole were seen. Gonadotropin levels were monitored for 6 months after reaching a normal level to insure a sustained remission.

The incidence of recurrent disease in this study population was 0.6%. All patients achieved complete remission for each episode of molar pregnancy. Recurrent molar pregnancy was associated with histologic evidence of increasing malignancy with later episodes. Despite a benign clinical course after evacuation with earlier moles, 5 of the 7 patients required chemotherapy to achieve remission in subsequent episodes. Metastatic disease was observed in only 1 patient. None of the patients had a normal viable pregnancy after two or more consecutive hydatidiform molar gestations. Previous reports also suggest that these patients have a reduced ability to achieve a normal pregnancy.

The etiology of trophoblastic tumors remains unclear. Once a patient has had a molar pregnancy, any future pregnancy must be regarded as being at high risk for the development of trophoblastic neoplasia, and subsequent gestations should be carefully monitored to detect recurrence.

▶ [This report provides helpful information concerning an unusual situation, recurrent molar pregnancy. The data suggest that persistent trophoblastic disease is common with recurrent mole and that subsequent successful pregnancy outcome is not. A problem with the latter statement is that we do not know how frequently women with two previous molar pregnancies try to achieve another pregnancy.] ◄

Acute Pulmonary Complications of Molar Pregnancy. Women with hydatidiform mole who experience acute pulmonary distress after uterine evacuation are at high risk for treatment complications. Leo B. Twiggs, C. Paul Morrow, and John B. Schlaerth[11-42] (Los Angeles) reviewed data on 128 patients with histologically proved hydatidiform mole who underwent evacuation in 1970–76. The preferred treatment was suction curettage under general anesthesia. Acute respiratory embarrassment was defined as abrupt onset of tachypnea at over 30 respirations per minute and hypoxemia, with a Po_2 below 80 mm Hg, associated with tachycardia after delivery of the molar pregnancy.

Twelve patients (9.4%) had acute, severe respiratory embarrassment during hospitalization. Symptoms began within 12 hours of evacuation, occurring in 11 patients within 4 hours. No patient required ventilatory aid other than supplemental oxygen, and all recovered completely. Three patients had hemoptysis. Arterial blood gas abnormalities resolved within 72 hours in all patients. Chest x-ray studies showed fluffy, patchy or alveolar infiltrates; in addition, 4 patients had a concomitant pleural effusion. Lung scans, done in 3 patients, disclosed multiple perfusion defects. Five patients were hypertensive, and in 4 the diagnosis of preeclampsia was made. Only 1 of the 12 study patients was not transfused; 4 received 6 or more units of blood.

Seven of the patients probably had trophoblastic embolization. Thyrotoxicosis developed in 1, and another patient had pulmonary edema

(11–42) Am. J. Obstet. Gynecol. 135:189–194, Sept. 15, 1979.

from overadministration of blood and fluids. The high risk of respiratory distress in molar patients having a uterus large for dates requires special precautions to avoid fluid overload. Central venous pressure monitoring is an important aid. If respiratory distress occurs, nasal oxygen and intravenous diuretic therapy are indicated. These patients are at a substantial risk of having invasive mole or choriocarcinoma.

▶ [This is a nice clinical report concerning the unusual, but not rare, pulmonary problems that can follow the evacuation of molar pregnancies. Patients with molar pregnancies may be anemic, hyperthyroid, and/or preeclamptic. Therefore, careful attention directed to their cardiovascular status is required. Most of the acute respiratory problems in this study were due to presumed trophoblastic embolization. These patient often look very ill, but usually improve markedly over a few hours with only supportive care. The authors suggest that these patients may be at increased risk for the development of persistent trophoblastic disease.] ◀

Methotrexate with Citrovorum Factor Rescue: Reduced Chemotherapy Toxicity in the Management of Gestational Trophoblastic Neoplasms. Single-agent chemotherapy has produced excellent remission rates in both nonmetastatic and metastatic gestational trophoblastic neoplasia (GTN), but optimal management has not been fully defined. Ross S. Berkowitz, Donald P. Goldstein, Miles A. Jones, Ann R. Marean, and Marilyn R. Bernstein[11-43] (Harvard Med. School) compared the systemic toxicity of methotrexate (MTX) used with citrovorum factor (CF) rescue (MTX-CF), MTX alone and actinomycin D (Act-D) in the treatment of GTN in 75 patients without metastatic disease. Twenty-five patients received each regimen. Methotrexate was given intramuscularly in a dose of 1 mg/kg every other day for 4 doses and CF in a dose of 0.1 mg/kg 24 hours after each dose of MTX. Methotrexate alone was used in a dose of 0.4–0.5 mg/kg daily for 5 consecutive days. Actinomycin D was given intravenously in a dose of 12–15 μg/kg daily for 5 consecutive days.

Only 1 patient treated with MTX-CF had thrombocytopenia or granulocytopenia, or both. Methotrexate alone and Act-D induced hematologic toxicity in 32% and 48% of patients, respectively. Hepatocellular dysfunction occurred in 20% of patients given MTX alone. Actinomycin D induced a generalized rash and marked alopecia in 24% and 52% of cases, respectively. Methotrexate-CF and MTX caused marked stomatitis in 16% and 20% of patients, respectively, and Act-D in 40% of patients.

Treatment of GTN with MTX-CF rescue resulted in less systemic toxicity than treatment with either MTX alone or Act-D in this study. Less hematologic and hepatic toxicity occurred with this regimen, despite a higher cumulative dose of MTX administered than in the MTX-only regimen. The use of MTX-CF rescue reduced the number of courses of chemotherapy necessary to induce remission and also minimized associated morbidity. However, this lowered morbidity may be related to the alternating-day administration of TMX-CF. In the absence of preexisting liver dysfunction, MTX with CF rescue is

(11–43) Cancer 45:423–426, Feb. 1, 1980.

the preferred chemotherapeutic regimen for the management of patients with GTN.

▶ [The adjunctive administration of citrovorum factor (tetrahydrofolic acid) blocks the systemic toxicity (particularly hepatic and hematologic) of methotrexate, enabling the use of higher doses of the chemotherapeutic agent. This study was retrospective and, unfortunately in a scientific sense, methotrexate was given every other day in the citrovorum factor rescue protocol and daily when used alone. Nonetheless, the data seem to indicate clearly the lower toxicity with the former therapy. Though efficacy was not addressed in this report, other studies have indicated the same high order of remission rate with methotrexate-citrovorum factor as with methotrexate alone.] ◀

Role of Operation in the Current Therapy of Gestational Trophoblastic Disease. The responsiveness of patients with gestational trophoblastic neoplasms (GTNs) to chemotherapy has reduced the role of operation in their management. Charles B. Hammond, John C. Weed, Jr., and John L. Currie[11-44] (Duke Univ.) reviewed the results of treatment of 257 patients with GTN, treated at one institution by the same group of physicians in 1966–1978. Choriocarcinoma or invasive mole or hydatidiform mole was diagnosed histologically in all cases. Patients with nonmetastatic disease were treated with intramuscularly administered methotrexate or actinomycin D, administered intravenously. Patients with metastatic disease and a "good" prognosis were managed similarly. Those with a "poor" prognosis now receive triple-agent MAC chemotherapy consisting of methotrexate, actinomycin D and chlorambucil, with courses repeated at 12- to 14-day intervals depending on toxicity.

An overall remission rate of 92% was achieved. All 139 patients with nonmetastatic disease had remission, as did all 55 with metastatic GTN and a "good" prognosis. The remission rate for "poor"-prognosis patients was 66%. Selected patients had surgical or x-ray therapy, or both, as well as chemotherapy. Hysterectomy, done coincident with the institution of systemic chemotherapy, significantly reduced the duration of hospitalization and the amount of chemotherapy used to achieve remission, regardless of whether metastases were present. Delayed excision of chemotherapy-resistant foci of GTN was also of benefit, but was less effective than primary operation. Surgery for other disease or for complications of GTN or its treatment was quite useful in stabilizing patients and permitting chemotherapy to be completed. Chemotherapy did not compromise wound healing.

Chemotherapy remains the single most effective method of treating trophoblastic disease, but surgery and irradiation may also be of use. With the use of all modalities, nearly complete control of this disease can be achieved.

▶ [Although the mainstay of treatment of malignant trophoblastic disease is chemotherapy, there remains a distinct place for surgery, as outlined in this report. The clearest indication is in the patient with locally invasive tumor in the uterus ("chorioadenoma destruens") which persists despite chemotherapy. Considerably less certain is the matter of elective initial hysterectomy (along with chemotherapy) in the older woman who does not want to retain the uterus. The authors *believe* this may improve the prognosis—all of their 32 patients treated this way for nonmetastatic or "good"

(11–44)   Am. J. Obstet. Gynecol. 136:844–858, Apr. 1, 1980.

metastatic disease were cured and seemed to need less hospitalization and fewer courses of chemotherapy—but this is not universally accepted.] ◄

Correlation Between Retinal and Pelvic Vascular Status: Determinant Factor in Patients Undergoing Pelvic Irradiation for Gynecologic Malignancy. The degree of arteriolar sclerosis in pelvic vessels is related to the incidence of radiation-related enteric and genitourinary tract injury. J. R. van Nagell, Jr., R. Kielar, E. S. Donaldson, E. C. Gay, D. F. Powell, Y. Maruyama, and J. Yoneda[11-45] (Univ. of Kentucky, Lexington) examined the relation between pelvic vascular status and retinal vessel changes in 48 patients admitted in 1972 to 1977 who underwent surgical exploration within 3 weeks of retinal examination. Arterial vessels less than 100 μ in diameter were evaluated in each organ removed. Half the patients were hypertensive or diabetic. Cervicovaginal vessels were evaluated in 42 cases.

No retinal or pelvic vascular abnormality was found in 92% of normotensive patients, but vascular changes were seen in the pelvic or retinal vessels of 87% of hypertensive or diabetic patients. An absolute correlation of grade of change was seen between the retinal and pelvic vessels in 74% of the cases, whether or not vascular disease was present. A marked difference between retinal and pelvic vascular findings was noted in only 1 patient. Overall correlation between vascular changes at the two sites was 0.88. Retinal vascular changes correlated significantly with changes in both the cervicovaginal vessels and bowel vessels. Correlation with changes in other pelvic organs such as the ovary and fallopian tube also was significant.

Funduscopy can provide useful information on the extent of vascular disease in structures normally present in the field of pelvic irradiation. Greater dose fractionation should be considered only for those tumor patients with severe sclerotic vascular changes, who are at the highest risk of acquiring radiation-related enteric complications.

► [This study demonstrates a very strong correlation between arteriolar sclerosis in retinal vessels and that in pelvic vessels. Patients with sclerotic pelvic vessels are presumably at increased risk for radiation complications. Thus, it appears that the gynecologic oncologist might utilize the ophthalmoscope in planning treatment regimens.] ◄

Fine-Needle Aspiration Cytology in Gynecologic Oncology: I. Diagnostic Accuracy. Fine-needle aspiration (FNA) cytology offers an alternative to surgical biopsy in many settings. Staffan R. B. Nordqvist, Bernd-Uwe Sevin, Mehrdad Nadji, Shirley E. Greening, and Alan B. P. Ng[11-46] (Univ. of Miami) reviewed preliminary experience with FNA cytology in 74 gynecologic patients who had a total of 77 aspirations, 46 of them from pelvic masses. Aspiration was done transvaginally or transrectally. Eight patients had transabdominal procedures. Seventeen samples were taken from subcutaneous lymph nodes, 5 from other subcutaneous sites, and 1 from a pleural metastasis. Comparison with surgical biopsy or autopsy findings was pos-

(11–45) Am. J. Obstet. Gynecol. 134:551–556, July 1, 1979.
(11–46) Obstet. Gynecol. 54:719–724, December 1979.

CORRELATION BETWEEN ASPIRATION CYTOLOGY AND SUBSEQUENT
HISTOLOGIC DIAGNOSIS

	Histology	
Cytology	Same	Different
Benign	21	2
Adenocarcinoma	20	1
Adenosquamous carcinoma	3	
Squamous cell carcinoma	8	
Undifferentiated carcinoma	1	
Histiocytic lymphoma	2	
Total	55	3

sible for 58 aspirations. Anesthesia was generally unnecessary. The Papanicolaou staining method was used routinely.

Ovarian cancer was confirmed in 8 of 9 cases. Thirty-four aspirations were done to establish or rule out primary malignant disease, and 43 were in patients with suspected recurrent metastatic disease or disease after treatment. There were no complications. The correlation between cytologic and histologic diagnoses is shown in the table. Absence of malignancy was confirmed in 21 of 23 aspirations with normal cytologic findings. A cytologic diagnosis of malignant disease was confirmed histopathologically in 35 cases; agreement on cell type was total in 34. In many cases of benign disease the specific histologic diagnosis was correctly predicted by FNA cytology.

Fine-needle aspiration cytology can differentiate benign from malignant ovarian tumors with great accuracy. The method is applicable to a variety of problems in gynecologic oncology. It is particularly useful in confirming or ruling out metastatic and recurrent disease. Laparotomy and other surgery has been avoided in several instances. No false positive results were obtained in this study, and with proper training and skill the false negative rate should be below 5%. Fine-needle aspiration cytology has also been useful as an adjunct in following irradiated patients with cervical and endometrial cancer. It may be useful in monitoring tumor responses to chemotherapy.

▶ [The authors of this study suggest that fine-needle aspiration cytology may well be useful in confirming the presence of metastatic or recurrent tumor, thereby eliminating the need for a surgical procedure prior to radiotherapy or chemotherapy in certain situations. In all 35 cases with a cytologic diagnosis of malignant disease, histologic specimens confirmed malignancy. Agreement as to cell type was found in 34 of the 35 cases. More work is needed, although this technique looks promising.] ◀

Computerized Tomography Applied to Gynecologic Oncology. Guy J. Photopulos, William H. McCartney, Leslie A. Walton, and Edward V. Staab[11-47] (Univ. of North Carolina) reviewed the first year's experience with computerized tomography (CT) in the evaluation of patients with gynecologic malignancy. Forty patients had pelvic CT examination, and 19 of these also had para-aortic CT scan-

(11–47) Am. J. Obstet. Gynecol. 135:381–383, Oct. 1, 1979.

ning. Most patients had carcinomas of the cervix and endometrium. Scans generally were made after injection of contrast medium. In 17 women, needle aspiration biopsy was directed by CT scanning. Most of the CT studies were done to detect possible recurrent malignancy. Prior to CT examination, 26 patients had received pelvic radiation and 16 had undergone hysterectomy.

The biopsies directed by CT scanning were uncomplicated; confirmation of metastasis obviated the need for surgery in 6 patients. Pelvic bone metastases were identified in 3. Bimanual examination and CT scanning each was incorrect 3 times in 32 verified evaluations of the central pelvis. The CT was incorrect at the pelvic wall in 5 instances and clinical evaluation in 9. The CT scan was incorrect in the para-aortic area in 4 patients and clinical examination in 8.

CT scanning appears to provide valuable differential diagnostic information and to clarify relationships between soft tissues and bony structures. It may help to distinguish both pelvic radiation fibrosis and conglomerate bowel from tumor. The CT scan is also useful in evaluating the pelvic wall and para-aortic regions. Further study with faster scanning methods is necessary to establish more clearly the role of this modality in evaluating pelvic cancer.

▶ [The ultimate role of CT scanning in gynecology in general or in gynecologic oncology in particular remains to be determined. Some role for this tool that has so remarkably altered practice in other areas of medicine seems assured. In this report, needle biopsies directed by the CT image were quite effective in identifying metastatic disease. This obviated the need for laparotomy in order to plan further therapy in some patients.] ◀

Ultrasonographic Versus Clinical Evaluation of a Pelvic Mass. R. David Reeves, Terrance S. Drake, and William F. O'Brien[11-48] (Natl. Naval Med. Center, Bethesda, Md.) compared the preoperative ultrasound and pelvic examination findings with the laparotomy findings in 72 women seen in 1977 and 1978 with a diagnosis of pelvic mass. Patients drank at least 24 oz of fluid before ultrasound study and refrained from voiding for 3 hours before examination.

Sixty-five patients (90%) had correct preoperative detection by both ultrasound and pelvic examination. Four patients had false negative results on ultrasound studies, and 3 had false positive results with pelvic examinations. Seven patients with normal ultrasound studies did not undergo laparoscopy. The accuracy of pelvic examination in detecting a pelvic mass was 95.6%, and that of ultrasound was 94.4%. Both preoperative studies were equally accurate in estimating lesion size and in detectng unilateral and bilateral lesions. Ultrasonography was significantly more accurate in determining the cystic or solid nature of the mass. Ultrasound study failed to do this in only 1 instance.

Ultrasonography is highly accurate in detecting and characterizing pelvic masses, but its routine use did not alter management in this series of patients suspected of having a clinically significant mass on physical examination. Routine preoperative ultrasonography is not

(11-48) Obstet. Gynecol. 55:551-554, May 1980.

indicated in such patients unless knowledge of the cystic or solid nature of the mass will alter management.

▶ [As extraordinarily valuable as ultrasonography has proved to be in obstetrics and gynecology, it seems to us that at times there is a danger of overreliance on the technique, even to the exclusion of pertinent clinical data. A case in point is the question of preoperative ultrasonography where a significant pelvic mass clearly exists. Our bias, which seems to be confirmed by the results of this report, is that the study represents unnecessary expense because the sonographic findings will not influence management. Ultrasonography is often of value in evaluating patients with a questionable mass or a mass of questionable significance and, as indicated by this study, can distinguish cystic vs solid nature more reliably than can physical examination.] ◀

12. Infections

Gynecologic Examination of Prepuberal Child With Vulvovaginitis: Use of Knee-Chest Position is described by S. Jean Emans and D. P. Goldstein[12-1] (Harvard Med. School). Vulvovaginitis is common among prepuberal girls because of such factors as suboptimal hygiene, use of harsh soaps and tight-fitting garments, and pinworm infestation. The vagina and cervix are visualized with the child in the knee-chest position, after inspection of the peritoneum with the child supine. The knee-chest position provides a good view without instrumentation. Specimens for wet preparations and cultures are then taken with the child supine. The rectal examination is done last, and usually only in girls with vaginal bleeding, abdominal pain, or an unusual history. A bimanual rectal abdominal examination is done with the child supine.

Thirty-six girls aged 2 to 11 years were seen for 38 episodes of vulvovaginitis in an 18-month period. The chief symptom was discharge. The vagina was successfully visualized in 32 girls. The causes of vulvovaginitis in this series were variable (table). A specific cause was identified in all 8 patients who reported a green discharge.

Visualization of the vagina in the knee-chest position is possible in most prepuberal girls. In this way pediatricians can readily and ade-

VULVOVAGINITIS IN PREPUBERAL GIRLS		
Etiology	Episodes	
	No.	Total
Nonspecific vaginitis		20
Escherichia coli or other Gram-negative organisms	10	
Normal flora*	10	
Specific vaginitis		18
Foreign bodies	5	
Candida	3	
Group A β streptococci	3	
Neisseria gonorrhoeae	2	
Staphylococcus aureus	1	
Haemophilus influenzae and *E coli*	1	
Trichomonas	1	
Herpes	1	
Cervical polyp	1	

*Two had recently used bubble bath.

(12–1) Pediatrics 65:758–760, April 1980.

quately examine the prepuberal girl and assess the cause of vulvovaginitis.

▶ [We will certainly try the knee-chest position as advocated here. Other important points are that a duration of symptoms of less than 1 month suggests a specific rather than nonspecific etiology, as does a green discharge, and 4 of 5 patients with a blood-tinged discharge had vaginal foreign bodies.] ◀

Natural History of Bacteriuria in Schoolgirls: Long-Term Case-Control Study. Jay Y. Gillenwater, R. Brent Harrison, and Calvin M. Kunin[12-2] followed 60 schoolgirls with bacteriuria and 38 matched controls for 9–18 years in an attempt to define more clearly the natural history of this condition. Bacteriuria was defined as 10^5 or more organisms per ml in 2 or more consecutive cultures. Patients and controls were matched for age, race and school. Episodes of bacteriuria were treated with an appropriate agent for 10–14 days.

Reflux was repaired in 5 of the 60 study subjects, and 2 underwent nephrectomy. One with atrophic pyelonephritis had reduced inulin clearance. Serum creatinine levels were slightly higher in the study group than in controls. Renal scarring or caliectasis was noted in 16 of the study patients but in no controls. Blood pressures were similar in the two groups. Five or more episodes of bacteriuria occurred in 21.7% of the study patients and in 2.6% of controls. Bacteriuria occurred during pregnancy in 63.8% of the study group and in 26.7% of controls. Urinary tract infection developed in 7 children (5 girls) of study patients, but in none of the children of controls. All the mothers had had considerable previous morbidity from recurrent urinary tract infections. All had normal urethral diameters.

Although bacteriuria in schoolgirls rarely leads to end-stage renal failure, it is not an entirely benign disease and should not be ignored. Bacteriuria may be the first clue to important underlying anatomic abnormalities or the start of a long-term course of recurrent symptomatic infections leading to complications of pregnancy. The nitrite test, with bacteriologic studies for confirmation, shows great promise in screening preschool girls for bacteriuria. It is necessary to develop therapeutic measures that prevent recurrent infection. Although long-term, low-dose prophylaxis is highly effective in girls, it does not appear to reduce recurrent infections appreciably after it is discontinued.

▶ [The numbers are not large, but they suggest that schoolgirls identified as being bacteriuric have subsequent problems. Several had urologic structural abnormalities identified; subsequent symptomatic urinary tract infections were common, especially in pregnancy. The prevalence of hypertension on follow-up was not increased over that in controls. End-stage renal failure did not develop in any of the study subjects. This may partly reflect their having been identified by the screening program. This identification permitted early surgical correction of structural abnormalities and vigorous treatment of subsequent urinary tract infections.] ◀

Periurethral Bacterial Flora in Women: Prolonged Intermittent Colonization with *Escherichia coli.* The chief problem in managing urinary tract infection in women is its tendency to recur frequently. Recurrences usually are related to reinfection by bowel flora. Calvin M. Kunin (Ohio State Univ.), Frank Polyak, and Eliza-

(12–2) N. Engl. J. Med. 301:396–399, Aug. 23, 1979.

beth Postel[12-3] (Univ. of Wisconsin) conducted a prospective study of matched premenopausal women to determine whether the periurethral flora is distinctive in women with recurrent urinary tract infections. Daily or alternate-day urine cultures were obtained for 6 to 12 months, as were daily records of sexual intercourse. Thirteen women with at least 2 culture-proved infections in the past year were compared with 18 control subjects with no past history of urinary tract infection. The groups were well matched for age, marital status, sexual activity, and contraceptive use.

Ten study subjects and 4 controls had significant bacteriuria during follow-up. Only 1 of the controls had symptoms of urinary tract infection, and all episodes in the control group cleared spontaneously. The study subjects had 33 bacteriuric episodes, 16 associated with symptoms. *Escherichia coli* was isolated on 17.7% of colonization days in study subjects and 11.4% in controls. Enterococci were isolated on 2.9% and 0.3% of colonization days, respectively. The mean time of colonization with *E. coli* did not differ in the two groups. Colonization periods did not correlate significantly with rates of intercourse. Periurethral colonization with the same organism preceded 29 of 31 episodes of significant bacteriuria in study subjects and 6 of 7 episodes in controls. Spontaneous cures were observed despite continued sexual intercourse.

It cannot be concluded that more prolonged carriage of enteric organisms in the periurethral region explains why certain women have recurrent urinary tract infections. Recurrence appears to be a chance phenomenon. Some women have recurrences even after long remissions, leaving the question of whether this is a unique constitutive or environmental characteristic of this group of women or whether a part of the same population simply remains at risk of acquiring significant bacteriuria.

▶ [Although periurethral colonization with a specific strain of a gram-negative organism typically preceded significant bladder bacteriuria with this organism in both case and control groups, the group with recurrent urinary tract infections was not more likely to have periurethral colonization with these organisms. Others have suggested that women with frequent urinary tract infections have a propensity for colonization in the periurethral area; this study does not support that view.] ◀

***Hemophilus vaginalis* Infection: Diagnosis and Treatment.** Women presenting with a vaginal discharge resulting from nonspecific infection have largely gone untreated. *Hemophilus vaginalis* is believed by many to be the causative agent of these disorders. Mukti N. Bhattacharyya and Brian M. Jones[12-4] investigated 4,263 women attending a specialty, family planning, or gynecologic clinic. The 3,241 patients in the specialty clinic underwent clinical examination, and the rest had laboratory investigations only. The laboratory studies were solely concerned with the isolation and identification of *H. vaginalis*.

A wet mount preparation and gram-stained smear were made. The wet mounts were examined for "clue cells," ie, squamous epithelial

(12–3) JAMA 243:134–139, Jan. 11, 1980.
(12–4) J. Reprod. Med. 24:71–75, February 1980.

cells covered by masses of bacteria. The gram-stained smear always corresponded with wet mount findings in these conditions. Masses of small, gram-variable coccobacilli were present; Döderlein's bacilli were absent. In a large percentage of clue cell-positive specimens, spermatozoa or their remnants were present.

The predominant symptom of *H. vaginalis* infection was a thin, offensive, homogenous gray and sometimes frothy discharge having a pH between 5.0 and 5.5. Vulvar and vaginal inflammation was rarely present.

Overall, 26% of the patients in the specialty clinics had *H. vaginalis* infection, compared to 8% from family planning clinics and 5% from the gynecology clinics.

The 582 patients infected solely with *H. vaginalis* were treated with ampicillin, ampicillin with probenecid, or sulfonamide vaginal tablets. In the successfully treated patients the discharge cleared and *H. vaginalis* was not isolated on repeat culture. Döderlein's bacilli were again present, and neither clue cells nor the masses of gram-variable organisms were seen.

When the male consorts of 68 women infected solely with *H. vaginalis* were examined and urine samples cultured, all tests were negative.

Of the infected women attending the specialty clinic, 41% reported no symptoms, although about half of them did in fact have an offensive discharge on examination. The others, 21% of the total, had no signs or symptoms.

Simple wet-mount microscopy, backed by a gram-stained smear, is reliable in detecting the presence of *H. vaginalis* infection.

▶ [Recently, the value of "clue cells" in the diagnosis of *H. vaginalis* infection and of topical sulfonamide therapy in the treatment of nonspecific vaginitis have both been questioned. The results of this large-scale study indicate reasonably close agreement between the presence of clue cells (epithelial cells whose surfaces are covered by masses of bacteria) and positive cultures for *H. vaginalis.* Many patients with *H. vaginalis* infection are asymptomatic. Although there were no placebo controls, 80% of 247 patients achieved a microscopic and bacteriologic cure after treatment with sulfonamide vaginal tablets.] ◀

Lack of Evidence for Cancer due to Use of Metronidazole. Experimental studies have shown metronidazole to be both carcinogenic and mutagenic, but no long-term studies of exposed patients have been reported. C. Mary Beard, Kenneth L. Noller, W. Michael O'Fallon, Leonard T. Kurland, and Malcolm B. Dockerty[12-5] (Mayo Clinic and Found.) assessed the risk for cancer development after the use of metronidazole to treat trichomoniasis in 771 women seen in 1960–69, in comparison with 237 women with vaginal trichomoniasis who did not receive the drug. A dose of 750 mg daily was given for 10 days; consorts also were treated. Both tablets and vaginal suppositories were prescribed.

Both groups had a median age of 25 years at the time trichomoniasis was diagnosed. Of 40 cancers diagnosed in the study group, 16 were carcinomas in situ of the cervix; there were no invasive cervical

(12–5) N. Engl. J. Med. 301:519–522, Sept. 6, 1979.

cancers. Excluding cervical carcinomas, there was no evidence that cancer developed more frequently in exposed women than in the general population. Observed and expected numbers of breast cancers were the same; however, there were 4 lung cancers, with 0.6 expected, all developing in women who smoked. Eleven cancer deaths occurred in the exposed population, with 7.1 expected on the basis of age-specific cancer death rates for white females in the United States population.

No appreciable increase in cancer was associated with metronidazole administration in this survey. Controlled clinical trials would appear to be ethical for metronidazole but, given the long latent periods of most cancers, such trials seem impractical. Further studies of the type reported are more reasonable alternatives.

▶ [This retrospective study has several drawbacks, which the authors acknowledge. Nonetheless, the lack of a demonstrated relationship between metronidazole exposure and an excess of subsequent malignancies is somewhat reassuring. We continue to use this most effective drug in the treatment of trichomoniasis.] ◀

Do Contraceptives Influence the Incidence of Acute Pelvic Inflammatory Disease in Women with Gonorrhea?

Gunnar Rydén, Lars Fåhraeus, Lars Molin, and Karin Åhman[12-6] (Univ. of Linkoping) examined the influence of various contraceptive methods on the incidence of pelvic inflammatory disease in 672 women seen in 1973–1977 with urogenital gonorrhea, confirmed by laparoscopy in all. Pelvic inflammatory disease was diagnosed in 87 women (12.9%). Two patients with uncomplicated gonorrhea were matched with each study patient. Uncomplicated gonorrhea was treated with pivampicillin and probenecid in a single oral dose. Patients with pelvic inflammatory disease were placed on bed rest, usually for 2 weeks, and given doxycycline monohydrate therapy.

Pelvic inflammatory disease was least frequent in women using hormonal contraception. Their incidence was 8.8%, compared with 23.5% for women using an intrauterine device, and 15.1% for those using neither of these. The incidence in patients using hormonal contraception was significantly lower than that in both the other groups. Gonococci were present in the cervix in nearly all patients with pelvic inflammatory disease but less often in women with uncomplicated gonorrhea who used intrauterine devices. No differences in sensitivity patterns of the gonococcal strains isolated were observed.

The low frequency of cervical gonococci found in women of the control group using intrauterine devices may support the suggested bacteriostatic property of copper ions, however, copper appears not to protect against ascending infection. Studies on the relation between sexually transmitted infection, such as that caused by *Chlamydia trachomatis,* and various contraceptive methods should be of great importance.

▶ [This study notes that among patients with positive gonorrhea cultures (from cervix, urethra, or rectum) the incidence of laparoscopically proved pelvic inflammatory disease was 23.5% in intrauterine device (IUD) users, 8.8% in oral contraceptive users, and 15.1% in users of neither. That the IUD should lead to increased risk of upper tract

(12–6) Contraception 20:149–157, August 1979.

infection is not surprising, though why hormonal contraception should be more "protective" than use of neither hormones nor IUD is less clear. Nearly all of the IUDs were copper in type, which is interesting in view of a reported antigonococcal action of copper in vitro.] ◄

► ↓ For a further consideration of the IUD-PID problem, read on. ◄

Intrauterine Contraceptive Device and Acute Salpingitis. Multifactor Analysis. George Flesh, John M. Weiner, Robert C. Corlett, Jr., Charles Boice, Daniel R. Mishell, Jr., and Rosalie M. Wolf[12-7] (Univ. of Southern California) compared data regarding 163 consecutive indigent women hospitalized with acute salpingitis and 222 women presenting to the minor trauma section of the emergency room.

The two groups were similar in age, number of live births, type of termination of last pregnancy, spontaneous abortions, frequency of intercourse, and methods of contraception other than intrauterine device (IUD). Four variates were significantly different between cases and controls: race, type of contraception, number of sex partners in the past year, and previous history of salpingitis. There were more blacks in the case group (49%) than among controls (19%) and more Spanish-Americans among controls (57%) than among cases (26%). Intrauterine devices were used by almost twice as many salpingitis patients (25%) as controls (14%). Two or more sexual partners were reported by 63% of the patients and 24% of controls. Previous episodes of salpingitis occurred in 42% of cases and 14% of controls. Differences in types of IUDs used by cases and controls were interesting but not significant: Lippes loop in 38% of cases and 48% of controls, copper devices in 27% of cases and 20% of controls, and Dalkon shield in 32% of cases and 16% of controls.

By combining the four individually significant variates, a series of subgroups emerged which were analyzed in a multiple linear logistic equation to give each subgroup an estimated probability for acquiring salpingitis (table). Each risk factor remained valid not only when applied to the study group as a whole, but also when applied to every possible subgroup of combined risk factors. This finding lays to rest the suspicion that these risk factors might be reflections of each other rather than independent factors.

Any study of IUD-related infection must examine at least three risk factors in addition to contraceptive use: race, previous history of salpingitis, and number of sexual partners. Clinicians working with lower socioeconomic populations should carefully consider whether to insert IUDs in women who have one or more of these risk factors.

► [The authors of this report are aware of the weaknesses inherent in this type of case-control analysis and of the potential biases in the data. For example, are patients with acute pelvic inflammatory disease (PID) more apt to be hospitalized if they have IUDs in situ than if they do not? Given this uncertainty, the results reported *suggest* that IUD users of low socioeconomic class are predisposed to hospitalization for acute PID. This predisposition cannot be explained away by a consideration of other identified risk factors.

In a related study also based on hospital admission for PID, Osser and colleagues

---

(12–7) Am. J. Obstet. Gynecol. 135:402–408, Oct. 1, 1979.

PROBABILITY OF PID IN SUBGROUPS DEFINED BY RISK FACTORS*

| | Risk factors | | | | Sample size in subgroup | | | |
Group	Black	IUD	Sex partner	Previous PID	Controls	Cases	Probability (%)	Relative risk
1	No	No	1	No	92	13	14	1.00
2	No	No	1	Yes	14	4	27	2.34
3	No	Yes	1	No	17	8	32	2.96
4	Yes	No	More	No	18	12	36	3.65
5	No	Yes	1	Yes	26	19	43	4.86
6	No	No	1	Yes	1	2	52	6.92
7	Yes	Yes	1	No	3	7	57	8.55
8	Yes	No	More	Yes	4	4	62	10.82
9	No	Yes	More	No	8	18	64	11.38
10	No	No	More	No	1	7	69	14.40
11	Yes	Yes	1	Yes	7	19	73	17.78
12	Yes	Yes	More	Yes	1	4	79	25.30
13	No	No	More	Yes	2	4	84	33.67
14	Yes	Yes	More	No	4	16	86	41.58
15	Yes	Yes	More	Yes	1	8	89	52.61
16	Yes	Yes	More	Yes	0	1	95	123.06
Total					199	146		

*Equation: -1.423 (black $- 1.3159$) $+ 1.271$ (IUD $- 1.1884$).
$+ 1.059$ (sex partners $- 1.4087$) $+ 1.555$ (previous PID $- 1.2580$).
Codes: Black: 1 = no; 2 = yes. Sex partners: 1 = one; 2 = two or more.
IUD: 1 = no; 2 = yes. Previous PID: 1 = no; 2 = yes.

(Lancet 1:386, 1980) concluded that PID risk was doubled in IUD users over that in age-matched controls. No relationship with parity was found.] ◄

Intrauterine Contraceptive Device Use and Pelvic Inflammatory Disease. Pelvic inflammatory disease is among the more common gynecologic disorders affecting women of childbearing age. David W. Kaufman, Samuel Shapiro, Lynn Rosenberg, Richard R.

Monson, Olli S. Miettinen, Paul D. Stolley, and Dennis Slone[12-8] studied the relationship between intrauterine contraceptive device (IUD) use and first episodes of pelvic inflammatory disease among sexually active women. The length of IUD use and types of IUD were also evaluated.

The study included the records of 44 women with first episodes of pelvic inflammatory disease and 259 control women with nongynecologic problems. Women who had an abortion or ectopic pregnancy in the 6 months prior to admission were excluded, as were pregnant patients. Every woman included had used either an IUD or an oral contraceptive in the month prior to admission.

Rates of current IUD use were higher among women with pelvic inflammatory disease in all age groups. The age-adjusted relative risk for IUD users was 6.5. The findings were not affected by such variables as religion, ethnic origin, marital status, educational level, or family income. Simultaneous adjustment for age and parity increased the relative risk estimate to 7.9.

The duration of IUD use was also relevant. The age-adjusted relative risk for those who had used IUDs continuously for at least 5 years was 12.9. The estimate of risk was 5.7 for women with less than 5 years of IUD use. The duration effect remained when women using the copper-7 IUD were excluded, because all had used the device for less than 5 years.

The type of IUD being used also seemed to influence the relative risk estimate. The relative risk for copper-7 IUD users was 3.8; for Lippes loop users, 7.9; for Saf-t-coil users, 9.2; and for Dalkon shield users, 12.3. When age and duration of use were taken into account, the risk to copper-7 users was consistently the least elevated.

This study suggests that women using IUDs have a rate of hospital admission for pelvic inflammatory disease which is approximately 7 times greater than the rate among oral contraceptive users.

▶ [This retrospective case-control study suggests that PID risk is increased somewhere between 3 and 13 times in IUD users, findings quite consistent with several other recent reports. What is new here is the suggestion (and it should be emphasized that it is only a suggestion) of a lower risk with copper devices than with others.] ◀

Cefoxitin as Single-Dose Treatment for Urethritis Caused by Penicillinase-Producing *Neisseria gonorrhoeae*. Penicillinase-producing *Neisseria gonorrhoeae* constitutes over 40% of isolates in some parts of the world. Most such strains are not eradicated by standard high-dose penicillin regimens. S. William Berg, Michael E. Kilpatrick, William O. Harrison, and J. Allen McCutchan[12-9] (San Diego) evaluated cefoxitin in the treatment of urethritis caused by penicillinase-producing *N. gonorrhoeae*. Military personnel were studied at a base where 41% of gonococcal urethritis had been caused by penicillin-resistant strains. Patients were treated with 2 gm cefoxitin intramuscularly, mixed with 0.5% lidocaine, or with 4.8 million units of procaine penicillin G in two simultaneous intramuscular injections. A 1 gm dose of probenecid was given before each antibiotic treatment.

(12–8) Am. J. Obstet. Gynecol. 136:159–162, Jan. 15, 1980.
(12–9) N. Engl. J. Med. 301:509–511, Sept. 6, 1979.

The 54 cefoxitin-treated and 53 penicillin-treated men were similar in age, duration of symptoms, past history of gonococcal urethritis and percentage of penicillinase-producing gonococci. All 54 cefoxitin-treated patients were cured, as were only 64% of the penicillin-treated patients. Those with penicillin-resistant isolates had a 77% failure rate with penicillin therapy. Five infections due to resistant strains were cured by penicillin. Penicillinase-producing strains usually were resistant to 20 μg of penicillin per ml, but they were sensitive to cefoxitin. Five patients had moderate pain at the cefoxitin injection site. No serious adverse effects were noted.

Cefoxitin appears to be an effective alternative to spectinomycin in the treatment of gonococcal urethritis caused by penicillinase-producing strains of *N. gonorrhoeae*.

▶ [Cefoxitin (a semisynthetic cephamycin), like spectinomycin, is an effective treatment for lower tract gonorrhea caused by penicillinase-producing strains.] ◀

Aseptic Arthritis After Gonorrhea. L. Rosenthal, B. Olhagen, and S. Ek[12-10] (Karolinska Hosp., Stockholm) sought to determine whether gonococcal infection plays a role in the pathogenesis of uroarthritis, including Reiter's syndrome, by comparing the clinical course and immunologic reactions to gonococcal antigen in 16 patients with postgonococcal aseptic arthritis and 14 with arthritis that followed nongonococcal urogenital infection. Twelve of the former had developed arthritis or severe arthralgia within 3 weeks of gonococcal urethritis. Mean age was 30.8 years, compared with 31.4 years for patients with nongonococcal urogenital infection. Diagnoses in this group included acute Reiter's disease of venereal origin, chronic uroarthritis, and pelvospondylitis. Fifty-eight healthy subjects were used as controls in the lymphocyte studies.

The clinical course of postgonococcal arthritis was not distinct from that of other forms of uroarthritis. Four patients had conjunctivitis, and 1 had keratodermia blenorrhagica. Five patients in the nongonococcal group had symptoms of conjunctivitis. *Chlamydia trachomatis* was isolated in 1 case. Antibiotics including penicillin had no dramatic effect on the articular symptoms. No leukocytosis was observed. The gonococcal complement fixation test was positive in 9 postgonococcal cases. Lymphocyte stimulation by gonococcal antigen was significantly greater in postgonococcal patients than in healthy controls. Cell reactivity also differed significantly between the two patient groups, but the nongonococcal group did not differ significantly from the control group.

The findings support the hypothesis that *Neisseria gonorrhoeae* may induce an aseptic arthritis, which sometimes presents as a complete Reiter syndrome. In many patients with gonorrhea who receive adequate penicillin therapy, gonococci may survive in the accessory glands or oviducts and induce an aseptic postinfectious, or "reactive," arthritis among those who are susceptible. This probably is an immune reaction in the joint similar to the arthritides that follow rheumatic fever and other infections.

▶ [Reiter's syndrome (urethritis, conjunctivitis, and aseptic arthritis) is generally con-

(12–10) Ann. Rheum. Dis. 39:141–146, April 1980.

sidered to include nongonococcal urethritis. *Mycoplasma* and *Chlamydia* organisms have been implicated. This report suggests that the urethritis may be due to gonococcal infection in some cases and that the clinical picture is similar regardless of the specific etiology of the urogenital infection. Therefore, in the view of the authors of this article, Reiter's syndrome does not necessarily mean nongonococcal urogenital infection. Conversely, arthritis occurring in a patient with gonorrhea may not necessarily indicate bacterial infection of the joint.] ◄

Genital *Chlamydia trachomatis* Infections in Patients with Cervical Atypia. *Chlamydia trachomatis* has received attention as an important agent in venereally transmitted urogenital infections, and cervical infection with this agent may be related to cervical atypia. Jorma Paavonen, Ervo Vesterinen, Bengt Meyer, Pekka Saikku, Jukka Suni, Esko Purola, and Eero Saksela[12-11] (Helsinki) determined the frequency of genital *C. trachomatis* infection prospectively in patients with cytologically verified cervical epithelial atypia. Studies were done in 177 women with a mean age of 33.2 years, seen over about 1 year with cervicovaginal smears that showed atypical cells of mild or moderate dysplasia (153 cases) or severe dysplasia (24 cases). Cervical and urethral samples were assessed for *C. trachomatis* using irradiated McCoy cells. Antibody to *C. trachomatis* was determined by microcomplement fixation and single-antigen immunofluorescence tests in 93 subjects.

Chlamydia trachomatis was isolated from 29 (16%) patients. Seventeen patients had the agent in both the cervix and the urethra, 7 in the cervix only, and 5 in the urethra only. Six of 24 patients with malignant changes harbored *C. trachomatis*. Antichlamydial complement fixation antibody was present in titers of 8 or above in 56% of the patients, compared with 17% of a control series. Immunofluorescence antibody was found in 81% of the patients and in 51% of the controls. No significant differences in antibodies against herpesvirus II or cytomegalovirus were observed.

This study showed an increased incidence of excretion of *C. trachomatis* from the urogenital tract in patients with cervical dysplasia, and an increase in antichlamydial antibodies. The long-term effects of the latent stage of host-parasite interactions are not known, and the present seroepidemiologic observations do not constitute proof of an etiologic role for *C. trachomatis*. It is possible that the high level of chlamydial seropositivity in patients with cervical atypia simply reflects a sexually more promiscuous population.

► [Chlamydiae are currently in vogue on the gynecologic infectious disease circuit. Since infection with these intracellular parasites can be venereally transmitted, it is not surprising that patients with cervical atypia were more likely to possess antibodies against *C. trachomatis* than were the control patients. Association does not mean causation, as the authors point out. We were somewhat surprised that antibodies to herpesvirus type II were not more common in the study patients compared with the controls.] ◄

Perihepatitis and Chlamydial Salpingitis. Perihepatitis, a complication of acute salpingitis, is characterized by sudden pain in the right upper part of the abdomen; in the acute stage, there is a localized peritonitis involving the anterior surface of the liver and adja-

(12–11) Obstet. Gynecol. 54:289–291, September 1979.

cent peritoneum. Chlamydial infection has been described in patients with peritonitis and perihepatitis. P. Wølner-Hanssen, L. Weström, and P.-A. Mårdh[12-12] (Univ. of Lund) describe 3 patients with salpingitis and perihepatitis with evidence of genital chlamydial infection. A fourth patient had salpingitis and symptoms suggesting Fitz-Hugh-Curtis syndrome, but the surface of the liver was normal at laparoscopy. None had evidence of gonococcal infection.

Girl, 14, a nullipara, had had low abdominal pain for 3 weeks which moved to the right upper quadrant 10 days earlier. Physical examination showed right upper-quadrant tenderness and liver enlargement, but no adnexal tenderness. An ultrasound scan of the gallbladder was normal, but the gallbladder was not seen at cholecystography. Laparotomy showed violin-string adhesions between the anterior capsule of the left hepatic lobe and the anterior abdominal wall, with a small abscess near the gallbladder. The fallopian tubes were red and swollen, and adhesions were present. The male partner had urethritis and was culture positive for *Chlamydia trachomatis,* but gonorrhea was not diagnosed. The patient received 100 mg doxycycline daily, and symptoms subsided within 12 days. Pelvic examination was normal 9 days later.

Chlamydia trachomatis is at least as common a cause of sexually transmitted genital infections as *Neisseria gonorrhoeae* and may be even more common in salpingitis associated with perihepatitis. Serologic evidence of *C. trachomatis* infection was obtained in all 4 patients, and *C. trachomatis* was found in cervical specimens from 3 patients, but not from the 1 tubal biopsy specimen. Young women with right upper-quadrant pain and signs of lower genital tract infection should have laparoscopy.

▶ [*Chlamydia trachomatis* has been implicated as an etiologic agent in acute salpingitis. These cases suggest, but do not prove, that the organism may be responsible for perihepatitis as well. The Fitz-Hugh-Curtis syndrome apparently can no longer be regarded as definitely indicating gonococcal infection.] ◀

In Vitro Susceptibility of Anaerobic Flora of Female Genital Tract to Ampicillin Compared to Spectinomycin. Pelvic inflammatory disease may be caused by anaerobic bacteria or the gonococcus. Haragopal Thadepalli, Vinh Toan Bach, David Webb, and Ira Roy[12-13] (Univ. of Southern California) compared the efficacy of two antibiotics, ampicillin and spectinomycin, against 370 clinical isolates of anaerobic bacteria from the female genital tract. The 136 strains of *Bacteroides* included 86 of *Bacteroides fragilis.* Other common isolates were *Peptococcus, Peptostreptococcus,* and *Clostridium* spp.

Spectinomycin inhibited 76% of the anaerobic isolates at 64 µg/ml, and also inhibited 78% of the *B. fragilis* strains. *Peptococcus* was highly susceptible to spectinomycin, but peptostreptococci were relatively resistant. At 128 µg/ml, spectinomycin inhibited 98% of all isolates. Ampicillin at 8 µg/ml inhibited 75% of all anaerobes and 75%–76% of strains of *Peptostreptococcus* and *Peptococcus.* Ampicillin was also effective against other gram-positive bacteria, but not against *B.*

(12–12) Lancet 1:901–904, Apr. 26, 1980.
(12–13) Chemotherapy 26:111–115, 1980.

fragilis. At 16 μg/ml, ampicillin was satisfactorily active against 78% of all anaerobes except *B. fragilis.*

It appears that both ampicillin and spectinomycin may have a place in the treatment of pelvic inflammatory disease. More anaerobes were susceptible to spectinomycin in this study than has been reported previously.

▶ [In view of the presumed polymicrobial nature of pelvic inflammatory disease, it seems reasonable to use a drug whose spectrum includes both aerobic and anaerobic organisms. This in vitro study indicates a better anaerobic action for spectinomycin than has been thought to be the case. Levels of 128 μg/ml, theoretically attainable with a dosage schedule of 8 gm/day, inhibited 92% or more of all anaerobes tested. Ampicillin, by contrast, at 16 μg/ml (attainable with 3.5 gm orally accompanied by 1 gm probenecid simultaneously) inhibited only 70% of *Bacteroides fragilis.*] ◀

False Positive Hemagglutination Inhibition Tests for Pregnancy with Tubo-ovarian Abscess. The hemagglutination inhibition (HI) test for human chorionic gonadotropin (hCG) has been in wide use since 1960, and many false positive test results have been reported. Edward Jacobson and Desider Rothe[12-14] (New York Hosp.-Cornell Med. Center) encountered eight false positive HI test results for pregnancy associated with tubo-ovarian abscess during the past 6 years. The Pregnosticon Accuspheres 2-hour qualitative test for pregnancy has been used during this time. Urine specimens were random collections submitted for immediate incubation. No false positive results were obtained in patients with acute salpingitis, pyosalpinx or perioophoritis, but tests in 8 of 42 patients with tubo-ovarian abscess (21%) had false positive results. All eight tests reverted to negative within 2 to 5 days after treatment. Abscess formation and the absence of pregnancy or teratoma were confirmed at operation in 5 patients.

Substances generated by pelvic inflammatory masses may interfere with immunologic assays for pregnancy, resulting in misdiagnosis or inappropriate management. False positive reactions have been attributed to many pharmaceutical agents, nonspecific inhibitors in the serum and urine, and the production of substances immunologically similar to hCG from nongestational sources. Various tumors have also been implicated, but inflammatory masses have rarely been suggested as a cause of a positive reaction to a pregnancy test. The overall occurrence of false positive reactions is low, making present conventional tests useful and accurate. A high rate of false positive HI reactions should, however, be considered when the nature of a pelvic inflammatory mass is assessed and when intrauterine or ectopic pregnancy is being ruled out.

▶ [Among 42 patients with tubo-ovarian abscesses in whom pregnancy tests were done, the results were falsely positive in 8 (5 of whom proved at surgery to not be pregnant), an amazingly high incidence. By way of explanation, the authors speculate that an acute-phase immunologic resection may produce something that is excreted in the urine and interferes in any of several hemagglutination-inhibition tests.] ◀

Pelvic Colonization with *Actinomyces* in Women Using Intrauterine Contraceptive Devices. Intrauterine devices (IUDs) are widely used for contraception by women in the United States. Pelvic infections and actinomycotic granules have been observed in associa-

---

(12–14) Int. J. Gynaecol. Obstet. 17:307–311, Jan.–Feb. 1980.

tion with all modern types of device. The species most often identified has been *Actinomyces israelii*. About 300 cases of pelvic actinomycosis have been reported. W. D. Hager, B. Douglas, B. Majmudar, Z. M. Naib, O. J. Williams, C. Ramsey, and J. Thomas[12-15] (Atlanta, Ga.) carried out a prospective case-control study of *Actinomyces* colonization or infection in IUD users. Fifty women who desired or required removal of their IUDs, in place for at least a month, were compared with 50 controls who had dysfunctional uterine bleeding. All subjects were aged 17 and over and were parous and sexually active. All patients with positive cultures had specimens evaluated by fluorescent antibody testing.

The two groups had similar past histories of pelvic inflammatory disease. *Actinomyces* organisms were isolated from 4 of 9 IUD patients aged 35 or over and from none of 29 controls. The overall rate of *Actinomyces*-like organisms was 8% in the IUD group. The difference from the comparison group approached significance at the 5% level. All 4 affected women were aged 40 or over and were multiparous. Three had had an IUD in place for at least 2 years. None had pelvic inflammatory disease at IUD removal, but 1 had cervicitis. The patients were managed by IUD removal only. Follow-up biopsies or Papanicolaou smears showed no evidence of *Actinomyces* infection after at least 1 month of follow-up.

Infection or colonization with *Actinomyces* organisms may occur in women using IUDs. Cervical cytologic study detected *Actinomyces* colonization in all culture-positive cases in this series. Patients with symptoms should have the IUD removed and should receive antibiotics providing both aerobic and anaerobic coverage. *Actinomyces* organisms are sensitive to both penicillin and tetracycline. Patients in whom *Actinomyces* organisms are identified on culture, biopsy, or smear and who have no evidence of pelvic infection should be considered for IUD removal and should have a follow-up biopsy or cytologic smear a month later.

▶ [Several recent reports have suggested an increased incidence of genital *Actinomyces* infections in IUD users, an association confirmed in this study that also illustrates the use of cytologic diagnostic techniques.] ◀

Single-Dose and Multidose Prophylaxis in Vaginal Hysterectomy: Comparison of Sodium Cephalothin and Metronidazole.

Abbreviated courses of prophylactic antibiotics have reduced febrile morbidity in connection with vaginal hysterectomy. Kamal A. Hamod, Michael R. Spence, Neil B. Rosenshein, and Michael B. Dillon[12-16] (Johns Hopkins Hosp.) attempted to determine whether a single preoperative dose of antibiotic can prevent infection after vaginal hysterectomy and whether metronidazole, effective against anaerobic bacteria, compares favorably with the broad-spectrum agent sodium cephalothin.

Subjects were 79 premenopausal patients, aged 20 to 44 years (mean, 28.58 years) who were undergoing vaginal hysterectomy for cervical intraepithelial neoplasia. Patients were assigned to three

(12–15) Am. J. Obstet. Gynecol. 135:680–684, Nov. 1, 1979.
(12–16) Ibid., 136:976–979, Apr. 15, 1980.

treatment groups: (1) cephalothin, 3 gm by intravenous minibottle as a single dose on call to the operating room; (2) 3 gm followed by 1 gm every 6 hours for eight subsequent doses; (3) metronidazole, 2 gm orally the night before operation.

There was no statistically significant difference between the three treatment groups with regard to age, weight, operating time, blood loss, and number of drugs given. The overall mean hospital stay was 6.2 days; it was not significantly different in the three groups. Fever indices were lower in the single-dose cephalothin group than in the other groups. Three patients (3.8%) had serious pelvic infection. Two patients given multidose cephalothin and 1 patient given metronidazole had vaginal cuff cellulitis; 1 of these had to be rehospitalized for drainage of a vaginal cuff abscess. No patient given a single dose of cephalothin had a pelvic infection.

A single dose of sodium cephalothin on call to the operating room appears to be adequate prophylaxis in vaginal hysterectomy. Prophylactic antibiotic administration beyond a single dose appears not to be warranted. The antibiotic need not necessarily be a broad-spectrum agent but one that has activity against either anaerobic or aerobic flora.

▶ [This report is representative of several recent publications suggesting efficacy of metronidazole for prophylaxis with vaginal hysterectomy. Although the "fever index" was somewhat lower with single-dose cephalothin than with metronidazole, on balance, the results were similar. Because cephalothin acts against aerobic bacteria and metronidazole against anaerobic organisms, this similarity implies that postoperative pelvic infections are polymicrobial and that agents directed against either are effective.

Somewhat different results were reported by Kuhn (Aust. N.Z. J. Obstet. Gynaecol. 20:43, 1980) in a double-blind study of tinidazole, a nitroimidazole derivative claimed to be more effective than metronidazole against *Bacteroides fragilis.* Prophylactic treatment before abdominal and vaginal hysterectomy had no significant effect on febrile morbidity, nor did drainage of the vaginal vault make any difference.] ◀

Serum Antibody Response to *Bacteroides fragilis* in Women with Abscesses Following Hysterectomy. B. Frank Polk, Dennis L. Kasper, Mervyn Shapiro, Ira B. Tager, Stephen C. Schoenbaum, and Paul R. Goldstein[12-17] (Boston) report a prospective study in which serologic data were collected to determine the role of *B. fragilis* in infectious complications after hysterectomy, particularly abscess formation.

Serum samples were collected from 53 women before hysterectomy and prior to discharge. The patients fell into one of five categories: (1) those with an uncomplicated postoperative course; (2) those with fever on at least 2 days postoperatively, excluding the first 24 hours; (3) those with wound infection; (4) those with pelvic cellulitis; and (5) those with a cuff or pelvic abscess.

Serum antibody to the capsular polysaccharide of *B. fragilis* was measured with a radioactive antigen binding assay.

Both baseline and final antibody concentrations of the five groups varied widely. When changes in antibody concentrations for each patient in the five groups were measured, significant differences among the groups were found. The mean antibody concentration rise in the

(12-17) Obstet. Gynecol. 55:163-166, February 1980.

abscess group (4.91 μg/ml) was significantly greater than the rise among patients with no complications (0.62 μg/ml), wound infection (1.90 μg/ml), pelvic cellulitis (0.63 μg/ml), or febrile episodes (0.95 μg/ml). The changes in antibody concentrations in these latter four groups were not significantly different from one another.

Of 5 patients who had an antibody concentration rise greater than 3.0 μg/ml but no abscess, 2 had pelvic inflammatory disease and 1 had a wound infection with two types of anaerobic gram-negative bacilli.

These data suggest that most cuff or pelvic abscesses which occur after hysterectomy are associated with increased production of antibody to *B. fragilis*. This organism, however, seems to be infrequently involved in other infectious complications of hysterectomy.

▶ [This is a somewhat different approach that confirms the important role of *Bacteroides fragilis* in posthysterectomy infectious complications, especially abscess formation.] ◀

13. Endocrinology

Correlation of Ultrasonic and Endocrinologic Assessment of Human Follicular Development. Accurate assessment of follicular growth and development is important in the investigation and management of infertile women, and noninvasive methods must be used. B. J. Hackelöer, R. Fleming, H. P. Robinson, A. H. Adam, and J. R. T. Coutts[13-1] assessed human ovarian follicular development by measuring peripheral plasma hormone levels and by ultrasonic visualization of the ovary in women apparently menstruating normally. Longitudinal ultrasound scans were made with an apparatus that had a 19-mm internally focused 3.5-MHz transducer; the full bladder technique was used. Hormone concentrations were measured by specific radioimmunoassays. Twenty-three cycles in 15 women were evaluated. Age range was 18 to 36 years.

The coefficient of correlation between mean plasma estradiol values and follicular diameter on day -5 to day 0 of normal cycles was 0.968. When individual paired data were subjected to multiple linear regression analyses, the coefficient of correlation was 0.771. No significant correlation was found between follicular diameters and 17α-hydroxyprogesterone values.

Ultrasound measurements of follicular diameter are of value in assessing follicular growth and development. Among patients in whom ovulation is induced with gonadotropins, the ultrasound technique may differentiate those in whom a single follicle has matured from others who are at risk of multiple ovulation. The management of women receiving either artificial insemination-husband or artificial insemination-donor might benefit from a knowledge of the exact stage of follicular growth, since accurate timing of insemination should improve the pregnancy rate.

Assessment of Ovulation by Ultrasound and Estradiol Levels During Spontaneous and Induced Cycles. Ovulation induction must be monitored carefully to reduce ovarian hyperstimulation syndrome, multiple ovulations, and multiple pregnancies. David H. Smith, Richard H. Picker, Michael Sinosich, and Douglas M. Saunders[13-2] (Royal North Shore Hosp., Sydney) assessed the value of ultrasound in monitoring ovulation induction.

Graafian follicle growth and subsequent ovulation were studied in 45 spontaneous menstrual cycles of 28 patients by estimation of plasma estradiol (E_2) levels and measurement of follicle size and number by ultrasound. Twenty cycles were in 13 apparently normal women undergoing artificial insemination with donor semen (control

(13–1) Am. J. Obstet. Gynecol. 135:122–128, Sept. 1, 1979.
(13–2) Fertil. Steril. 33:387–390, April 1980.

group). Twenty cycles were in 11 infertile women given 50 mg clomiphene citrate daily for 5 days, starting on cycle day 5. Five cycles were in 4 infertile patients receiving human pituitary gonadotropin (hPG). Follicle size was measured by B-mode gray-scale ultrasound, with use of a 3.5-MHz transducer. Patients were examined daily from day 10 of each cycle.

Only one follicle cyst was present in 19 of the 20 cycles in the control group. The mean follicle diameter was 2.55 cm, and the mean peak E_2 levels was 1,523.1 pmoles/L. Four pregnancies occurred in this group. In 1 cycle with two graafian follicle cysts, no pregnancy occurred.

Six pregnancies occurred in the clomiphene-treated patients. The mean estradiol level with only one follicle present was significantly above that in control cycles. No difference in follicle size was noted. In 1 hPG-treated patient with five large follicles, the ovulatory dose of human chorionic gonadotropin was withheld because of a high E_2 level.

There was no difference between pregnant and nonpregnant cycles in all groups studied as judged by peak estradiol levels or graafian follicle diameters. No conceptions have occurred in patients with a peak estradiol level less than 950 pmoles/L and a follicle diameter of less than 1.5 cm.

Ultrasound measurement of follicle diameter and estimation of E_2 level are complementary studies in monitoring ovulation induction.

▶ [This article and the preceding one describe an exciting new use for ultrasound—visualization of the developing follicle. Both studies noted a very close correlation with estradiol levels. Ultrasound gives additional information since a given estradiol level could reflect either a single mature follicle or multiple immature follicles. This technique seems particularly promising as an adjunct to ovulation induction; indeed, in one case of Smith and associates, human chorionic gonadotropin was withheld for fear of multiple pregnancy when five large follicles were seen. Ultrasound might even be useful in timing coitus or insemination in infertility patients.

Follicular growth was also measured ultrasonically by Renaud and colleagues (Fertil. Steril. 33:272, 1980). The average growth rate was 3 mm/day to a maximum diameter of 2.7 ± 0.3 cm on the day prior to disappearance.] ◄

Morphology of Hemostasis in Menstrual Endometrium. G. C. M. L. Christiaens, J. J. Sixma, and A. A. Haspels[13-3] (Univ. of Utrecht) used light and electron microscopy and immunofluorescence to evaluate the endometrium in 9 uteri, removed during the first 72 hours of normal menstruation, to assess the morphological features of hemostasis in menstrual endometrium. Most hysterectomies were done because of genital prolapse. All the patients were under age 46 years and had had regular cycles and normal menses. None had used hormonal medication for the past two cycles, and recent cervical smears were normal.

Stromal disintegration and vessel lesions without any hemostatic reaction were seen during premenstrual spotting. Blood extravasation was prominent in the functional endometrium for up to 20 hours after onset of menstrual bleeding. The vessels were partly or totally sealed by intravascular thrombi functioning as hemostatic plugs. The

(13–3) Br. J. Obstet. Gynaecol. 87:425–439, May 1980.

thrombi contained various amounts of platelets and fibrin and were shed with the tissue. New plugs were seen to have formed upstream in the same vessels. Most functional endometrium had desquamated 20 hours after onset of bleeding. Few thrombi or none were seen from 20 to 72 hours after the start of menstrual bleeding. Extravasation, disintegration, shedding, and plug formation moved gradually toward the deeper layers until the basal endometrium was reached at about 20 hours.

The findings suggest that hemostasis in menstrual endometrium may be due to adherence of the vessel lips. In contrast to skin wounds, unplugged vessels are seen with endometrial lesions, and the plugs are entirely intravascular and are much smaller. Probably, differences in prostaglandin content of these tissues are important.

▶ [This study suggests that different mechanisms of hemostasis are operative at different times during menstruation. In the first day, intravascular platelet and fibrin plugs are found in the functional endometrium. After this endometrium is shed from the basal layer, plugs are no longer seen. Hemostasis then apparently depends on vaso-constriction and on endometrial regeneration.] ◀

Effects of Exercise on the Serum Concentrations of FSH, LH, Progesterone, and Estradiol. It has been reported that intense training can interfere with the normal menstrual cycle. A. Bonen, W. Y. Ling, K. P. MacIntyre, R. Neil, J. C. McGrail and A. N. Belcastro[13-4] (Dalhousie Univ.) examined the effects of 30 minutes of bicycle exercise at 74.1% of maximal VO_2 on hormonal responses in 10 young women with an average age of 21.1. Eight had never used oral contraception and 2 discontinued oral contraception before the study. Six tests were done in the luteal phase and 3 during the menses. The lactate level at the end of exercise was 94.8 mg/100 ml.

The serum progesterone increased on exercise, as did the estradiol level. Increments of 37.6% and 13.5%, respectively, were observed. The LH level fell slightly at the end of exercise, largely because of a marked fall in 1 subject tested on the day of the LH surge. Increments in progesterone were more marked at higher exercise intensities. Estradiol changes were more marked when exercise exceeded 60% of maximal oxygen uptake in the luteal phase. Estradiol levels increased on exercise during the luteal phase but not during menses. Increments in progesterone during these two phases were comparable. The FSH/LH ratio increased during menses but not during exercise in the luteal phase of the cycle.

Heavy exercise in untreated subjects provoked significant increments in ovarian hormones. No such increments are noted in trained subjects exercising at the same absolute work loads. Pituitary hormones were not altered by exercise in the present study.

▶ [These results are interesting. Why should estradiol and progesterone levels increase with intense exercise? It seems unlikely that ovarian secretory rates should be increased, but perhaps metabolic clearance rates might diminish by, for example, lowering of blood flow to the site(s) of clearance (ie, the liver). The increase in ovarian hormone levels was not seen when the subjects were retested after training but, unfortunately, these observations were confounded by the occurrences of menstrual irregularity.] ◀

(13-4) Eur. J. Appl. Physiol. 42:15–23, September, 1979.

Human Chorionic Gonadotropin-Like Material: Presence in Normal Human Tissues. Braunstein et al. (1975) described a human chorionic gonadotropin (hCG)-like material in extracts of normal human testis, and Chen et al. (1976) found such material in pituitary tissue and urine from a patient with Klinefelter's syndrome. Yoshio Yoshimoto, Ada R. Wolfsen, Frank Hirose, and W. D. Odell[13-5] (Univ. of California, Los Angeles) have used a radioreceptor assay for gonadotropin and a β-chain radioimmunoassay for hCG to demonstrate hCG-like material in all normal human tissues evaluated. The activity was completely absorbed by a hCG-antibody affinity column, and was shown to possess altered carbohydrate content in studies in which the material failed to bind to concanavalin A-Sepharose affinity columns. More than 90% of placental hCG was bound to concanavalin A in control studies, whereas placental hCG rendered carbohydrate-free failed to bind to concanavalin A.

Carbohydrate-free hCG is cleared rapidly from the circulation, and has little or no biologic potency in vivo. It appears that the hCG-like material present in normal tissues has the protein structure of hCG, but probably little or no bioactivity in vivo. The trophoblastic cell appears not to be unique in its ability to synthesize hCG, but can glycosylate hCG, transforming a ubiquitous cellular protein into a hormone. It might be better to term hCG "human cellular gonadotropin." The hCG-like material observed in tissue extracts is not an artifact of assay procedures, and is not LH or the free β-chain of hCG.

▶ [Human chorionic gonadotropin is a glycoprotein. Apparently the protein portion can be synthesized by most (maybe all?) human tissues. It is the ability of the trophoblast to add carbohydrate to this protein that transforms it into a hormone. We are not looking at latent genetic information in other tissues, but the protein itself. Does this phenomenon apply to other glycoprotein hormones as well?] ◀

Practical Value of Progestogen Challenge Test, Serum Estradiol Estimation or Clinical Examination in Assessment of Estrogen State and Response to Clomiphene in Amenorrhea. M. G. R. Hull, U. A. Knuth, M. A. F. Murray, and H. S. Jacobs[13-6] compared the results of the progestogen challenge test with those of serum estradiol-17β (E₂) determination and clinical assessments of the estrogen status of the lower genital tract in 246 amenorrheic women. Twenty-three patients had primary and 223, secondary amenorrhea. The menstrual response to oral medroxyprogesterone acetate, given in a dose of 5 mg daily for 5 days, was assessed in 225 subjects. Serum E_2 was measured in 154 subjects, and clinical assessment was carried out in 183 cases.

Clomiphene was given for 5 days to 188 patients, starting a week after administration of progestogen. Ovulation was diagnosed if the serum progesterone level was at least 25 nmoles/L 12 days after clomiphene was administered and if menstruation occurred 5 to 10 days after the blood sample was obtained.

Values of E_2 were useful only when they were below 150 pmoles/L, when they indicated that ovulation was very unlikely to occur after

(13–5) Am. J. Obstet. Gynecol. 134:729–733, Aug. 1, 1979.
(13–6) Br. J. Obstet. Gynaecol. 86:799–805, October 1979.

administration of clomiphene. Clinical assessments also were only useful in predicting failure to ovulate with clomiphene. The progestogen challenge test predicted both ovulatory and anovulatory responses to clomiphene. Only 4% of patients with absent or scanty bleeding after administration of progestogen ovulated, and repeat treatment with clomiphene did not increase the rate of ovulation. After a normal menstrual response to progestogen, 39% of the patients ovulated in the first clomiphene cycle using only 50 mg daily. The rate was 55% if 100 mg was given, and 75% after treatment for three cycles.

The progestogen challenge test was more useful than E_2 measurement or clinical assessment of estrogen status for determination of the estrogen state of amenorrheic women in this study.

▶ [This study compared three indices of estrogen status—clinical findings, serum E_2 level, and progestogen challenge test—in relation to clomiphene response in amenorrheic patients. The last was by far the most useful predictor. Only 5 of 131 patients (4%) with absent or scant bleeding following medroxyprogesterone acetate, 5 mg daily for 5 days, ovulated with clomiphene whereas normal menstrual bleeding after the progestogen challenge identified patients with a 75% chance of clomiphene response. In this case, the simplest test apparently turns out to be the best.] ◀

Premenstrual Spotting: Its Association with Endometriosis but Not Luteal Phase Inadequacy. Recent reviews have suggested that premenstrual spotting is a sign of luteal phase inadequacy and suggestive of deficient progesterone production. Anne Colston Wentz[13-7] (Univ. of Tennessee) has observed that spotting is common in patients found to have endometriosis and is rare in those with luteal phase inadequacy. Thirty-two patients with infertility for more than a year were identified as having luteal phase insufficiency on the basis of two endometrial biopsies more than 2 days out of phase in two different cycles. Twenty-three patients with pelvic endometriosis were also evaluated.

Only 2 of the 32 patients with luteal phase inadequacy had premenstrual spotting. Laparoscopic examination was normal in 1, and the other conceived on progesterone supplementation before laparoscopy. Eight of the 23 patients with endometriosis reported premenstrual spotting of 3 or more days. Five had endometrial histologic findings in phase with the next menses, suggesting luteal phase adequacy. One patient had a polypoid endometrium treated by curettage. Two patients did not have biopsies. Two patients with endometriosis were found to have short cycles but not premenstrual spotting. In both, endometrial biopsies were in phase with the next menstrual period.

These findings do not substantiate an association of premenstrual spotting with luteal phase inadequacy. Premenstrual spotting was associated with endometriosis in about one third of patients in this study, and it may provide a clinical clue to this diagnosis. Patients ultimately found to have endometriosis have an incidence of luteal phase inadequacy of below 5%, about that expected for the population at large.

▶ [We had always assumed that premenstrual spotting might indicate inadequate lu-

(13–7) Fertil. Steril. 33:605–607, June 1980.

teal function. Not so, according to Wentz. Premenstrual spotting may, however, be a tip-off to the presence of endometriosis. The mechanism involved is not readily apparent.] ◄

Practical Approach for Evaluation of Women With Abnormal Polytomography or Elevated Prolactin Levels. Leon Speroff, Richard M. Levin, Ray V. Haning, Jr., and Nathan G. Kase[13-8] reviewed experience with 60 patients seen from 1976 to 1978 with abnormal polytomographic findings, elevated serum prolactin concentrations, or both. Mean age was 27.2 years. Eighteen patients had transsphenoidal microsurgical removal of microadenomas, and 1 had craniotomy. Three patients received postoperative irradiation because complete removal was impossible. Nine patients with empty sellae are being followed. Two patients are on thyroid replacement therapy.

Fifty-seven patients had thinning of cortical bone on polytomography, and 23 had expansion of the sellar floor also. The highest prolactin concentrations were in patients presenting with amenorrhea and galactorrhea. Two of 24 patients with amenorrhea only had normal polytomographic findings but elevated prolactin concentrations. All 16 patients with amenorrhea and galactorrhea had abnormal polytomograms. Their mean prolactin concentration was 107.7 ng/ml. One of 8 patients with galactorrhea only had a normal polytomogram and a prolactin value of 115 ng/ml. Twelve patients presenting with anovulation and infertility had a mean prolactin concentration of 30.4 ng/ml. Three patients in this group had abnormal polytomograms and normal prolactin values.

Clinical features in these cases do not always correlate with the prolactin concentration. Visual field examination is not a useful screening procedure, but evaluation of thyroid function is important. Computed tomographic scanning contributes little to the evaluation of these patients. With a prolactin concentration above 100 ng/ml, a normal polytomogram does not rule out tumor, and an air study should be performed. If the sella is enlarged but the prolactin value is normal, transsphenoidal surgery should be performed after pneumoencephalography. If both the polytomogram and the prolactin value are normal, annual evaluation is adequate. The authors have become less aggressive in recommending operation, particularly in view of the efficacy of high-dosage bromocriptine therapy in reducing the size of large pituitary tumors.

► [This paper provides excellent practical advice on evaluation of patients with amenorrhea-galactorrhea. Do prolactin and thyroid function tests in all cases and polytomography in those with high prolactin, galactorrhea, or failure of progesterone withdrawal bleeding. Of 57 patients with abnormal polytomograms, 20 (35%) had *normal* prolactin levels and 5 of these patients had pituitary tumors confirmed at surgery. This "false negative rate" for serum prolactin is much higher than our own experience and the literature would indicate.

In an interesting report, Vaughn and associates at Duke University (Am. J. Obstet. Gynecol. 136:980, 1980) described 2 cases of hyperprolactinemia with radiographic evidence of prolactinoma that regressed spontaneously.] ◄

(13–8) Am. J. Obstet. Gynecol. 135:896–906, Dec. 1, 1979.

Estrogenic Response in Women With Amenorrhea During Treatment With Human Menopausal Gonadotropin With and Without Simultaneous Administration of Bromocriptine. The physiologic role of prolactin in the human ovary has not been fully elucidated. Suppression of ovarian function appears to be due to an inhibitory effect of elevated prolactin levels at the hypothalamic-pituitary level, but a direct effect of prolactin on the ovary cannot be excluded.

Steen Larsen and Ejvind Honoré[13-9] (Odense Univ.) examined the estrogenic responses of amenorrheic women under treatment with human menopausal gonadotropin (hMG), with or without the prolactin inhibitor bromocriptine. Six women aged 27 to 36 years, 2 with primary amenorrhea and 4 with secondary amenorrhea of 5 to 14 years' duration, all of whom wished to conceive, were studied in four consecutive hMG treatment cycles. When used, bromocriptine dosage was 2.5 mg twice daily along with hMG from the first day of the cycle.

All patients except 1 with a low basal follicle-stimulating hormone (FSH) and a limited response to gonadotropin-releasing hormone had increased excretion of estrogens when bromocriptine was given along with hMG. Levels of estradiol-17β were also increased. In 1 patient, the dose of hMG had to be reduced. Serum prolactin levels increased slightly throughout the treatment cycles without bromocriptine, but were low in cycles during which bromocriptine was administered. Serum progesterone levels were low before and during hMG therapy and were equal in the two types of treatment cycles. Menstrual bleeding occurred in all cycles 12 to 14 days after hCG administration. There were no signs of overstimulation or other side effects. No pregnancies occurred.

The results suggest that both normal and elevated serum prolactin levels can have a direct inhibitory effect on the ovary and that FSH may be necessary for formation of prolactin receptors in the ovary.

▶ [A comment in the 1980 YEAR BOOK (p. 392) suggested that the effects of prolactin on the ovary were not limited to the corpus luteum. The present study lends support to this view. Anovulatory patients with normal or elevated prolactin levels being treated with human menopausal gonadotropin responded to adjunctive treatment with bromocriptine by increasing estrogen secretion. This suggests that prolactin has an inhibiting effect on the ovarian follicle as well as on the corpus luteum.] ◀

Induction of Ovulation in Women With Hyperprolactinemic Amenorrhea Using Clomiphene and Human Chorionic Gonadotropin or Bromocriptine. Significant hyperprolactinemia is often associated with anovulation and amenorrhea, and it appears that hyperprolactinemia causes anovulation, though the mechanism is uncertain. Ewa Radwanska, Hugh H. G. McGarrigle, Valerie Little, Daphne Lawrence, Spiros Sarris, and Gerald I. M. Swyer[13-10] (Univ. College Hosp., London) compared the use of clomiphene followed by human chorionic gonadotropin (hCG) with that of bromocriptine in 29 infertile amenorrheic women with hyperprolactinemia. The women, aged 20 to 38 years, had had amenorrhea for an average of

(13–9)   Fertil. Steril. 33:378–382, April 1980.
(13–10)   Ibid., 32:187–192, August 1979.

3.8 years. Plasma prolactin concentrations exceeded 60 ng/ml. Two patients with sellar enlargement received radiotherapy for pituitary tumor. Fourteen patients had previously received clomiphene without effect. Clomiphene was given orally in incremental doses of 100 to 200 mg daily for 5 days, followed by 5,000 IU of hCG given intramuscularly 8 to 10 days after clomiphene withdrawal and again a week later. Bromocriptine was given in incremental doses of 2.5 to 15 mg daily until adequate ovulatory function appeared to be restored.

All but 2 of 21 patients given clomiphene and hCG therapy ovulated, and 12 of them had 17 pregnancies. Six conceptions occurred in the first course of therapy. The pregnancies were uncomplicated. Eight patients who failed to conceive subsequently received bromocriptine therapy, and 3 conceived. Six of 8 patients given bromocriptine therapy only conceived within one to seven treatment cycles. The overall pregnancy rate in the series was 73%.

It appears that bromocriptine therapy restores ovulation in women with hyperprolactinemic amenorrhea by a mechanism different from that operative during clomiphene-hCG therapy. Suppression of prolactin appears to be unnecessary for successful induction of ovulation. Clomiphene and hCG could be conveniently used to induce ovulation in this setting, and resistant patients could be given bromocriptine.

▶ [Hyperprolactinemic amenorrhea generally fails to respond to clomiphene but, as indicated by this study, clomiphene-hCG seems to have a very high success rate, as high, in fact, as bromocriptine. United States labeling requirements state that bromocriptine is not indicated for infertility because of concerns about its administration after conception. For those wishing to follow this injunction, clomiphene-hCG offers a reasonable alternative.

Similar results were found in a study by McGarrigle and colleagues abstracted in the 1980 YEAR BOOK, page 363.] ◀

Prolactin-Secreting Pituitary Adenomas: Association With Multiple Endocrine Neoplasia, Type I. Cryer and Kissane, in 1974, postulated the occurrence of prolactinomas in patients with established multiple endocrine neoplasia, type I syndromes (MEN I). Johannes D. Veldhuis, Joseph E. Green, III, E. Kovacs, Thomas J. Worgul, Frederick T. Murray, and James M. Hammond[13-11] (Milton S. Hershey Med. Center, Hershey, Pa.) observed the evolution of multiple extrapituitary neoplasms of endocrine gland origin in 2 patients who presented with prolactin-secreting pituitary adenomas. The tumors were either present concurrently or evolved sequentially. The pedigree of one family exhibited autosomal dominant transmission of tumors of the pituitary, parathyroids, and pancreatic islet cells. Evidence for familial multiple endocrine tumors was not obtained in the other case.

These cases and studies of three other MEN I prolactinomas, with a review of the literature, indicate that a prolactin-secreting adenoma may be the first manifestation of MEN I, with concurrent or sequential tumor evolution. Endocrine tumors may occur in an autosomal dominant pattern in affected families. The ultrastructural findings do not distinguish isolated prolactinomas from those occurring in pa-

(13–11) Am. J. Med. 67:830–837, November 1979.

tients at risk of MEN I. Serum calcium determinations and a detailed family history are recommended in all cases of prolactinoma. Serum prolactin concentration should be measured in members of families with the MEN I syndrome. The cost-effectiveness of extensive biochemical screening for MEN I in patients with prolactinoma but no incriminating family history requires further clarification.

▶ [The association between the syndrome of multiple endocrine neoplasms and prolactinomas demonstrated by the three cases in this report has clear implications for the gynecologist. A patient with a prolactinoma should have a detailed review of endocrine systems carried out, a careful family history taken, and perhaps the serum calcium level measured as well.] ◀

Effect of Pregnancy and Lactation on Pituitary Prolactin-Secreting Tumors. There is concern that bromocriptine therapy given to induce ovulation may accelerate the growth of prolactin-secreting pituitary tumors through an increase in estrogen levels. Arturo Zárate, Elías S. Canales, Mucia Alger, and Gerardo Forsbach[13-12] (Mexico City) reviewed experience with 14 women with amenorrhea-galactorrhea syndrome due to pituitary microadenoma, in whom pregnancy followed the administration of bromocriptine. The diagnosis was based on sellar roentgenograms and a serum prolactin level above 100 ng/ml. No patient had had surgery or radiotherapy. The duration of symptoms ranged from 2 to 19 years. Hirsutism and obesity were not present, and neuro-ophthalmologic examinations showed no abnormalities. Bromocriptine was begun in a dose of 2.5 mg twice daily.

Galactorrhea disappeared within 3 to 8 weeks of the start of bromocriptine therapy. Serum prolactin levels decreased to normal in 10 women after 3 to 4 weeks of therapy. All patients conceived within 6 months. Three women conceived before the reinitiation of menses, 8 to 12 weeks after the start of bromocriptine therapy. No neuro-ophthalmologic abnormalities developed during pregnancy and no patient had clinical evidence of tumor enlargement. All pregnancies were uneventful. Sellar x-ray films taken at 3-month intervals during pregnancy showed no signs of tumor growth. All pregnancies were single births. Patients nursed their infants for at least 6 months without any problems. No patient had spontaneous menses during lactation. Three patients again received bromocriptine because they wished to conceive; 2 had uneventful full-term pregnancies and 1 is in wk 25 of a normal gestation. Sixteen healthy infants have been delivered to date.

Infertile patients with pituitary microadenomas can be allowed to conceive on bromocriptine therapy alone if they are carefully supervised during pregnancy. Whether long-term bromocriptine therapy inhibits further growth or causes regression of prolactin-secreting tumors remains unclear.

Effect of Pregnancy on Suspected Pituitary Adenomas After Conservative Management of Ovulation Defects Associated with Galactorrhea. Alan B. Shewchuk, G. David Adamson, Pierre

(13–12) Acta Endocrinol. (Copenh.) 92:407–412, November 1979.

Lessard, and Calvin Ezrin[13-13] (Univ. of Toronto) report their experience with 30 patients having ovulation defects and galactorrhea, who conceived after medical therapy.

Meticulous prepregnancy evaluation included sellar tomography, ophthalmologic examination, and endocrine and metabolic assessment. Pituitary function and reserve were evaluated. All patients were considered to have a possible pituitary prolactinoma, whether or not it could be demonstrated, and were advised of the possible complications of pregnancy associated with occult or overt pituitary tumors.

All patients received at least three cycles of clomiphene citrate with or without human chorionic gonadotropin. The 26 patients in whom ovulation or conception failed to occur received bromoergocryptine to suppress galactorrhea and hyperprolactinemia. Three patients were given bromoergocryptine and clomiphene citrate concomitantly.

All patients received routine prenatal care and were instructed to report the occurrence of headache, visual symptoms or polyuria. Two patients had spontaneous abortions; 1 patient with a macroadenoma underwent elective abortion. Perimeter visual field examination and sellar tomography were repeated at 36 weeks and at 8 weeks post partum. Lactation was suppressed with a preparation containing testosterone enanthate benzilic acid, estradiol dienanthate, and estradiol benzoate (Lactostat) or bromoergocryptine.

Elevated serum prolactin levels were found in 18 of 21 anovulatory patients and 3 of 4 sporadically ovulating patients, but in none of 5 patients with luteal phase defects. This suggests a relationship between degree of ovulation defect and basal prolactin levels in these patients. However, no relationship was seen between size or change in shape of the pituitary fossa and degree of ovulation defect or basal prolactin level.

Of 27 patients who carried a pregnancy to viability, 18 were reevaluated at 36 weeks' gestation. Pituitary fossa tomograms were unchanged in 16 and showed only minor asymptomatic enlargement in 2.

The sudden development of diplopia occurred in 1 patient at 7 weeks' gestation followed by a right third nerve palsy shortly afterward. Carotid angiography demonstrated a right-sided suprasellar mass, which was removed by transsphenoidal adenectomy. The remainder of the pregnancy was uneventful.

The 27 pregnancies resulted in 29 live infants, all of whom did well. Obstetric complications occurred in 10 women.

Five of the 8 patients who were taking Lactostat had sella turcica enlargement at 8 weeks post partum; all 8 had recurrence of amenorrhea-galactorrhea and hyperprolactinemia. Bromoergocryptine was used to suppress lactation in the other patients. With this regimen, 14 patients resumed ovulatory cycles; repeat sellar tomography in 13 patients showed no pituitary fossa enlargement.

▶ [The controversy continues regarding optimal treatment—surgical or medical—of

(13–13) Am. J. Obstet. Gynecol. 136:659–666, Mar. 1, 1980.

the prolactinoma patient who plans to conceive. This report and the preceding article by Zárate et al. indicate that drug therapy is *generally* safe. There was no clinical or radiographic evidence of tumor growth in any of the 14 subjects in the Zárate series or in 16 of 18 patients in the Shewchuk series. However, 2 patients in the latter group had minor asymptomatic enlargement and, more importantly, 1 other patient had acute symptomatic enlargement at 7 weeks' gestation. Thus, the frequency of adverse effects seems to be low but, nonetheless, some risk exists. Lactation suppression with estrogen was associated with puerperal enlargement in 5 of 8 patients, and on this basis it certainly seems clear that bromocriptine, and not estrogen, should be used to prevent lactation.] ◄

Cytotoxic-Induced Ovarian Failure in Women With Hodgkin's Disease: I. Hormone Function. Severe seminiferous tubular failure has been observed in men treated with cyclic combination chemotherapy for advanced Hodgkin's disease. Ramona M. Chapman, Simon B. Sutcliffe and James S. Malpas[13-14] (St. Bartholomew's Hosp., London) evaluated fertility and hormonal status in 41 young women treated for advanced Hodgkin's disease in 1969–77. All but 1 had received standard MVPP (mechlorethamine hydrochloride, vinblastine sulfate, procarbazine hydrochloride and prednisolone) therapy; 1 had received 1 course of MVPP and 9 courses of chlorambucil-VPP therapy. Twenty-one women had received MVPP as maintenance therapy, or other agents for relapse after MVPP. Seven patients were still receiving chemotherapy at the time of evaluation. At the end of the study the median age was 30 years, and the group had received no chemotherapy for a median of 36 months.

Only 7 patients (17%) appeared to have unaltered ovarian function. Ovarian function had failed in 20 patients; gonadotropin levels were elevated and estradiol levels were in the postmenopausal range. All but 3 of these 20 patients had postmenopausal symptoms. Ovarian function in 14 women was failing. These patients exhibited a wide spectrum of ovarian dysfunction and irregular menses. There generally were inadequate luteal phase progesterone levels, elevated follicle-stimulating hormone levels, or elevation of both follicle-stimulating hormone and luteinizing hormone. Estradiol levels were widely variable in this group. Progressive ovarian failure was noted during 16 months of follow-up. At the end of the study, ovarian function in only 5 women was functioning. Ovarian biopsies indicated a reduction in numbers of primordial follicles.

Progressive ovarian failure with severe estrogen deficiency and a lack of libido is observed in women treated successfully for advanced Hodgkin's disease. Thyroid disease and hyperprolactinemia must be ruled out in these women. Cyclic estrogen-progestogen therapy is instituted early in patients with erratic ovarian function who do not wish to conceive and in symptomatic women with complete ovarian failure. It remains unclear whether suppression of ovulation during the course of chemotherapy has any protective effect against the development of ovarian failure.

► [Intensive combination chemotherapy of Hodgkin's disease and other lymphomas can produce long-term remissions and cures unheard of a few years ago. That such therapy can have undesirable side effects on gonadal function is indicated by these

(13–14) JAMA 242:1877–1881, Oct. 26, 1979.

findings of an astonishingly high frequency of ovarian failure subsequent to treatment with a combination of various types of antineoplastic agents. The resultant symptoms included amenorrhea, hot flushes, irritability, and other components of the menopausal syndrome. These same authors, in a companion paper (JAMA 242:1882, 1979), found a high incidence of loss of libido and disruption of marital relationships. The message seems clear that young women receiving this type of chemotherapy should be observed carefully for menopausal symptoms, and hormonal replacement should be utilized as needed.] ◄

Menopausal Flushes: Neuroendocrine Link With Pulsatile Luteinizing Hormone Secretion. R. F. Casper, S. S. C. Yen and M. M. Wilkes[13-15] (Univ. of California, San Diego) studied 55 flush episodes in 6 postmenopausal women. Blood samples were obtained from each woman at intervals of 12 to 15 minutes for a study period of 8 to 10 hours.

Fig 13–1.—Mean (±SE) serum LH, FSH (follicle-stimulating hormone), and PRL (prolactin) concentrations measured before, during, and after the 55 episodes of flushes. Onset of each flush is set at time t = 0, and the data are expressed as the difference from this reference point. Serum LH concentration is significantly elevated (P < .0001) immediately after onset of the flush, and the elevation lasts for at least 45 minutes. A small but significant (P = .016) parallel increase in serum FSH occurred, with no associated change in serum PRL concentration. Data analysis was by analysis of variance and Student's t test for paired data. (Courtesy of Casper, R. F., et al.: Science 205:823–825, Aug. 24, 1979.)

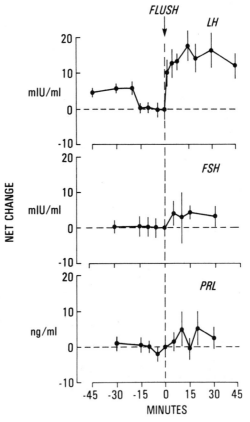

Onset of each of the 55 flushes was characterized by a sudden intense sensation of heat, accompanied by perspiration, at first centered on the face and then becoming generalized. Mean flush duration was 2.7 minutes. Associated with the flushes were a mean increase in finger temperature of 7.5 F and a mean increase in pulse rate of 9 beats per minute.

Flushes and luteinizing hormone (LH) pulses were closely synchronized. Frequency of LH pulses was $54^{1}/_{2}$ to 120 minutes (mean, $73^{1}/_{2}$ minutes). A total of 66 LH pulses and 55 flushes occurred during the study. Thus, LH pulses were not always accompanied by flushes. However, a flush was never seen without an LH pulse. Onset of the flushes coincided with the initial rise in circulating LH at the time of an LH pulse (Fig 13–1). A small rise in serum follicle-stimulating hormone was also found, but there was no associated change in serum prolactin level. During the 30 minutes before and the 30 minutes after a flush, there were no significant changes in levels of plasma catacholamines (dopamine, norepinephrine or epinephrine).

Because pulsatile LH release results from episodic secretion of LH releasing factor by the hypothalamus, these findings suggest a link between the neuroendocrine mechanisms that initiate such episodic secretion and those responsible for onset of flush episodes.

▶ [The study adds important information to our understanding of the menopausal flush. YEAR BOOK readers may remember that reports abstracted in earlier editions failed to identify the biochemical hallmarks of this phenomenon. The present work suggests that there is a clear temporal association between the flush and pulsatile LH secretion. Since flushes can occur in hypophysectomized women, LH per se is not essential. The authors suggest that central adrenergic neuronal activity results both in the flush and in the release of LH releasing factor. The LH pulses, therefore, indirectly reflect the central adrenergic activation.

Similar findings of a correlation between pulsatile LH release and the menopausal hot flush (reflected in increased skin temperature) were reported by Meldrum and associates (J. Clin. Endocrinol. Metab. 50:685, 1980). Levels of adrenal steroids and progesterone rose shortly after the flush.] ◀

Effects of Estrogens on Sleep and Psychologic State of Hypogonadal Women. Many postmenopausal women report improved sleep and general well-being while taking estrogens. Isaac Schiff, Quentin Regestein, Dan Tulchinsky and Kenneth J. Ryan[13-16] (Boston) compared the effects of estrogen and placebo on sleep and psychologic status in 16 hypogonadal women, aged 31–65 years, seen in a menopause clinic. Eight had been postmenopausal for 2–22 years, and 8 had undergone oophorectomy for benign gynecologic disease. Only 10 had vasomotor symptoms. Either low-dose estrogen or placebo was administered. The daily dose of conjugated estrogens was 0.625 mg.

A 31% fall in serum follicle-stimulating hormone and a 19% fall in luteinizing hormone occurred after 1 month of estrogen therapy. The incidence of hot flushes decreased significantly. No marked changes in psychometric test scores were evident with estrogen administration. The time to sleep onset was reduced with estrogen therapy, and more rapid eye movement sleep was observed. Psychologic intactness, as estimated clinically, correlated positively with latency to sleep onset.

(13–16)   JAMA 242:2405–2407, Nov. 30, 1979.

Estrogens improved sleep patterns in these postmenopausal women. However, although the drug caused them to be less outwardly aggressive, they were more inwardly hostile, as reflected by psychologic test results. Further studies of the effect of estrogens on sleep should take psychologic differences among patients into account. Clinical ratings should be used to estimate psychologic intactness.

▶ [Various forms of sleep disturbance are often included in the long list of symptoms composing the "menopausal syndrome." This controlled double-blind crossover study indicates that estrogen replacement may influence some aspects of sleep—the time required to fall asleep and time spent in rapid eye movement sleep. The most marked effect of estrogen, however, occurred in patients whose Minnesota Multiphasic Personality Inventory scores indicated substantial elements of defensiveness and denial, suggesting a compounding effect of psychologic state. All in all, the effects of hormone replacement on sleep appear to be much less clear than those on more "biologic" indices such as hot flushes or gonadotropin suppression.] ◀

Relation Between the Karyopyknotic Index and Plasma Estrogen Concentrations After the Menopause. The karyopyknotic index (KPI), or percentage of superficial squamous cells with pyknotic nuclei, excluding parabasal squamous cells, is a popular means of assessing the degree of estrogenic proliferation of vaginal epithelium.

Anne R. Morse, J. D. Hutton, H. S. Jacobs, M. A. F. Murray, and V. H. T. James[13-17] (St. Mary's Hosp., London) examined the relation between the KPI and plasma estrogen concentrations in 44 women who consented to uterine aspiration and who had not received estrogen or progestogen therapy for 3 months. All had serum gonadotropin levels in the menopausal range. The mean age was 56 years, and the mean time since the last period was 7.4 years. A lateral vaginal wall smear for determination of the KPI was obtained at the time of uterine cavity aspiration; at least 500 cells were counted. Estrogen levels were determined by radioimmunoassay.

Thirty-eight women with adequate samples and without prolapse were included in the statistical analysis. A highly significant correlation was found between the KPI and plasma estradiol concentrations, but no significant correlation between the KPI and plasma estrone concentrations.

The degree of proliferation of the vaginal epithelium in postmenopausal women is correlated with the plasma estradiol level, but not with the plasma estrone concentration. The findings are in accord with the view that estradiol is the biologically important estrogen. The KPI may be a valuable aid in management of postmenopausal women, especially those requiring estrogen therapy.

▶ [In this study of postmenopausal women, the degree of maturity of the vaginal epithelium correlated significantly with estradiol levels but not with estrone values, supporting the generally held view that estradiol is substantially more potent biologically. The mechanism of this difference is unknown; perhaps it involves differential affinity of estrogen receptors.] ◀

Intravaginal Administration of Conjugated Estrogens in Premenopausal and Postmenopausal Women. Estrogen administration to postmenopausal women restores the vaginal mucosa to a pre-

(13–17) Br. J. Obstet. Gynaecol. 86:981–983, December 1979.

menopausal condition. Intravaginal applications of estrogen-containing creams often are used in cases in which oral administration is contraindicated. Mirjam Furuhjelm, Erva Karlgren, and Kjell Carlström[13-18] (Stockholm) attempted to determine whether daily intravaginal applications of 0.625 mg of conjugated estrogens for 2 weeks to postmenopausal women can restore the vaginal mucosa to a premenopausal state. Premarin cream was used in 12 healthy women with a mean age of 64.5 years. Biopsy specimens were taken from the vaginal wall just before treatment began and after 15 days.

Marked atrophy was present before treatment in half of the patients. After 2 weeks of treatment, the mucosa was nearly identical to that seen in normal premenopausal women. Similar results were obtained in 5 women with slight to moderate atrophy. A woman with no signs of atrophy initially showed marked signs of keratinization after treatment. A rapid rise in unconjugated immunoreactive serum estrogen and total estrone levels was noted in 4 of 5 postmenopausal subjects. By contrast, in premenopausal patients vaginal estrogen cream was not associated with increases in serum immunoreactive estrogen or total estrone levels.

Two weeks of daily therapy with 0.625 mg of intravaginal conjugated estrogens appears to be sufficient to restore an atrophic vaginal mucosa to a premenopausal state in postmenopausal women. The vagina appears to possess a built-in mechanism of protection against overdosage from local estrogens. If this is so, it will be possible to treat urethritis and colpitis by vaginal estrogen applications in cases in which systemic treatment is contraindicated. A study of the effect of long-term vaginal estrogen therapy on serum levels in postmenopausal women is in progress.

▶ [Several recent studies have demonstrated that absorption of vaginally applied estrogen is considerable. These observations indicate that measurable absorption occurs through atrophic mucosa but not through the previously estrogenized vagina, which makes sense morphologically.] ◀

Use of Progestogen Challenge Test to Reduce Risk of Endometrial Cancer. The risk of endometrial adenocarcinoma has been shown to be increased with estrogen replacement therapy, but reduced when a progestogen is prescribed with estrogen. Some postmenopausal women who produce adequate endogenous estrogens may be among those at the greatest risk of developing endometrial carcinoma. R. Don Gambrell, Jr., Fred M. Massey, Tristan A. Castaneda, Aldonna J. Ugenas, Corrine A. Ricci, and Jean M. Wright[13-19] (Wilford Hall USAF Med. Center, Lackland AFB, Texas) reviewed 4 years' experience with the progestogen challenge test (PCT), designed to identify women at the greatest risk of endometrial cancer. The test is administered by giving either 5 mg of Norlutate or 10 mg of Provera for 10 days. The progestogen is continued for 10 days each month as long as withdrawal bleeding ensues.

By 1978, over 90% of oral estrogen users were also receiving a progestogen. Endometrial adenocarcinoma was diagnosed in 17 patients,

(13–18) Int. J. Gynaecol. Obstet. 17:335–339, Jan.–Feb. 1980.
(13–19) Obstet. Gynecol. 55:732–738, June 1980.

INCIDENCE OF ENDOMETRIAL CANCER AT WILFORD HALL USAF MEDICAL CENTER, 1975 TO 1978

Therapy group	Patient-years of observation	Patients with cancer	Incidence (per 100,000)
1 Estrogen–progestogen users	5323	3	56.4*
2 Estrogen users	2228	8	359.1†
3 Estrogen vaginal cream users	910	1	109.9
4 Progestogen or androgen users	397	0	—
5 Untreated women	2014	5	248.3
Total	10,872	17	156.4

*$P < .05$ (difference between group 1 and group 5).
†$P < .01$ (difference between group 1 and group 2).

for an incidence of 156/100,000 women annually (table). The incidence figures were 56.4 for estrogen-progestogen users and 248.3 for untreated women, a significant difference. The incidence among women using oral estrogens only was 359.1/100,000 women. The difference between estrogen users and estrogen-progestogen users was also significant. Only 1 cancer occurred among users of estrogen vaginal cream, and none occurred among users of progestogen or androgen. Eleven of the 17 patients with carcinoma were oral estrogen users. Mean duration of estrogen therapy was 6.9 years, closely similar to that for all estrogen users. In 7 patients hyperplasia was diagnosed before endometrial cancer was detected. Progestogen therapy has usually reversed hyperplastic endometrium to normal or atrophic endometrium.

Use of the PCT can reduce the risk of endometrial cancer in both estrogen-treated postmenopausal women and women with increased amounts of endogenous estrogens. It appears that at least ten days of progestogen therapy each month or menstrual cycle are necessary effectively to prevent or treat most endometrial hyperplasias that may lead to neoplasia.

▶ [The addition of cyclic progestins to therapy with estrogen in menopausal women was associated with a decreased risk of the development of endometrial cancer. The authors advocate a 10-day course (eg, medroxyprogesterone acetate 10 mg/day) each month. Their suggestion of screening asymptomatic patients not receiving estrogens with progesterone challenge tests is an interesting one. Presumably, withdrawal bleeding would indicate that more than atrophic endometrium is present and that histologic sampling is indicated.] ◀

Noncontraceptive Estrogens and Myocardial Infarction in Young Women. Noncontraceptive estrogens have been increasingly used as replacement therapy after premenopausal hysterectomy with bilateral oophorectomy and are still advocated as prophylaxis against coronary artery disease in women. Lynn Rosenberg, Dennis Slone, Samuel Shapiro, David Kaufman, Paul D. Stolley, and Olli S. Miettinen[13-20] examined the relation between noncontraceptive estrogen use and nonfatal myocardial infarction (MI) in 477 women aged 30 to 49 years with first infarctions and 1,832 hospital controls.

Little evidence of an effect was obtained. The estimated relative

(13–20) JAMA 244:339–342, July 25, 1980.

risk of acute MI for women using noncontraceptive estrogens in the past month, allowing for potential confounding factors, was 1.0. The estimate for women who had discontinued the use of estrogen more than a month previously was 1.2. No association was evident in various subgroups such as women who smoked heavily and those with no apparent predisposition to MI. A large majority of past estrogen users had taken preparations containing conjugated estrogens, mostly in doses of 1.25 mg or less. Risk estimates did not vary consistently with duration of estrogen use.

It appears that noncontraceptive estrogens neither increase nor decrease the risk of MI appreciably in young women. Caution in their use, however, is warranted in view of other hazards, which include endometrial cancer and possibly gallbladder disease and breast cancer.

▶ [Noncontraceptive estrogen use (chiefly for menopausal symptoms) in young women does not increase their risk of myocardial infarction, according to this study.] ◀

Postmenopausal Estrogens Protect Against Fractures of Hip and Distal Radius: Case-Control Study. Estrogens given after menopause have beneficial effects on bone thickness and density and on vertebral osteoporosis, but their efficacy in preventing major limb fractures is unknown. Tom A. Hutchinson, Stanley M. Polansky, and Alvan R. Feinstein[13-21] (Yale Univ.) conducted a retrospective case-control study of the protective effect of estrogens against postmenopausal fractures of the hip and distal radius in a population of 2,609 women, aged 40 or older, seen on an orthopedic service during 1974–1977. Patients admitted specifically for vertebral compression fracture were not included. Controls and patients with fractures were matched for age and race. Estrogen users were women who had taken at least 0.3 mg or an unknown dose of conjugated estrogen for 6 months or longer, starting after menopause.

Analysis of data on estrogen use in 157 matched case-control pairs gave an odds ratio for "protection" of 1.5. If "exposure" was defined as starting estrogens within 5 years of menopause, the ratio rose to 2.6. With estrogen use ascertained from interviews of 80 case-control pairs, the ratio was 3.0, rising to 3.8 for exposure starting within 5 years of menopause. A blind review of lateral chest x-ray films showed the prevalence of osteoporosis to be 32% in fracture cases and 15% in controls.

These findings constitute epidemiologic evidence for the view that exogenous estrogens protect against postmenopausal osteoporosis. Since case-control methods can be used to test for benefits as well as risks, this approach may be helpful in assessing the effects of other important therapeutic agents.

▶ [The retrospective "case-control" method that has been used to express the relative risk associated with a particular type of drug (eg, use of oral contraceptives and death from thromboembolism or use of exogenous estrogens and endometrial cancer) is employed here to describe the relative benefit of postmenopausal estrogen use concerning hip and forearm fractures. These results are consistent with the current view that exogenous estrogens help protect against the development of osteoporosis.] ◀

(13–21) Lancet 2:705–709, Oct. 6, 1979.

Relationship of Fasting Urinary Calcium to Circulating Estrogen and Body Weight in Postmenopausal Women. An association of osteoporosis with slender body habitus has been suggested, and circulating estrogen levels vary with body weight. Anthony M. Frumar, David R. Meldrum, F. Geola, Issa M. Shamonki, Ivanna V. Tataryn, Leonard J. Deftos, and Howard L. Judd[13-22] attempted to determine whether reduced endogenous estrogen production could contribute to the more frequent development of osteoporosis in slender postmenopausal women. Studies were done in 40 healthy postmenopausal women and 20 women in the early follicular phase of their menstrual cycles. None had received estrogen in the past month. Studies were redone in 10 postmenopausal women after daily oral administration of 10 μg of ethinyl estradiol for 30 days. Serum hormone levels were measured by radioimmunoassays.

Circulating estrogen levels correlated with percent ideal weight in postmenopausal women. Both estradiol and estrone levels correlated positively with this index of obesity. Slender body habitus was associated with lower circulating estrogen levels. Estrogen levels were not significantly related to age, time since menopause, or height. The urinary calcium-creatinine (Ca/Cr) ratio correlated negatively with percent ideal weight and also with body weight. Significant negative correlations were found between the Ca/Cr ratio and both estradiol and estrone levels. The Ca/Cr ratio was higher in postmenopausal than in control subjects. The ratio decreased significantly with estrogen therapy in postmenopausal subjects, to a level similar to that seen in normal premenopausal women.

These findings suggest that increased body weight and its effects on endogenous estrogen metabolism influence urinary calcium excretion. The lower amount of circulating estrogen present in slender patients may be a factor in the increased urinary calcium excretion observed and in the more frequent occurrence of osteoporosis in slender postmenopausal women.

▶ [This study extends considerably our knowledge of the pathophysiology of postmenopausal osteoporosis. The fasting urinary calcium-creatinine ratio (an index of bone resorption) correlated negatively with body weight which, in turn, correlated positively with serum estrogen levels. Thus, it appears that overweight women are protected from osteoporosis by virtue of their higher estrogen levels from peripheral aromatization of androgens. A therapeutic implication is that slender women might be especially appropriate candidates for estrogen replacement. However, the estrogen-osteoporosis story is more complicated than might be thought, as indicated by the following article.] ◀

Adrenal Steroids and the Development of Osteoporosis in Oophorectomized Women. S. C. Manolagas, D. C. Anderson (Univ. of Manchester), and R. Lindsay[13-23] (Glasgow) explored the possibility that the wide variation in bone loss observed in oophorectomized women might be due to differences in adrenal androgens or their biosynthetic pathways. Eighteen women, 10 with very fast and 8 with very slow bone loss, were evaluated. Serum levels of nine adrenal steroids were measured under basal conditions and after overnight

(13–22) J. Clin. Endocrinol. Metab. 50:70–75, January 1980.
(13–23) Lancet 2:597–600, Sept. 22, 1979.

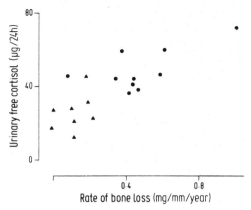

Fig 13–2.—Urinary free cortisol excretion in relation to rate of bone loss for fast *(circles)* and slow *(triangles)* losers. (Courtesy of Manolagas, S. C., et al.: Lancet 2:597–600, Sept. 22, 1979.)

suppression followed by acute corticotropin stimulation. Five women who had received mestranol in a mean daily dose of 28.4 μg for 3 to 7 years were also studied. Bone density was assessed by photon absorption measurements made at the midpoint of the third metacarpal of the right hand.

Urinary free cortisol excretion was significantly higher in fast bone losers (Fig 13–2). Estrogen-treated patients had values similar to those of slow bone losers. No differences were found between fast and slow bone losers in plasma values for the other adrenal androgens or in basal concentrations of estrogens, dehydroepiandrosterone, sex hormone-binding globulin, or corticosteroid-binding globulin. Estrogen-treated patients had higher basal plasma cortisol values than both untreated groups and higher sex hormone-binding globulin values. There were no significant group differences for eight of the nine adrenal steroids tested during corticotropin stimulation after dexamethasone suppression. Fast bone losers had lower cortisol values than slow bone losers.

The findings indicate that it is unlikely that endogenous adrenal androgens or estrogens have a major role in protecting against postoophorectomy or menopausal osteoporosis, despite the beneficial effect of estrogen replacement therapy. There is, however, positive evidence for direct effects of glucocorticoids on bone. Cytoplasmic receptors for glucocorticoids seem to mediate a glucocorticoid-dependent inhibition of bone growth. The osteolytic effect of these hormones may be due in part to sensitization of bone to the potent resorbing effects of 1,25-dihydroxycholecalciferol, whose receptors are regulated by glucocorticoids, at least in the rat.

▶ [Although exogenous estrogen seems to retard bone loss postmenopausally, no statistically significant differences in plasma estrogens between "fast" and "slow" bone losers were found in this study. Likewise, androstenedione levels did not distinguish the fast losers from the slow losers. Urinary free cortisol levels were higher in the fast losers, but, paradoxically, their plasma cortisol response to adrenal stimulation was less than that of the slow losers.

Other studies, in contrast, have shown a relationship between osteoporosis and low levels of estrone and androstenedione (eg, Marshall, D. H., et al.: Br. Med. J. 2:1177). The question remains open.

Yet another possibility involves growth hormone. Rico and associates (Arch. Intern. Med. 139:1263, 1979) found a decreased GH response to levodopa in osteoporotic patients compared to normal subjects. Could this be mediated through estrogen (since older literature suggests that estrogen raises basal GH levels) or is it independent of sex hormones?] ◄

Steroid Production and Responsiveness to Gonadotropin in Isolated Stromal Tissue of Human Postmenopausal Ovaries. It is generally accepted that the postmenopausal ovary is constantly exposed to high levels of endogenous gonadotropins, and it has been assumed that steroid biogenesis in the stromal compartment is stimulated by these hormones. Bo L. Dennefors, Per Olof Janson, Folke Knutson, and Lars Hamberger[13-24] (Univ. of Göteborg) examined production of steroids in specimens of stroma from postmenopausal women and tested their responsiveness to human chorionic gonadotropin (hCG) in an in vitro system.

An ovary was taken from each of 15 postmenopausal women aged 53 to 78 years who were undergoing laparotomy for various gynecologic disorders. All were more than 2 years postmenopausal, and none had received radiotherapy or estrogen therapy in the past 6 months. Cortical stromal specimens were incubated for 4 hours in Krebs' bicarbonate buffer containing 5.5 mM glucose and 1% bovine serum albumin.

Normal postmenopausal stroma produced measurable amounts of androstenedione, estradiol, and progesterone in vitro. Specimens with stromal hyperplasia produced larger amounts of androstenedione and estradiol. Androstenedione was the predominant steroid in both groups of specimens. Addition of hCG led to significant increase in cyclic adenosine monophosphate formation in specimens of stromal hyperplasia.

Androstenedione was the chief steroid produced by ovarian stromal tissue in these studies, but an aromatizing capacity of stromal tissue is apparent from the not negligible production of estradiol observed. Preserved responsiveness to gonadotropin is apparent in ovarian stromal hyperplasia. Ovaries with stromal hyperplasia react differently from atrophic ovaries, and they may play a role in pathogenesis of endometrial hyperplasia and endometrial cancer through producing larger amounts of androgens and estrogens than normal ovaries.

► [The postmenopausal ovary is far from atrophic, as evidenced by this in vitro study demonstrating appreciable endocrine synthesis by ovarian stroma. Androstenedione was the major hormone produced, as has been shown previously, but nearly as much estradiol was made also, and the rates for both were doubled in ovaries with stromal hyperplasia over those with normal histology. According to current concepts, stromal hyperplasia is thought to predispose to endometrial cancer by increased secretion of androstenedione which is aromatized to estrogens in peripheral tissues. Perhaps the stromal hyperplasia patient is at double jeopardy because of increased ovarian estrogen synthesis as well.

In a related study with somewhat different results, Schenker and colleagues (Cancer 44:1809, 1979) measured estradiol and testosterone levels in ovarian vein and peripheral blood in postmenopausal women. Testosterone was fourfold higher in ovarian

(13–24) Am. J. Obstet. Gynecol. 136:997–1002, Apr. 15, 1980.

blood whereas estradiol levels were similar, leading the authors to conclude that the postmenopausal ovary makes testosterone but not estradiol.] ◄

Correlation of Hyperandrogenism With Hyperinsulinism in Polycystic Ovarian Disease. George A. Burghen, James R. Givens, and Abbas E. Kitabchi[13-25] (Univ. of Tennessee) report new evidence indicating that hyperandrogenism correlates with hyperinsulinism in obese patients with polycystic ovarian disease (PCOD). Eight such patients and 6 obese control subjects were evaluated. The patients were aged 17–43 and ranged from 121% to 263% above ideal body weight. The control subjects were significantly more obese. No patients were taking any medications, including oral contraceptives.

The patients with PCOD showed significantly higher levels of plasma testosterone and androstenedione, LH/FSH ratios, basal insulin levels, and glucose sums than control subjects. Only 3 study patients and 1 control subject, however, had glucose sums greater than 580 mg/dl. Study patients showed higher plasma glucose levels than controls during oral glucose tolerance testing. Plasma insulin was significantly increased both basally and after oral glucose administration. The insulin response areas during glucose tolerance testing correlated significantly with testosterone levels but not with androstenedione levels.

This study showed a striking positive correlation between hyperandrogenism and hyperinsulinism in PCOD with relatively mild glucose intolerance. The abnormalities are not due to simple obesity. Relative insulin resistance appears to be present in these patients. The findings imply a relationship between hyperandrogenism and insulin resistance in patients with PCOD.

► [This study notes a correlation between androgen levels and insulin, both in the basal state and in response to an oral glycemic stimulus. In addition, PCOD patients had a tendency to higher glucose levels with oral glucose tolerance tests than did obese non-PCOD subjects. Before leaping to the conclusion that androgens lead to insulin resistance or in some other way impair carbohydrate metabolism, it is well to remember that (at least to our knowledge) there is no known sex difference in insulin levels or clinical diabetes. Nevertheless, perhaps we should include some type of glucose tolerance testing in the evaluation of patients with PCOD.] ◄

Estrogen-Androgen Balance in Hirsutism. Chung H. Wu[13-26] (Univ. of Pennsylvania) studied blood samples from 35 hirsute women, aged 18 to 27 years, who had oligomenorrhea or secondary amenorrhea and who responded to progesterone injection by uterine withdrawal bleeding, in 9 age-matched nonhirsute women with menstrual disorders, and in 10 age-matched normal women with normal ovulatory cycles as controls.

Follicle-stimulating hormone (FSH), luteinizing hormone (LH) and steroid hormones (testosterone, androstenedione, estradiol, estrone, and progesterone) were measured by radioimmunoassay. The percentage of free fraction of estradiol and testosterone was determined by equilibrium dialysis at 37 C. The percentage of testosterone-estradiol-binding globulin-bound fraction of estradiol and testosterone was estimated by the specific steroid displacement-charcoal adsorption tech-

(13–25)   J. Clin. Endocrinol. Metab. 50:113–116, January 1980.
(13–26)   Fertil. Steril. 32:269–275, September 1979.

nique. The binding capacity of plasma testosterone-estradiol-binding globulin was measured by the modified Scatchard plot method. The estradiol-testosterone ratios of concentrations and the binding factors were also studied.

Weight (but not height) of hirsute women was significantly higher than that of normal women. In hirsute women, levels of plasma LH, testosterone, androstenedione, and estrone were significantly elevated, with some correlation with degree of hirsutism. In the 44 women with menstrual disorders with or without hirsutism, plasma testosterone concentrations, including free, index, and total, correlated positively with degree of hirsutism (table). Estradiol-testosterone ratios of concentration also suggested a similar, but negative, correlation. The percentage of free estradiol increased more than the percentage of free testosterone when the percentage of testosterone-estradiol-binding globulin-bound estradiol decreased more than the percentage of testosterone-estradiol-binding globulin-bound testosterone in hirsute women. The estradiol-testosterone ratios of the percentage of free and testosterone-estradiol-binding globulin-bound fractions showed no correlation with degree of hirsutism. The testosterone-binding capacity of plasma testosterone-estradiol-binding glob-

CORRELATION ANALYSIS BETWEEN ENDOCRINE FACTORS AND DEGREE* OF HIRSUTISM IN 44 WOMEN WITH MENSTRUAL DISORDERS

Endocrine parameter	Correlation coefficient	Statistical analysis
Free T	+0.464	$P < 0.01$
T index	+0.638	$P < 0.01$
Total T	+0.446	$P < 0.01$
% Free T	+0.153	NS
% TeBG-bound T	−0.229	$P < 0.05$
T binding capacity	−0.348	$P < 0.01$
Free E_2	+0.192	NS
E_2 index	+0.185	NS
Total E_2	+0.197	NS
% Free E_2	+0.254	$P < 0.01$
%TeBG-bound E_2	−0.266	$P < 0.01$
E_2 binding capacity	−0.221	NS
E_2:T ratios		
Free	−0.199	NS
Index	−0.150	NS
Total	−0.190	NS
% Free	+0.123	NS
% TeBG-bound	−0.145	NS
Binding capacity	−0.047	NS
Androstenedione	+0.414	$P < 0.01$
Estrone	+0.292	$P < 0.01$
Progesterone	+0.244	$P < 0.01$
LH	+0.001	NS
FSH	+0.112	NS
Weight	+0.217	$P < 0.05$
Height	−0.203	NS

*Degrees of hirsutism are numerically assigned as 0, 1, 2, and 3 for none, mild, moderate, and severe hirsutism, respectively.

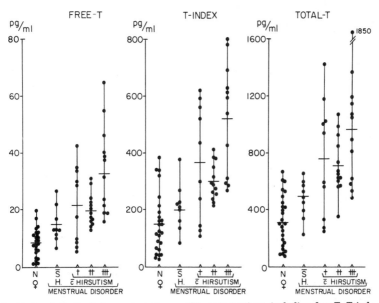

Fig 13–3.—Individual plasma testosterone *(T)* concentrations, including free T, T index, and total T, in normal women and women with menstrual disorders, with or without associated hirsutism. Horizontal lines indicate mean levels; vertical lines include the ranges. (Courtesy of Wu, C. H.: Fertil. Steril. 32:269–275, September 1979.)

ulin decreased in hirsute women and was also correlated significantly with degree of hirsutism. The elevated plasma testosterone concentrations (including free, index and total concentrations) in hirsute women overlapped significantly with those of normal women (Fig 13–3), thus failing to discriminate each other.

▶ [In a special article in the 1979 YEAR BOOK pages 311 to 334, Strickler and Warren indicated that hirsute women could be clearly separated from normal women on the basis of their respective plasma levels of free (unbound) testosterone. In the present report, although testosterone levels were positively correlated with the severity of the hirsutism, some overlap with normal women existed. No specific level of either free or total testosterone clearly distinguished normal from hirsute women. The differential effects of estradiol and testosterone on testosterone-estradiol-binding globulin concentrations and the different affinity of testosterone-estradiol-binding globulin for estradiol and testosterone help illustrate the complexity of the situation.] ◀

New Therapeutic Approach to Hirsute Patient. Andrée Boisselle and Roland R. Tremblay[13-27] (Laval Univ., Ste-Foy, Que.) evaluated spironolactone, an aldosterone antagonist causing antiandrogenic side effects, in hirsute women. Ten healthy women aged 20–35 years were given 50 mg spironolactone daily for 1 week. Six hirsute females aged 10–25 years, in whom no cause of hirsutism was known, received spironolactone for 6 months. The patients were within 15–25% of ideal body weight and had fairly regular menstrual cycles. They had not used oral medications for the past few months.

A slight but significant acceleration of the metabolic clearance rate of plasma testosterone was noted in normal women given spironolac-

(13–27) Fertil. Steril. 32:276–279, September 1979.

tone. The total testosterone level was reduced. In the hirsute women a 50% reduction in the blood production rate of testosterone was noted after 6 months of spironolactone therapy. Urinary 17-ketosteroid excretion was reduced by 50% after 6 months of therapy. Urinary 17-hydroxysteroid excretion was not altered. The growth of existing hair slowed, and no progression of coarsening or darkening of hair was noted during treatment. Subsequently, similar clinical results were obtained in 25 other women with idiopathic or adrenal-ovarian hirsutism.

It is suggested that spironolactone, in addition to its effect on androgen biosynthesis, can compete in vivo for intracellular androgen receptor sites in human skin. Spironolactone and canrenone should be considered antiandrogenic agents. Their clinical use in hirsute patients should prove to be useful.

▶ [This preliminary report suggests that spironolactone, an aldosterone antagonist, may be helpful in the treatment of hirsutism. The drug decreased the blood production rate of testosterone and diminished urinary 17-ketosteroid excretion. The authors describe an inhibition of testosterone effects at the end-organ level as well. More study is needed, but perhaps spironolactone can be used to advantage along with either corticosteroids or oral contraceptives in the therapy of this condition which is so distressing to many women.] ◀

Partial Adrenocortical Hydroxylase Deficiency Syndrome in Infertile Women. Adrenocortical dysfunction has been implicated in the androgen excess leading to acne and hirsutism in some women. Michael D. Birnbaum and Leslie I. Rose[13-28] (Hahnemann Med. College) studied 18 infertile women with clinical evidence of excess androgen production who wished to conceive. The women had been unable to conceive after a year and were younger than age 30 or had been unable to conceive after 6 months if they were older than age 30. Women with secondary infertility were selected after having attempted to conceive for 6 months. All patients had facial acne, facial hirsutism, or both, and clinical evidence of ovulatory dysfunction. Eight patients were oligomenorrheic, but none was amenorrheic. Treatment was with 5 mg of prednisone twice daily. Unresponsive patients received 50 mg of clomiphene citrate daily for 5 days, starting on day 5 of the menstrual cycle.

All patients had elevated excretion of pregnanetriol, tetrahydro compound S, or both in response to ACTH. Ten women conceived on glucocorticoid suppression therapy, 5 of them within 2 to 3 months after the start of treatment. Seven of the 8 unresponsive women had other significant infertility factors; 6 had infertile husbands. Four of the 8 patients given clomiphene therapy conceived, all within two cycles of combined clomiphene-prednisone therapy. Both patients with evidence of a luteal phase defect conceived during clomiphene therapy.

Women in whom adrenocortical suppression does not restore totally normal ovarian function probably have prolonged chronic anovulation and a complete disorder of the hypothalamic-pituitary-ovarian axis that has become self-perpetuating. Clomiphene treatment is necessary in these women, besides glucocorticoid suppression therapy.

(13–28) Fertil. Steril. 32:536–541, November 1979.

▶ [In most gynecologic patients with evidence of hyperandrogenism, the ovary is the source of excess hormone production. Indeed, some authors have concluded that the adrenal is seldom, if ever, responsible for the syndrome. This paper takes a contrary view, based on ACTH stimulation studies of 18 women with presumed partial adrenocortical hydroxylase deficiency. It is impressive that ten of the patients conceived while receiving corticosteroid suppression alone and most of the remainder had some additional reason for their infertility.] ◀

Relief of Dysmenorrhea With the Prostaglandin Synthetase Inhibitor Ibuprofen: Effect on Prostaglandin Levels in Menstrual Fluid. The etiology of primary dysmenorrhea remains poorly understood, and current treatment of the condition with analgesia is unsatisfactory. Recent studies have suggested that prostaglandin (PG) synthetase inhibitors may be of value in the treatment of dysmenorrhea. W. Y. Chan, M. Yusoff Dawood, and Fritz Fuchs[13-29] (Cornell Univ. Med. College) performed a double-blind crossover study of ibuprofen (Motrin), a PG synthetase inhibitor, in 7 dysmenorrheic patients during 23 menstrual cycles. All the subjects were nulliparous and had a history of primary dysmenorrhea starting within a year of menarche. The age range was 23 to 25 years. All had regular menstrual cycles. Patients took 400 mg of ibuprofen or a placebo four times daily, starting 3 days before the expected onset of menses and continuing through 3 days after onset.

Ibuprofen was given during seven cycles in the 5 evaluable subjects. Patients with severe dysmenorrhea usually had higher levels of menstrual PG than nondysmenorrheic controls. Good to excellent relief of menstrual cramps and symptoms associated with dysmenorrhea occurred in cycles where ibuprofen was given, compared with placebo cycles. A reduction in menstrual PG release also was associ-

Fig 13–4.—Relationship between severity of dysmenorrhea and levels of menstrual PG released in treatment and nontreatment cycles of a dysmenorrheic patient. Open bars show daily global assessment of dysmenorrheic symptoms by the patient, on a scale of 0 (no pain) to 10 (maximum pain). Hatched bars show levels of menstrual PG released during the corresponding period. (Courtesy of Chan, W. Y., et al.: Am. J. Obstet. Gynecol. 135:102–108, Sept. 1, 1979.)

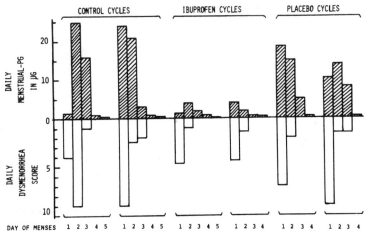

(13–29) Am. J. Obstet. Gynecol. 135:102–108, Sept. 1, 1979.

ated with ibuprofen administration. Individual subjects showed close correlation between the severity of menstrual pain and the level of menstrual PG released during the corresponding period (Fig 13–4).

Patients with severe primary dysmenorrhea often have increased release of PG into the menstrual fluid, which can be effectively suppressed by ibuprofen administration, with marked relief from symptoms of dysmenorrhea. The PG synthetase inhibitor must be given a few days before onset of menstruation to inhibit effectively endometrial PG production. No side effects were noted in the present subjects.

▶ [A number of recent studies have documented the therapeutic efficacy of prostaglandin inhibitors in primary dysmenorrhea, and this carefully done study appears to represent the "nail in the coffin" as far as a relation between prostaglandins and this common gynecologic complaint is concerned. The daily level of bioassayable prostaglandins in menstrual fluid exhibited a close correlation with symptoms and was suppressed threefold to fourfold with ibuprofen (Motrin), a synthetase inhibitor. It is worthy of note that the medication was initiated three days prior to onset of menses.

In a related study, Kajanoja and Vesanto (Acta Obstet. Gynecol. Scand. [Suppl.] 87:87, 1979) compared naproxen and indomethacin in primary dysmenorrhea. Efficacy was similar but fewer side effects accompanied naproxen.] ◀

▶ ↓ Not all reports are so favorable about the therapeutic efficacy of prostaglandin inhibitors. For a contrary voice, read on. ◀

Flurbiprofen in Management of Dysmenorrhea. Primary spasmodic dysmenorrhea is common in nulliparas. Prostaglandins have been implicated in dysmenorrhea, and inhibitors of prostaglandin synthetase have been suggested for patients with this incapacitating condition. J. R. Pogmore and G. M. Filshie[13-30] compared the analgesic effect of the potent prostaglandin synthetase inhibitor flurbiprofen with that of aspirin and placebo in 41 patients, using a double-blind, triple-crossover design. The dosage of flurbiprofen was 50 mg every 6 hours, and that of aspirin was 500 mg every 6 hours. The active agents and placebo were used in 3 consecutive menstrual periods.

Pain relief did not differ significantly with any of the treatments. Fourteen patients reported side effects with all treatments including placebo. No significant differences in blood loss were observed.

Flurbiprofen, unlike the fenamates, does not antagonize the action of prostaglandins directly once they are present, which could explain why no significant analgesic effects were obtained in this study of dysmenorrheic subjects. The issue may be clarified by evaluating flurbiprofen given a few days before the start of the menstrual period.

▶ [Flurbiprofen, a prostaglandin synthetase inhibitor, was no more effective than the placebo in this study. However, flurbiprofen does not antagonize preformed prostaglandins, and perhaps efficacy would be improved by premenstrual administration of the drug.] ◀

Effect of Acetylsalicylic Acid, Paracetamol, and Placebo on Pain and Blood Loss in Dysmenorrheic Women was evaluated by Torun Janbu, Per Løkken, and Britt-Ingjerd Nesheim[13-31] (Univ. of Oslo). Over 50% of women have dysmenorrhea affecting their daily activities. Acetylsalicylic acid, a prostaglandin synthesis inhibitor,

---

(13–30) Br. J. Obstet. Gynaecol. 87:326–329, April 1980.
(13–31) Acta Obstet. Gynecol. Scand. [Suppl.] 87:81–85, 1979.

appears to be active in dysmenorrhea, but may contribute to menor-rhagia. The present study compared this agent with paracetamol and placebo in a double-blind crossover trial in 30 women with fairly constant dysmenorrhea and no history of peptic ulcer disease. The age range was 21–27 years. All women were nulliparous. Two used oral contraception. Both active drugs were used in a dose of 0.5 gm four times daily for three days, starting with onset of menstruation.

No significant differences in pain relief were noted with aspirin, paracetamol, and placebo. Satisfactory relief was obtained in 21 of 90 menstrual periods—in 8 with paracetamol, in 7 with aspirin, and in 6 with placebo. No drug significantly affected the amount of menstrual blood loss. Thirteen women reported side effects in 16 menstrual periods. These effects occurred on 4 occasions when aspirin was used, on 6 occasions when paracetamol was used, and 6 times when placebo was used. One woman taking acetylsalicylic acid reported cardialgia. All other reported effects belong to the symptomatology of dysmenorrhea.

Acetylsalicylic acid and paracetamol were not significantly more effective than placebo in relieving severe dysmenorrhea in this study. Acetylsalicylic acid did not appear to increase menstrual blood loss.

▶ [Aspirin, by virtue of its antiprostaglandin effect, should alleviate dysmenorrhea but, in view of its anticoagulant action, might aggravate menorrhagia. In this controlled, double-blind crossover study, it was no different from placebo on either count. Could the apparent lack of benefit reflect the fact that treatment was not initiated until menstrual bleeding began or is the relative impotency of aspirin responsible?

Quite different results were found by Haynes and associates (Int. J. Gynaecol. Obstet. 17:567, 1980), who measured menstrual blood loss with and without mefenamic acid in women with menorrhagia. Oral mefenamic acid treatment (500 mg 4 times daily for the first 3 days of heavy menstruation) caused a reduction in menstrual blood loss from a mean of 137 ml to one of 76 ml.] ◀

14. Infertility

During the Infertility Survey, at Which Period Do You Feel Endoscopy Is Indicated? This question is discussed by J. F. Hulka, Robert Israel, and Jerome Jay Hoffman.[14-1] Hulka thinks that laparoscopy is indicated if any pathologic condition of the tubes is discovered at hysterosalpingography, unless ovulation problems must be resolved. If a male factor problem alone is present, laparoscopy is done at the fourth well-timed cycle of donor insemination. In other cases laparoscopy is done if the couple has been infertile for a year or longer. Fewer than half of patients will have laparoscopy with this approach, and those examined will quite often be found to have luteinized unruptured follicles.

Israel believes that endoscopy is indicated at the end of the routine infertility survey. In the ovulatory patient, a preovulatory fractional postcoital test and follicular phase hysterosalpingogram precede laparoscopy. If the results are normal, three months should elapse before laparoscopy is undertaken. In the anovulatory patient who bleeds after progesterone, ovulation induction should be achieved before postcoital testing and subsequent laparoscopy can be performed effectively. A hysterosalpingogram can be made if pregnancy has been ruled out or while clomiphene is being given, or immediately after treatment before ovulation.

Hoffman states that a modified Rubin test should be done after the preliminary workup. Hysterosalpingography should be done if carbon dioxide passage does not occur or is difficult. If an oviduct block is seen, ovulatory function should be evaluated before laparoscopy is undertaken. Laparotomy is preferably delayed after laparoscopy if fertility is the goal. Endoscopy is necessary when sterilization has been achieved by laparoscopic coagulation. Laparotomy may be done without endoscopy after a Pomeroy procedure if a minimal amount of tube has been excised, without the fimbriae, or if clips or bands have been used.

▶ [Three experts answer a pertinent question. Their view is "later" rather than "earlier." We agree. Often pregnancy will occur in the meantime, obviating the expense and risks (minimal, to be sure) of laparoscopy. Hulka suggests that the operation be performed 2–5 days after a presumed ovulation in order to look for a luteinized unruptured follicle (cf. 1979 YEAR BOOK, p. 387).] ◀

Endometrial Biopsy in the Evaluation of Infertility. The luteal phase defect (LPD) found in about 3% of infertile subjects has been associated with infertility, recurrent miscarriage, and occult miscarriage. Anne Colston Wentz[14-2] (Univ. of Tennessee) performed 210 endometrial biopsies as part of infertility evaluations in 149 patients.

(14–1) Int. J. Fertil. 25:1–4, 1980.
(14–2) Fertil. Steril. 33:121–124, February 1980.

Biopsies were scheduled within 2 to 3 days of the expected menses. A biopsy was obtained only to date the endometrium to diagnose LPD.

The initial biopsy was in phase in 92 patients (61.7%) and out of phase in 44 (29.5%). In 13 patients it could not be classified. Six of 31 second biopsies in patients with out-of-phase initial biopsies were in phase. Twenty-two patients had a luteal defect by biopsy criteria. Four of 12 patients with in-phase initial biopsies who had a repeat study had an out-of-phase biopsy, two in association with the start of clomiphene therapy. Clomiphene therapy was comparably frequent in patients with in-phase and out-of-phase biopsies. Three of 8 patients with a history of two or more first-trimester abortions had LPD. Three of 22 patients with a diagnosis of LPD based on two biopsies out of phase by more than 2 days in two cycles were hyperprolactinemic. Biopsies were done in the cycle of conception in 10 patients; 9 patients have been delivered normally, and 1 had an ampullary ectopic pregnancy. There were no "failed" biopsies in this series.

The overall incidence of LPD in this series, detected by late luteal phase endometrial biopsy in otherwise unselected infertility patients, was 19%. This reflects the bias of a patient population selected to include a high percentage of patients with menstrual and ovulatory dysfunction and some with miscarriages. The endometrial biopsy is a safe means of providing histologic evidence of normal endometrial development. Whether identification of patients with LPD will increase fertility after treatment remains to be seen. Biopsy of all patients presenting with infertility appears to be the most reasonable means of diagnosing LPD.

▶ [From this large series of endometrial biopsies, several important conclusions can be drawn regarding this test in infertile patients. The frequency of endometrium "out of phase" (ie, 2 or more days' lag) in two cycles was 19%. Previous suggestions that luteal phase deficiency is more likely with clomiphene-induced ovulation were not confirmed. There was no interference with pregnancy in 10 women in whom biopsy was done during the cycle of conception. Important technical points include obtaining fundal, as opposed to lower-segment, endometrium and doing the biopsy within 3 days of expected menses. Unfortunately, no information is given regarding the treatment or subsequent course of patients with abnormal endometrial histology.] ◀

Luteal Phase Deficiency and Infertility: Difficulties Encountered in Diagnosis and Treatment. Uncertainty concerning the importance of luteal phase defects as a cause of female infertility is closely related to problems in diagnosis. Thomas Annos, Irwin E. Thompson, and Melvin L. Taymor[14-3] (Harvard Med. School) examined the consistency of the measures used to diagnose luteal phase deficiency in 14 patients seen for infertility in 1978 and 1979. The criteria evaluated included basal body temperature (BBT), endometrial biopsy, and progesterone concentration. Prolactin and LH concentrations were measured at the time of progesterone determination. A total of 29 cycles were evaluated. Patients received treatment with 25-mg progesterone vaginal suppositories twice daily, from 3 days after the BBT rise until the menses, or clomiphene citrate in a starting dosage of 50 mg daily, from cycle day 5 to cycle day 9. Clomiphene

(14–3) Obstet. Gynecol. 55:705–710, June 1980.

dosage was increased to 100 mg after 4 cycles, if the earlier dosage was unsuccessful.

A shortened luteal phase was observed in 11 of the 29 cycles. Only 4 of these cycles showed consistent abnormalities on the endometrial biopsy and BBT chart, besides those in progesterone concentration. Only one abnormality was apparent in 2 cycles. The endometrial biopsy and progesterone concentration were discrepant in 6 of the 11 cycles. Prolactin was normal in all cycles with a shortened luteal phase. Luteinizing hormone was undetectable in 3 of 11 cycles at the time of endometrial biopsy. Six of 18 cycles with a normal luteal phase showed endometrial biopsy, BBT, and progesterone abnormalities. Seven other cycles had abnormalities in two of these, and 5 cycles had one abnormality. Five pregnancies have occurred, with 1 early pregnancy loss. Three patients conceived while on clomiphene therapy and 2 while using progesterone vaginal suppositories.

Endometrial biopsy appears to be the essential part of the evaluation. Clomiphene citrate should be considered for treatment, especially of those patients with a short luteal phase. Altered prolactin metabolism appears to represent only a small part of the pathogenesis of luteal phase deficiency.

▶ [The difficulties associated with the diagnosis and therapy of the deficient luteal phase in infertility are well illustrated by this report. The endometrial biopsy and blood progesterone results were consistent in 15 cycles and discordant in 14. Only 1 of the 14 patients consistently had both tests abnormal in subsequent cycles. Both vaginal progesterone and clomiphene were moderately effective therapies. Although other recent studies have suggested that hyperprolactinemia is frequent in patients with luteal insufficiency, only 1 patient in the present series had an elevated serum prolactin.] ◀

Increased Pregnancy Rate with Oil-Soluble Hysterosalpingography Dye. Hysterosalpingography is frequently performed for diagnostic purposes in infertility patients, but a therapeutic component has been observed. This has been attributed to mechanical lavage by the tube, stimulation of tubal cilia, and lysis of peritoneal adhesions, and possibly to use of oil-soluble dye contrast medium.

Alan H. DeCherney, Hilton Kort, Jay B. Barney, and Gregory R. DeVore[14-4] (Yale Univ.), in a prospective study during 1973 to 1978, evaluated 339 patients who underwent hysterosalpingography, 177 with use of an oil-soluble contrast medium and 162 with use of a water-soluble medium. With fluoroscopic visualization, either 10 ml of meglumine diatrizoate (Renografin-60) or 3 to 5 ml ethiodized oil (Ethiodal) was injected into the uterus and tubes.

The overall follow-up was 85%, with a minimum follow-up of 4 months. The pregnancy rate was significantly higher when oil-soluble contrast medium was used (29% vs. 13%). The most significant differences were in the groups with unexplained fertility and male-factor infertility. Rates for patients with both primary and secondary unexplained infertility were higher with oil-soluble medium. Adverse effects were not noted with the use of oil-soluble contrast medium.

Patients in this series with unexplained primary or secondary infertility and those with male-factor infertility had a significantly

(14–4) Fertil. Steril. 33:407–410, April 1980.

higher pregnancy rate when oil-soluble contrast medium instead of water-soluble contrast medium was used for hysterosalpingography. Initially, hysterosalpingography should be done with a small amount of water-soluble contrast medium to determine whether the fallopian tubes are patent. If they are, oil-soluble contrast medium should be used therapeutically. The only contraindication to use of oil-soluble medium may be promotion of granulomatous disease, but this appears to occur only in diseased tubes in which absorption of dye and spillage are retarded.

▶ [This report suggesting improved pregnancy rates following the use of an oil-soluble vs. a water-soluble dye for hysterosalpingography is provocative. The authors describe their study as a "random, prospective" one. These words are misused. Assignment of patients to one dye vs. the other depended on physician preference and there are clear differences between the two groups (eg, 31% of patients in the water-soluble group underwent major surgical procedures vs. 2% of the oil-soluble group). The results in the "unexplained infertility" groups do seem to favor the oil dye, but a prospective study with true random assignment is needed to clearly resolve this issue. Salpix, a water-soluble but viscous dye, should be included in such a study.] ◀

Febrile Morbidity Following Hysterosalpingography: Identification of Risk Factors and Recommendations for Prophylaxis.

Inflammatory reactions are the most serious and most common complications of hysterosalpingography (HSG). Paul G. Stumpf and Charles M. March[14-5] (Univ. of Southern California) reviewed the records of 448 consecutive healthy women who underwent HSG from 1976 to 1978. A total of 464 examinations were performed. Mean age was 27.4 years. Infertility was the indication for HSG in 62% of cases. Documented episodes of pelvic inflammatory disease had occurred in 23% of patients, and another 8% had had an illness compatible with possible pelvic infection. Pelvic examination was normal in three fourths of patients. About one-third received oral antibiotic prophylaxis, usually with ampicillin.

At least 9 patients had possible inflammatory reactions after HSG, and 1 was hospitalized. Fourteen patients (3.1%) met criteria for pelvic infection and were hospitalized. Treatment was with penicillin or a cephalorosporin and an aminoglycoside, and either clindamycin or chloramphenicol. One patient required hysterectomy and salpingo-oophrectomy. The HSG was abnormal in all patients with definite pelvic infection. Nine patients with infection had received ampicillin or tetracycline prophylactically in conjunction with HSG. Twelve of the 14 infected patients had been examined for infertility. Only 1 of 12 patients who wished to conceive has done so.

It is recommended that HSG not be performed in women at high risk of infection. The procedure is safe in women at lowest risk. In those at intermediate risk, the risk-benefit ratio of the study must be carefully weighed, and antibiotic prophylaxis with anaerobic coverage should be considered.

▶ [This report serves to remind us that latent pelvic inflammatory disease may become blatent pelvic inflammatory disease as a result of hysterosalpingography. Previously documented pelvic infection and a recent adnexal mass or tenderness were important predictors. The erythrocyte sedimentation rate was not helpful in identifying patients

(14-5) Fertil. Steril. 33:487-492, May 1980.

likely to have problems. The prophylactic use of broad-spectrum antibiotics did not prevent flare-ups in these patients.] ◄

Immunologic Infertility: I. Cervical Mucus Antibodies and Postcoital Test. Human sperm has immunogenic potential and, in susceptible women, sperm antigens may elicit antibodies against sperm-specific or coating antigens and lead to infertility. Kamran S. Moghissi, Anthony G. Sacco and Katherine Borin[14-6] (Wayne State Univ.) determined the incidence of sperm antibodies in cervical mucus and serum in infertile women and whether or not a postcoital test can indicate the presence of cervical mucus or circulating sperm antibodies. Studies were done in 172 infertile couples. Sperm-agglutinating antibodies (SAA) and sperm-immobilizing antibodies (SIA) were assayed in the serums and cervical mucus of the study women and in 18 control subjects.

Sperm antibodies were found in the cervical mucus of 25.6% of the infertile women and in the serums of 12.7% of females and 6.4% of males. No sperm antibodies were found in the cervical mucus of control subjects. Only 4.7% of subjects had both serum and cervical mucus antibodies; only cervical mucus antibodies were present in 20.9% of cases. Antibodies were present significantly more often in couples with unexplained infertility than in those with explained infertility. The presence and number of live spermatozoa in cervical mucus collected for postcoital tests were significantly related to the presence of SAA and SIA in cervical mucus and serum. Both types of antibody in cervical mucus and SAA in female serum correlated negatively with an endocervical postcoital test, whereas sperm mobility correlated positively.

The appearance of SAA and SIA in cervical mucus is not related to their presence or titer in the serum. The postcoital test is a reliable screening method where sperm antibodies are suspected of existing in cervical mucus and to a lesser extent in the serum. Sperm antibodies should be suspected in cases with consistently negative or poor postcoital tests when both the semen and cervical mucus are of high quality. The findings can be confirmed by in vitro sperm penetration tests or sperm-cervical mucus contact tests. The cervix may be an important local site of sperm antibody synthesis.

► [Few questions are as controversial as that regarding immunologic causes of infertility. This informative study may help explain some of the contradictions in the literature. There was a poor correlation between serum and cervical mucus with respect to presence of sperm antibodies. Sperm antibodies were found in cervical mucus of one fourth of the women with "unexplained infertility" and in none of the fertile controls. These observations suggest that the cervix itself might be the site of antibody production. Of practical importance is the generally good correlation between the Sims-Hühner postcoital test and cervical antibody studies. As we interpret the results, if a patient has a good or excellent endocervical postcoital test score (>10 sperm per high-power field), the chance of her having antibodies anyplace are only 25% (15/60) and that of cervical mucus antibodies, only 17% (9/54). On the other hand, among patients with a negative or poor endocervical postcoital test result (<5 sperm per high-power field) 57% had antibodies. While these odds are respectable, they are far from certain.] ◄

(14–6) Am. J. Obstet. Gynecol. 136:941–950, Apr. 1, 1980.

Treatment of Cervical Factor With Combined High-Dose Estrogen and Human Menopausal Gonadotropins. Either thick, tenacious cervical mucus or extremely scant mucus may respond to treatment with high-dose estrogen, but such therapy usually suppresses ovulation. Jerome H. Check[14-7] (Thomas Jefferson Univ.) reports 2 cases in which pregnancy occurred with high-dosage conjugated estrogen therapy and concomitant treatment with human menopausal gonadotropins (hMG).

Woman, 36, with infertility for $1\frac{1}{2}$ years, had both a cervical factor and an ovulation defect and had only one patent tube. Oligospermia responded to clomiphene therapy. The patient ovulated on clomiphene citrate therapy, but the mucus at midcycle was extremely thick and viscous, and attempts to improve it with up to 5 mg of conjugated estrogens daily on days 10 to 16 failed, even with adjunctive tetracycline therapy. Clomiphene was then stopped, and the patient was given 0.2 mg of diethylstilbestrol on days 5 to 16, but the mucus remained thick. On treatment with 5 mg of estrogens only for 2 weeks, excellent mucus developed but ovulation did not occur. The patient then received hMG for 3 cycles, but the cervical mucus remained thick. On treatment with 5 mg of estrogens and 1 ampule of hMG daily, besides human chorionic gonadotropin (hCG), the patient conceived during the second treatment cycle. Ultrasound study showed a single viable fetus.

The other patient had had secondary infertility for 3 years, and cervical mucus was absent. She ovulated in the first cycle of combined therapy and conceived in the second treatment cycle. A single viable fetus was demonstrated.

The use of hMG with high-dosage estrogen therapy permits ovulation despite pituitary suppression. Treatment with hMG is continued until a good postcoital test is achieved. This approach should be used only after all other therapy has failed, because of the risks of hyperstimulation and multiple births. In the future it may be feasible to perform estradiol assay while the patient is taking conjugated estrogens alone and again when she is taking hMG and estrogens together to guide hCG therapy.

▶ [What can be done for infertile patients whose scanty thick cervical mucus responds only to doses of estrogen that are so high that ovulation is inhibited? Treat them with sufficient estrogen and induce ovulation, if necessary, with hMG-hCG, according to this report.] ◀

Current Experience With a Standardized Method of Human Menopausal Gonadotropin-Human Chorionic Gonadotropin Administration. Ewa Radwanska, John Hammond, Mary Hammond, and Pamela Smith[14-8] (Univ. of North Carolina, Chapel Hill) reviewed experience in treatment of 26 infertile women with ovulatory disorders, who had failed to respond to treatment with clomiphene and human chorionic gonadotropin (hCG), in which a standardized human menopausal gonadotropin (hMG)-hCG regimen was used. Three to 8 ampules of hMG (Pergonal) were given on days 1, 3, and 5, with 10,000 IU of hCG on day 8 of the regimen (Fig 14-1). Treatment began on cycle days 4 to 8 in menstruating women. The hMG preparation contained 75 IU each of FSH and LH. A second hCG in-

(14-7)   Fertil. Steril. 33:562–563, May 1980.
(14-8)   Ibid., pp. 510–513.

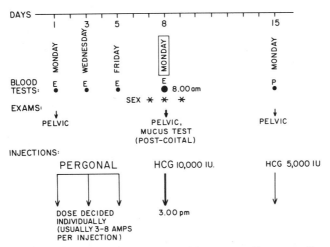

Fig 14–1.—Clinical protocol, standardized hMG-hCG treatment. *E,* estrogen; *P,* progesterone. (Courtesy of Radwanska, E., et al.: Fertil. Steril. 33:510–513, May 1980.)

jection of 5,000 IU was sometimes given a week after the first injection. Usually hCG was withheld if the estrogen concentration on day 8 exceeded 2,000 pg/ml.

Of 39 cycles completed in the 26 patients, 22 were considered to be adequately stimulated. In 7 cycles with estrogen concentrations above 1,500 pg/ml but with no clinical evidence of hyperstimulation, hCG was injected. Eight pregnancies have occurred; 6 patients conceived in the first cycle of therapy. Five of these patients had an initial diagnosis of amenorrhea. Inadequate response to treatment was usually followed by a higher dose of the hMG preparation. Four patients had excessive responses, with ovarian cystic enlargement, and hCG was withheld. Other probable infertility factors were present in 12 cases. Eight of the 16 patients with good postcoital findings and good hormonal findings conceived. Two pregnancies aborted spontaneously in the first trimester.

A standardized 1-3-5 regimen of Pergonal, with hCG injected on day 8 when ovarian stimulation is adequate but not excessive, offers a fairly effective alternative to other methods of inducing ovulation in clomiphene-resistant anovulatory patients. Ovulation was induced in 96% of patients in this series. A good postcoital test was a favorable prognostic sign.

▶ [As the authors of this article point out, this alternate-day hMG schedule is a convenient one, especially for patients who must travel a fair distance for care.] ◀

Use of Human Gonadotropins for Induction of Ovulation in Women With Polycystic Ovarian Disease. Ovarian wedge resection is an invasive means of inducing ovulation in patients with polycystic ovarian disease (POD) and gives variable results. Chun Fu Wang and Carl Gemzell[14-9] (SUNY, Downstate Med. Center) under-

---

(14–9) Fertil. Steril. 33:479–486, May 1980.

took to induce ovulation with human gonadotropins in 41 infertile women with POD. A total of 77 treatment cycles of human menopausal gonadotropin (hMG)-human chorionic gonadotropin (hCG) were administered after the patients had failed to ovulate or conceive on clomiphene therapy. Gonadotropin treatment was begun after a spontaneous menstrual period or a progesterone-induced flow, with 2 ampules of hMG (75 IU each of FSH and LH per ampule). The dose was increased by a factor of 0.3 to 0.5 if the plasma estradiol concentration did not rise after 4 or 5 days. When the estradiol concentration reached 600 to 800 pg/ml, hCG was given in a dose of 5,000 or 10,000 IU, 24 to 48 hours after the last injection of hMG. If the ovaries were not enlarged, a second dose of 5,000 IU was given a week later.

Average patients age was 28.7 years. Eleven patients had had ovarian wedge resections. The rate of conception was 65.9%; 2 patients conceived twice. The results were comparable with those obtained in another group of anovulatory patients. Three patients developed severe ovarian hyperstimulation. Two of them delivered at term and 1 aborted at 7 weeks' gestation. A patient with mild hyperstimulation was operated on for ectopic pregnancy, but she also had an intrauterine pregnancy and delivered at term.

Treatment with hMG-hCG is a safe, effective, nonoperative means of inducing ovulation in women with POD who have failed to respond to clomiphene therapy. Daily estrogen determinations are necessary to avoid hyperstimulation, multiple births, or both. The multiple pregnancy rate in this series was 36.3% and the abortion rate was 24.1%.

▶ [These patients with polycystic ovarian disease (rather loosely defined) who did not conceive with clomiphene therapy were treated with hMG-hCG. The ovulation and pregnancy rates were high, but hyperstimulation occurred in 12% of cycles even with daily plasma estradiol monitoring. The authors think this is due, in part, to the active ovaries in these patients with follicles in various stages of function and development.

Ten of the 41 patients were hyperprolactinemic. A trial of bromocriptine therapy prior to gonadotropin use would seem reasonable in this circumstance.] ◀

Relationship of Weight to Successful Induction of Ovulation with Clomiphene Citrate. Marguerite K. Shepard, Jose P. Balmaceda, and Connie G. Leija[14-10] (Univ. of Texas, San Antonio) administered clomiphene citrate to 117 anovulatory, euthyroid, estrogen-primed patients from 1972 to 1978. All patients were oligomenorrheic or amenorrheic, desired pregnancy, and had been infertile for at least 1 year. Sixty-two patients ovulated and conceived, ovulated in at least three treatment cycles, or failed to respond to a maximum dosage of 250 mg of clomiphene daily. The starting dosage was 50 mg, given on days 5 to 9 of a progestin-induced cycle. The dosage was subsequently increased by 50-mg increments each cycle until ovulation occurred or the maximum dose was reached.

Fifty patients (80.6%) ovulated, and 47 of them conceived, for an overall conception rate of 75.8%. Five pregnancies ended in spontaneous abortions, and 1 in an unexplained intrauterine fetal death at

(14–10) Fertil. Steril. 32:641–645, December 1979.

36 weeks. One patients was lost to follow-up; the rest delivered viable infants. About one fourth of ovulations and pregnancies occurred at clomiphene dosages of 150 mg or more. Nonresponders were significantly heavier than responders at all clomiphene dosages. The difference was significant at the 0.01 level for the 50- and 100-mg dosages. Other variables such as age, parity, duration of infertility, and oral contraceptive use did not differ significantly between responders and nonresponders.

Body weight may be a critical factor in estrogen-primed women given clomiphene therapy to induce ovulation. It might be logical to start treatment at dosages higher than 50 or 100 mg, depending on weight, in obese patients. In a selected population, pregnancy rates approaching normal can be achieved with clomiphene therapy.

▶ [This interesting report points out an inverse relationship between body weight and ovulation inducibility with clomiphene. Clomiphene's mode of action is not understood fully, but current theories all involve some type of competition with estrogen for estrogen receptors in the hypothalamus. Obese women are known to have increased levels of estrone, arising from peripheral conversion of androstenedione, so it may be that they require higher clomiphene doses to compete successfully. In any event, the clinical implication is that in fat patients it may be necessary to go higher than the usual dosage limit of 100 or 150 mg per day.] ◀

New Aspects of Pathophysiology of Endometriosis and Associated Infertility.
Endometriosis remains an enigmatic condition, its cause still debated. P. R. Koninckx, P. Ide, W. Vandenbroucke, and I. A. Brosens[14-11] (Univ. of Louvain) collected peritoneal fluid at laparoscopy from women with primary or secondary infertility. The centrifuged sediment was stained by the Papanicolaou technique, and the supernatant was assayed for several hormones. Viable endometrial cells were present as often in women without pelvic endometriosis as in affected women, most often during the follicular phase. No differ-

---

PROGESTERONE CONCENTRATION (NG/ML) IN PERITONEAL FLUID IN WOMEN WITHOUT ENDOMETRIOSIS AND IN WOMEN WITH MILD AND MODERATE ENDOMETRIOSIS

Day of Menstrual Cycle	Endometriosis	
	Absent	Present
2-9	3.4 (2.2–5.4)* [2]†	5.2 (2.8–9.6) [*f*3]
10-14	2.1 (0.8–5.2) [3]	4.1 (11.8–9.5) [*f*3]
14-18		
Ovulation stigmata absent	—	45.4 (31.9–64.8) [*f*7]
Ovulation stigmata present	144.9 (113.9–184.4) [8]	154.9 (113.2–216.0) [13]
19-20		
Ovulation stigmata absent	28.2 (20.9–38.0) [6]	23.0 (19.6–27.0) [*f*9]
Ovulation stigmata present	87.0 (61.2–123.6) [9]	76.4 (12.7–460.1) [*f*3]

*Numbers in parentheses indicate mean$_{log}$ (mean − 1 SD, mean + 1 SD).
†Numbers in brackets indicate number of experiments.

(14–11) J. Reprod. Med. 24:257–260, June 1980.

ences were found in total protein, steroid hormone-binding globulin, or transcortin values, and the concentrations of progesterone (table) and estradiol-17β did not differ significantly in the two groups. Both progesterone and estradiol-17β concentrations increased sharply after ovulation in women with ovulatory cycles, but not in those with unruptured luteinized follicles.

The endometrial cells in peritoneal fluid are probably derived from retrograde menstruation, not from endometriotic lesions. Presumably implantation of endometrial cells is normally prevented by the specific steroid hormone environment. Endometriosis may develop when this mechanism fails—when an unruptured luteinizing follicle is formed. This process may be better elucidated by determining local steroid hormone concentrations in peritoneal fluid than by determining plasma hormone concentrations. Infertility may be the cause rather than the result of endometriosis, through the unruptured luteinized follicle syndrome. Ovarian endometriosis, however, can cause infertility.

▶ [An interesting speculation (unruptured luteinized follicles → endometriosis + infertility), but a speculation nonetheless.] ◀

Sex Steroid Levels During Treatment of Endometriosis. Danazol, a synthetic derivative of ethisterone, has proved remarkably successful in the treatment of endometriosis, and may also restore fertility. Jack S. Hirschowitz, Norman G. Soler, and Jacobo Wortsman[14-12] (Southern Illinois Univ., Springfield) evaluated ovarian function in 19 women with endometriosis during prolonged danazol therapy. Sixteen patients presented with dysmenorrhea, 12 with infertility, and 6 with pelvic masses. Sixteen patients had galactorrhea before or during treatment. Endometriosis was considered mild in 9 cases, moderate in 4, and severe in 6. Danazol was given in a dose of 200 mg twice daily for 3 months to patients with mild disease, and in a dose of 400 mg twice daily for 9 months to the others.

Mean FSH levels did not change during danazol therapy, and the fall in the mean LH level was not significant. Serum prolactin concentrations decreased insignificantly with treatment. Both estradiol and testosterone levels increased significantly during danazol therapy, and all patients but 1 had abnormally high levels at some time. No clinical manifestations of these elevations were observed. High correlation was noted between the levels of estradiol and testosterone. Serum progesterone levels fell from 6.8 to 1.6 ng/ml during danazol therapy and returned to 5.2 ng/ml after treatment.

In most patients the disease remitted clinically within 3 months of the start of therapy. Only 3 patients had significant disease after 9 months of treatment. Conception has not occurred on follow-up for up to 5 months.

Danazol is not an antigonadotropic agent in the doses used in the present study. The increases in estradiol and testosterone observed may be due to an increase in sex-binding globulins. Hormone levels must be interpreted cautiously in patients who receive danazol.

(14–12) Obstet. Gynecol. 54:448–450, October 1979.

▶ [Danazol has proved to be very effective in treating endometriosis, yet its mechanism of action remains obscure. In this study, estradiol and testosterone levels more than doubled with danazol therapy, whereas FSH and LH were unaffected, which would seem to contradict the theory of an antigonadotropic action. The authors found no effect on their assays by adding danazol but it is conceivable that some metabolite(s) of the drug could be "read" as sex steroids, causing a false elevation in measured levels. The authors speculate that the effect may be on sex hormone-binding proteins, which could also account for elevated hormone measurements without clinical effect.

In a related study, Laurell and Rannevik (Postgrad. Med. J. 55 (Suppl. 5):40, 1979) measured 25 plasma proteins of hepatic origin in patients before and during danazol therapy. The observed changes were interpreted as indicating a competitive action on the hepatocyte receptor. The same results were reported by the same authors (perhaps reflecting the same subjects!) in another publication (J. Clin. Endocrinol. Metab. 49:719, 1979).

For another use of danazol—mastodynia—see Chapter 17, "Breast Diseases," in this YEAR BOOK.] ◀

Heritable Aspects of Endometriosis: I. Genetic Studies.

Joe Leigh Simpson, Sherman Elias, L. Russell Malinak, and Veasy C. Buttram, Jr.[14-13] examined the heritability of endometriosis in a series of 123 patients with histologically proved disease, who were operated on between 1971 and 1978. The mean age of the subjects interviewed was 30 years. The rate of involvement of sisters over age 18 years was 5.8%, and 8.1% of mothers were affected (table). One of 2 monozygotic twin subjects had a concordantly affected cotwin. Only 1% of the husbands' sisters and 0.9% of their mothers were affected. Two second-degree relatives and 5 third-degree relatives of the propositi were affected. Endometriosis was severe in 62% of the familial group and in 23% of the nonfamilial group.

The findings confirm the familial nature of endometriosis. Postulation of either a single autosomal recessive or a single autosomal dominant gene is unattractive, but it is also possible that endometriosis is several diseases, one form being inherited as the result of a single mutant gene and the others resulting from nongenetic factors or from different genes. Further studies elucidating inherited factors may help identify susceptible persons, by pedigree data and biologic markers, early in their reproductive years.

▶ [Several reports appearing over the past 40 years have pointed out a familial ten-

PROPORTIONS OF RELATIVES WITH ENDOMETRIOSIS*

	Relatives of patients with endometriosis	Relatives of patients' husbands ‡
Female sibs†	9/152 (5.8%)	1/104 (1.0%) [χ^2,1 df,p < 0.05]
Mothers	10/123 (8.1%)	1/107 (0.9%) [χ^2,1 df,p < 0.025]
All first-degree relatives	19/276 (6.9%)	2/211 (0.9%) [χ^2,1 df,p < 0.005]

*One patient had both an affected sib and an affected mother, whereas 18 had only 1 affected first-degree relative.
†Two patients were monozygotic twins; 1 of the 2 had a concordantly affected sib.
‡df: Degrees of freedom.

(14–13) Am. J. Obstet. Gynecol. 137:327–331, June 1, 1980.

dency to endometriosis. Whether this represents a genetic predisposition or simply a reflection of similarities in social, educational, and economic factors has never been clear. The results of this study, in which the incidence of the disease in first-degree relatives of endometriosis patients was 7%, give some insight. The controls were female siblings of the husbands of women with endometriosis and thus should be reasonably comparable with respect to these characteristics. Since the control incidence was only 1%, it certainly appears that some form of genetic inheritance is involved. The argument is further strengthened by a companion paper (Am. J. Obstet. Gynecol. 133:332, 1980) by the same authors (albeit in different order) in which the clinical characteristics of the same patient population are described. Among patients with an affected first-degree relative, endometriosis was graded as severe in 61%, compared with only 24% in whom there was no affected first-degree relative.] ◄

Perineal Endometrioma in Episiotomy Incisions: Clinical Features and Management. Implantation and growth of viable endometrial cells into fresh episiotomy incisions at vaginal delivery can occasionally result in development of a perineal endometrioma. Ernestine Hambrick, Herand Abcarian, and Durand Smith[14-14] (Abraham Lincoln School of Medicine) encountered 4 patients, aged 23 to 34 years, who developed endometriomas at an episiotomy site 19 months to 11 years post partum. All had periodic symptoms coinciding with the menstrual cycle. Pain and pruritus were associated with a tender mass at the episiotomy site and were most marked just before and after onset of menstrual bleeding. A tender swelling was present beneath the distal part of the incision in each patient. Two patients did well after complete excision of the lesion. One had medroxyprogesterone injection into residual endometrioma after incomplete excision because of involvement of the anal sphincter. One patient had recurrent symptoms after what was thought to be a complete excision and has been placed on oral contraception.

Occasional cells from the zona basalis may be expelled during placental separation, and it is these cells that are capable of replicating the endometrial lining. If viable zona basalis cells are implanted into a receptive site such as a fresh episiotomy incision, they may function as though still within the uterine cavity, with resultant formation of an endometrioma. Complete excision of perineal endometriomas should be curative.

► [Although we have seen endometriosis in an abdominal scar after cesarean section, we do not recall observing it in an episiotomy. In these 4 cases, the cardinal symptom was perineal pain and tenderness with menstruation; complete excision was curative.

In a related publication, Chatterjee (Obstet. Gynecol. 56:81, 1980) reported 17 cases of scar endometriosis (12 after hysterotomy abortion, 1 after low-segment cesarean section, 1 after puerperal sterilization, and 3 in the episiotomy after vaginal delivery.) Again, the most common symptom was painful swelling of the scar at time of menses. Oral progestational therapy was ineffective but surgical excision cured all cases.] ◄

Male Hyperprolactinemia: Effects on Fertility. The role of prolactin in male reproduction is unclear. Shmuel Segal, Haim Yaffe, Neri Laufer, and Menashe Ben-David[14-15] (Hebrew Univ.-Hadassah Med. School) detected hyperprolactinemia in 7 (4%) of 171 infertile men attending a male infertility clinic. These 7 patients received bromocriptine in an initial dosage of 2.5 to 5 mg daily, which was

(14-14) Dis. Colon Rectum 22:550–552, Nov.–Dec. 1979.
(14-15) Fertil. Steril. 32:556–561, November 1979.

rapidly increased to 7.5 to 400 mg daily until normal serum prolactin concentrations returned. One hypogonadal patient also received human menopausal gonadotropin and human chorionic gonadotropin therapy.

Three hyperprolactinemic men were impotent, 3 were infertile, 2 were hypogonadal, and 2 had galactorrhea. Serum prolactin concentrations were 39 to 1,200 ng/ml. Five patients had low or low-normal serum testosterone concentrations; 3 of them had normal LH values. Concentrations of FSH were normal except in the 2 hypogonadal patients. Three patients had sellar enlargement but normal visual fields. No patient had fathered a child. All had difficulties with ejaculation, and 2 were aspermic. Two other patients were oligospermic. Sperm motility was impaired in 4 patients with normal sperm counts or oligospermia. Bromocriptine therapy reduced prolactin concentrations in all patients in dosages of 5 to 10 mg daily. Three impotent patients reported improved sexual potency and libido. Galactorrhea ceased in the affected patients. Sperm activity and quality improved, and 2 patients with low counts showed improvement in the counts. One of the hypogonadal patients had erections and became able to ejaculate, but he remained aspermic. The other patient responded to combined bromocriptine and gonadotropin therapy. Serum testosterone concentrations rose significantly in 3 patients during bromocriptine therapy. Nausea and headache were prevented by giving the drug in four divided daily doses.

Bromocriptine therapy gave satisfactory results in all men with hyperprolactinemia in this study. Combined therapy with bromocriptine and gonadotropins was helpful in treatment of hypogonadotropic hypogonadism with hyperprolactinemia.

▶ [This collection of 7 cases calls attention to hyperprolactinemia in male infertility, indicating that serum prolactin levels should be included in the workup of infertile men. The underlying causes appear to be multiple, and a thorough investigation requires determination of gonadotropins, testosterone, and thyroid hormones and testicular biopsy. All subjects improved with bromocriptine, though 1 required hMG and hCG as well.] ◀

Effects of Bromocriptine on Prolactin and Testosterone Levels in Male Impotence. Male hypogonadism may be associated with elevated plasma prolactin concentrations, and males with hyperprolactinemia are usually impotent and may have oligospermia or azoospermia. A. A. Pierini, I. Sinay, S. Lederman, S. Damilano, J. A. Moguilevsky, and B. Nusimovich[14-16] (Buenos Aires) examined the effects of bromocriptine, which reduces plasma prolactin concentrations, in 20 patients aged 26 to 56 years with impotence of unknown cause. Each had loss or decrease of libido and loss or partial loss of erections. Bromocriptine was given for 1 month in a dosage of 5 mg daily by mouth, alternating with placebo.

Potency improved on bromocriptine therapy in ten patients, with complete erections, a full increase in libido, and a coital frequency of about twice a week. Hormone measurements also improved. Six of these patients were hyperprolactinemic, and all had low testosterone

(14–16) Int. J. Fertil. 24:214–216, 1979.

concentrations. Bromocriptine reduced prolactin values to normal and increased testosterone concentrations to normal. The ten unresponsive patients had normal prolactin and testosterone values. Bromocriptine also reduced prolactin concentrations in this group. Six responsive patients again were impotent during placebo administration and again had abnormal hormone values.

Half the patients in this study responded to bromocriptine therapy with improved sexual potency. Several experiments have shown an important relation between prolactin concentrations and androgenic function. Even some patients in this study with normal prolactin values had improved sexual potency when given bromocriptine. The response of impotence to bromocriptine therapy may be conditioned by changes in prolactin secretion that affect androgenic function. Basal testosterone concentrations may be predictive of the therapeutic response.

▶ [These results seem almost too good to be true. Exactly half of these 20 impotent men had low testosterone levels which, along with their impotence, improved with bromocriptine, whereas the other half had normal testosterone and did not benefit from therapy.] ◀

Artificial Insemination with Donor Semen Mixed with Semen of the Infertile Husband. The practice of mixing an oligoasthenospermic husband's semen with that of a donor before insemination (AIM) has been criticized, since such semen may contain antibodies that could interfere with normal sperm function. Stanley Friedman[14-17] (Tyler Med. Clinic, Inc., Los Angeles) conducted a prospective study to determine the effect of oligospermic semen on donor's sperm in vivo in 227 patients who began donor insemination in 1974 and were followed up to 1976. Not more than 0.1 ml of fresh oligospermic semen was mixed with about 1 ml of thawed donor semen. Postinsemination testing was begun in 1977 in patients having AIM.

Ninety conceptions occurred in the original study group of 227, and 5 further pregnancies occurred on longer follow-up. Thirteen of 34 couples who initially requested AIM conceived in this manner. Seven who failed to conceive changed to donor insemination (AID), and 2 conceived. Of 193 having AID alone, 80 conceived. Conception rates did not differ significantly between the AID and AIM groups. The success of AIM did not appear to be related to the motility of the husband's sperm, but more pregnancies occurred with sperm counts of more than 5 million. In 19 women having postinsemination testing, there was no evidence of any harmful effect of oligospermic semen on normal sperm.

This study does not disprove the suggestion that seminal fluid from some infertile men may harm normal donor sperm, but this effect is not a common occurrence. A normal PIT does not eliminate the possibility of an adverse interaction between normal and abnormal semen. More needs to be known of what happens to seminal fluid in vivo. At present, potential harmful effects do not outweigh the bene-

(14–17) Fertil. Steril. 33:125–128, February 1980.

fits to be gained from permitting AIM or intercourse in couples who request AID.

▶ [Arguments in favor of mixing husband semen with donor specimens or advising coitus by the infertile couple around the time of donor insemination are mainly psychologic in nature. By permitting the possibility, however slight, of fertilization by the husband's sperm, the technique may be more acceptable to some couples. On the other hand, objections have been raised on immunologic grounds (ie, sperm antibodies in the ejaculate of some infertile men). In this study, the pregnancy rate did not vary between "mixed" and "pure" donor inseminations nor was there any evidence of interference in a subset of patients having postinsemination testing. However, the dropout rate did not seem to be lessened by mixing husband with donor semen. These results imply that there are no harmful effects of adding husband semen and/or permitting intercourse in conjunction with donor insemination.] ◀

15. Contraception

Prospective, Randomized Study of Oral Contraceptives: Effect of Study Design on Reported Rates of Symptoms was investigated by Prem P. Talwar (Lucknow, India) and Gary S. Berger[15-1] (Univ. of North Carolina). Data were obtained from a study of 500 women performed in 1976 and 1977 to assess the effects of changing from oral contraceptive pills containing 50 μg of estrogen to pills with 30 or 35 μg of estrogen. General and specific inquiries concerning side effects were compared in a subsample of 100 subjects who were telephoned twice during a contraceptive cycle. For another 100 subjects, responses to specific inquiries made on days 12 and 23 of each cycle were compared with responses to an inquiry on day 28 about symptoms occurring any time in the cycle.

Asking subjects about specific symptoms led to the reporting of higher rates of side effects than did general inquiries about side effects. Events of short duration were less likely to be reported on general inquiry into side effects, and symptoms were reported less often as the interval between the symptom and the telephone contact increased. The one-contact-per-cycle schedule yielded consistently lower rates of side effects than the two-contacts-per-cycle schedule.

Differences in reported rates of oral contraceptive side effects may be due in part to the ways in which data are collected. Future reports on side effects of oral contraceptives should specify the type of contraceptive used and its dosage, the duration of use when symptoms were assessed, the frequency of contact with subjects, and the mode of inquiry.

▶ [These results are not surprising. In assessment of side effects of oral contraceptives, the rate of reported symptoms varied with the frequency of inquiry and the specificity of the questioning. These methodologic considerations probably account for much of the variation reported in incidence of side effects.] ◀

Randomized, Double-Blind Study of Two Combined Oral Contraceptives Containing the Same Progesterone, but Different Estrogens is reported by the Task Force on Oral Contraceptives of the World Health Organization, the members of which were Suporn Koetsawang, A. V. Mandlekar, Usha R. Krishna, V. N. Purandare, C. K. Deshpande, S. C. Chew, Rosilind Fong, S. S. Ratnam, L. Kovacs, S. Zalanyi, A. Tekulics, M. Briggs, M. A. Belsey, P. E. Hall, and R. A. Parker.[15-2] A multicenter, double-blind study was undertaken of two oral contraceptives containing the same dose of norethisterone acetate and either ethinyl estradiol or a mixture of estradiol and estriol. Both contraceptives contained 3 mg of norethisterone ac-

(15–1) Contraception 20:329–337, October 1979.
(15–2) Ibid., 21:445–459, May 1980.

MENSTRUAL SYMPTOMS

Complaint	Number of women reporting symptom after admission	
	3mg NEA + 4mg E2 + 2mg E3	3mg NEA + 50µg EE
Total women in study	458	467
All menstrual complaints†	217 (47.4%)	100 (21.4%)
Amenorrhea †	70 (15.3%)	20 (4.3%)
Irregular bleeding†	48 (10.5%)	21 (4.5%)
Light bleeding	48 (10.5%)	33 (7.1%)
Prolonged bleeding	8 (1.7%)	8 (1.7%)
Spotting*	38 (8.3%)	14 (3.0%)

*$P < .01$.
†$P < .001$.
NEA, norethisterone acetate; EE, ethinyl estradiol; E_2, estradiol; E_3, estriol.

etate. One contained 50 µg of ethinyl estradiol and the other, 4 mg of estradiol plus 2 mg of estriol per tablet. Tablets were begun on cycle day 5 and used with a 7-day interval between medication cycles. Healthy subjects aged 18 to 38 years at 4 centers in Asia and Europe were included in the trial and followed for up to 15 treatment cycles.

The contraceptive containing "natural" estrogens was used by 458 and the other by 647 subjects. All 7 pregnancies occured at 1 center; 4 were in subjects using the synthetic estrogen product. Menstrual problems, not general medical symptoms, accounted for the greater number of symptoms in subjects using the natural estrogen product (table). The only significant group difference in nonmenstrual symptoms was for skin problems. Bleeding in the first 3 cycles was clearly more frequent with the natural estrogen product. At cycles 9 to 12, both infrequent bleeding and amenorrhea were more frequent in this group than in subjects using the synthetic estrogen product.

Both these oral contraceptives were found to be highly efficient, with failure rates of about one per 100 women per year. Menstrual problems were frequent with the natural estrogen product, making it much less suitable for general use in family planning programs than combinations containing synthetic estrogens. Reformulation of the natural estrogen product might lead to more satisfactory results.

▶ [Since the side effects and complications of oral contraceptives are generally thought to reflect the estrogenic component, there is considerable theoretical appeal in an agent containing "natural" estrogen. In this study comparing ethinyl estradiol with estradiol and estriol, the efficacy was similar but, unfortunately, the incidence of abnormal bleeding was substantially higher with the natural than with the synthetic preparation.] ◀

Prolonged Amenorrhea and Oral Contraceptives. A "postpill amenorrhea" syndrome reportedly occurs in 0.2% to 2.64% of former oral contraceptive users. George Tolis, Doree Ruggere, David R. Popkin, James Chow, Mark E. Boyd, Alberto De Leon, Andre B. Lalonde, Antoine Asswad, Meyer Hendelman, Vincent Scali, Robert Koby,

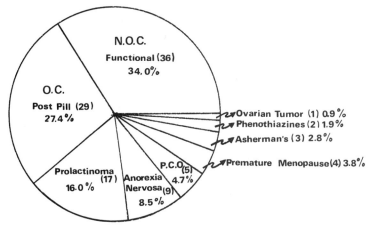

Fig 15–1.—Diagnoses in 106 consecutive patients referred for prolonged (more than one year) secondary amenorrhea. *P.C.O.,* polycystic ovarian disease; *O.C.,* oral contraceptive use; *N.O.C.,* no oral contraceptive use. (Courtesy of Tolis, G., et al.: Fertil. Steril. 32:265–268, September 1979.)

George Arronet, Boris Yufe, Frederick J. Tweedie, Paul R. Fournier, and Frederick Naftolin[15-3] (McGill Univ.) examined 106 consecutive women referred for secondary amenorrhea lasting more than 1 year. Of these, 65 had "functional" amenorrhea, 17 had prolactinomas, and 24 had various specific causative factors (Fig 15–1).

Among the 65 women with functional amenorrhea, 29 had amenorrhea directly after discontinuation of oral contraceptive use, and 36 had never used oral contraceptives. There was no difference between the two groups in incidence of prior menstrual irregularity; in levels of resting serum estrone, estradiol, luteinizing hormone, follicle-stimulating hormone, and prolactin; or in response to medroxyprogesterone acetate, clomiphene citrate, or luteinizing hormone-releasing factor.

Among the 17 women with prolactinomas, 8 had a history of prior oral contraceptive use, and 9 did not. With the exception of elevated serum prolactin levels, there were no significant differences in biochemical tests or in history of oral contraceptive use between the 17 patients with prolactinomas and the 65 with prolonged "functional" amenorrhea.

The lack of historical or biochemical differences between oral contraceptive users and nonusers indicates homogeneity between groups and does not support the existence of a "postpill" syndrome which is separable from prolonged amenorrhea occurring in the absence of oral contraceptive use.

▶ [The authors of this report point out that their data cannot tell us whether "postpill" amenorrhea is any more common than secondary amenorrhea that develops unrelated to recent oral contraceptive use, since we do not know the denominators. However, the findings do suggest that the amenorrhea that can follow the discontinuation of oral contraceptives is not distinctive in terms of basal hormone levels or of response to provocative testing. Again, the point is made that withdrawal bleeding to a progestin

(15–3) Fertil. Steril. 32:265–268, September 1979.

challenge does not rule out a prolactinoma (3 of 7 patients with documented tumors bled in response to Provera).] ◀

Probability of Side Effects With Ovral, Norinyl 1/50, and Norlestrin 1. Unpleasant side effects are the reasons most often cited by patients for discontinuing oral contraception. Gary S. Berger, David A. Edelman, and Prem P. Talwar[15-4] examined the side effects caused by Norinyl 1/50, Norlestrin 1, and Ovral, each assigned to 160 healthy women who had not used hormonal contraception for at least 3 months. None had contraindications to oral contraceptive use. Side effects were assessed over 3 cycles of oral contraceptive use.

The occurrence of symptoms in any of the first 3 cycles of use is shown in Table 1 and the probability of symptoms occurring in sub-

TABLE 1.—PERCENT OF WOMEN REPORTING SYMPTOMS IN ANY OF FIRST THREE CYCLES

Symptom	Ovral % (N=150)	Norinyl % (N=145)	Norlestrin % (N=147)	p-Value*
Acne	70.7	70.3	63.9	NS
Breast discomfort	63.3	67.5	59.9	NS
Nausea	61.3	52.4	58.5	NS
Abdominal bloating	47.3	44.8	52.4	NS
Headache	53.3	44.1	44.2	NS
Fatigue	49.3	48.2	38.2	NS
Depression	44.7	45.5	38.1	NS
Irritability	47.3	37.9	37.4	NS
Vaginal discharge	40.0	45.5	34.7	NS
Breakthrough bleeding	16.6	46.0	51.7	<0.01

*NS, not significant; P > .05.

TABLE 2.—CONDITIONAL PROBABILITIES OF SYMPTOMS IN SUBSEQUENT CYCLES OF OVRAL

Symptom	Probability of Symptom Given Presence of Symptom in the First Cycle		Probability of Symptom Given Absence of Symptom in the Previous Cycle	
	2nd Cycle	3rd Cycle	2nd Cycle	3rd Cycle
Acne	0.59	0.35	0.31	0.14
Breast discomfort	0.60	0.29	0.18	0.06
Nausea	0.47	0.23	0.20	0.09
Abdominal bloating	0.59	0.39	0.19	0.15
Headache	0.33	0.20	0.19	0.15
Fatigue	0.33	0.18	0.19	0.09
Depression	0.36	0.16	0.12	0.08
Irritability	0.52	0.29	0.23	0.04
Vaginal discharge	0.43	0.23	0.15	0.09
Breakthrough bleeding	0.20	0.13	0.09	0.07

(15-4) Contraception 20:447–453, November 1979.

sequent cycles of Ovral in Table 2. Women were contacted every 2 weeks and specifically asked about each symptom. Breakthrough bleeding was significantly less frequent with Ovral. The probability of side effects recurring in the second and third cycles declined significantly from the second to the third cycle for all three agents. The chance of a side effect occurring in a given cycle was less if it had not occurred in previous cycles.

The high rates of side effects observed in this study undoubtedly are related to the frequent questioning of subjects about specific side effects. Few significant differences were found in the patterns of side effects caused by the different oral contraceptive preparations. The findings support the clinical view that side effects occurring when oral contraceptive use is begun should not prohibit its continuation, because most effects will subsequently cease.

▶ [The frequency of symptoms relates to the method of ascertainment, as discussed previously. The essential point here is the documentation of the clinical impression that side effects tend to diminish with continued use. Since side effects are the reasons patients most often quit the pill, it is important for us to be certain that our patients understand the temporary nature of most of these. Time is the great healer.] ◀

Serum Copper and Zinc in Hormonal Contraceptive Users. Serum copper levels have been found to be high in women using combined oral contraceptives, but any changes in serum zinc levels are unclear. Krishnamurthy Prema, Baru Anantha Ramalakshmi, and Soma Babu[15-5] (Indian Council of Med. Res., Hyderabad, India) examined serum copper and zinc levels in undernourished Indian women using various hormonal contraceptives. The contraceptives used included combination pills containing 150 μg of *d*-norgestrel and 30 or 50 μg of ethinyl estradiol, injections of 100 mg of dihydroprogesterone acetophenide (DHPA) and 5 mg of estradiol enanthate (EE), intravaginal rings containing 60 to 78 mg of *d*-norgestrel and 30 to 40 mg of estradiol, injections of 150 mg of depomedroxyprogesterone acetate (DMPA) every 3 months, or injections of 20 mg of norethindrone enanthate (NET) every month. The 148 women using no contraception were compared with 150 using a combination pill, injectable DHPA + EE, or an intravaginal ring; 17 using DMPA; and 22 using NET.

Control subjects had a mean serum copper level of 111 μg/dl and a mean serum zinc level of 110 μg/dl, with considerable variations in both levels between individuals. Use of combined estrogen-progestogen contraceptives resulted in a rise in serum copper levels and a fall in serum zinc levels, regardless of the drug, dosage, or route of administration. Peak serum copper levels were reached after 3 months. The lowest serum zinc levels were reached within 2 weeks. Urinary excretion of copper and zinc was similar to that seen in control subjects. With injectable progestogens, serum zinc levels decreased, but serum copper levels remained unchanged.

The physiologic implications of changes in serum copper and zinc levels in women using hormonal contraceptives are unknown. Decreased serum zinc levels are reported to result in increased platelet

(15–5) Fertil. Steril. 33:267–271, March 1980.

aggregation and stickiness and increased serotonin release. If changes in platelet function play a role in inducing venous thrombosis, the use of progestogens may not be without some risk.

▶ [In this study, hormonal contraception was found to influence metabolism of the trace minerals copper and zinc in such a way as to raise the serum copper level and lower the serum zinc level without any effect on urinary excretion. Elevation in serum copper level, which also occurs in pregnancy, is thought to reflect an estrogen stimulation of ceruloplasmin synthesis, and the finding of this study that it did not accompany progestin-only treatment is consistent with such an hypothesis. Less clear is the explanation of a decline in serum zinc level which accompanied both estrogen-progestin and progestin-only treatments. Observations such as these suggest conception might best be postponed for a time after hormonal contraception in order to allow for recovery of the metabolic "aberrations." However, epidemiologic studies have generally failed to indicate any adverse effects of pregnancy immediately following oral contraception, so the risk may be more theoretical than real.] ◀

Incidence of Hyperprolactinemia During Oral Contraceptive Therapy was determined by J. Victor Reyniak, Michael Wenof, José M. Aubert, and John J. Stangel[15-6] (New York Med. College). The goal was to learn whether a rationale exists for performing periodic prolactin assays in women on oral contraceptives as a possible means of preventing hyperprolactinemic disorders. A total of 123 women with a mean age of 25.5 years were studied. Nearly 85% were parous. Mean duration of contraception was 25.8 months. Thirty-six subjects took preparations containing 80 or 100 μg of estrogen, 52 used 50-μg preparations, and 35 used preparations containing 20 or 30 μg of estrogen. Prolactin was measured by radioimmunoassay between days 5 and 20 of medication cycles.

Prolactin concentrations were elevated in 38 women (30.9%), and 4.1% had marked elevations (table). Neither the dose of oral contraceptive nor the duration of therapy influence the occurrence of moderate and marked hyperprolactinemia. The findings were not altered by adjusting for differences in the numbers of patients at various dosages.

An impressive number of women exhibit elevated prolactin concentrations during oral contraception. No relation with dose was apparent within the therapeutic range of currently used preparations, and the duration of therapy appeared to play no role in promoting hyperprolactinemia. The prognostic value of the hyperprolactinemia that occurs during oral contraception is difficult to assess. Periodic prolac-

SERUM HUMAN PROLACTIN (hPRL) LEVELS DURING ORAL
CONTRACEPTIVE THERAPY IN 123 WOMEN

hPRL level	No. of patients
Normal (2.2–20 ng/ml)	85(69.1%)
Mild (21–40 ng/ml)	26(21.1%)
Moderate (41–60 ng/ml)	7(5.7%)
Marked (≥ 61 ng/ml)	5(4.1%)
Total	123(100%)

(15–6) Obstet. Gynecol. 55:8–11, January 1980.

tin measurement might be of value in women who elect steroid contraception to identify those who may be at risk of developing hyperprolactinemic disorders.

▶ [The results of this study are clear-cut. Hyperprolactinemia is not unusual in patients taking the pill (31% prevalence) and is independent of the dose of estrogen or the duration of therapy. We agree with the authors' call for a longitudinal study of this phenomenon, but do not think evidence exists to support routine screening for hyperprolactinemia in women on the pill. Patients with "postpill" amenorrhea should have prolactin determinations performed, as should other patients with nonphysiologic amenorrhea.] ◀

Effect of Rifampicin on Pharmacokinetics of Ethinyl Estradiol in Women was investigated by D. J. Back, A. M. Breckenridge, Francesca E. Crawford, J. M. Hall, M. MacIver, M. L'E. Orme, P. H. Rowe, Eileen Smith, and Margaret J. Watts[15-7] (Univ. of Liverpool).

The combination of antituberculosis medication and oral contraceptive steroids has been associated with breakthrough bleeding and a higher risk of accidental pregnancy. This study examines the effects of rifampicin on the plasma concentration of ethinyl estradiol in 7 women.

Each woman took a single tablet of Minovlar (50 μg ethinyl estradiol and 1 mg norethindrone acetate) near the end of her course of rifampicin therapy and 1 month after discontinuing the rifampicin. Plasma concentrations of ethinyl estradiol were measured by radioimmunoassay. One patient who was taking Minovlar was studied when she began rifampicin therapy.

The area under the plasma ethinyl estradiol versus time curve was 1,014 ± 317 pg/ml × hour during rifampicin therapy. This was increased significantly to 1,747 ± 218 pg/ml × hour after rifampicin was discontinued. The terminal half-life of ethinyl estradiol was also increased significantly after stopping rifampicin, from 2.9 ± 0.8 hour to 6.3 ± 1.4 hour.

In 1 patient the plasma ethinyl estradiol and follicle-stimulating hormone (FSH) levels were measured over two cycles of Minovlar. The ethinyl estradiol concentration began to fall 8–12 days after starting rifampicin, from approximately 50 pg/ml. After the first cycle, it seemed to fall no further than 20–30 pg/ml. Plasma FSH concentrations rose to a peak in the second cycle of Minovlar. The sex hormone-binding globulin capacities in the seven women were significantly greater during rifampicin therapy than after it.

The effects of rifampicin on ethinyl estradiol pharmacokinetics are consistent with induction of the microsomal enzymes which metabolize ethinyl estradiol.

These data indicate that oral contraceptive steroids taken concomitantly with rifampicin are likely to be less effective. Thus, in most women taking rifampicin, it is unwise to use oral contraceptives as the sole method of birth control.

▶ [An apparent decrease in efficacy of oral contraceptives in patients on antituberculous therapy with rifampicin has been suggested by several reports. This pharmacokinetic study suggests a possible mechanism. Blood levels of ethinyl estradiol, expressed as area under the concentration-time curve following a single oral dose, were

(15–7) Contraception 21:135–143, February 1980.

significantly lower during rifampicin treatment than those measured a month after the drug was stopped. Presumably, the mechanism involves induction of hepatic enzymes metabolizing ethinyl estradiol. The message for the clinician is that oral contraceptives may not be effective in conjunction with this antituberculous drug.] ◄

Pregnancy Attributable to Interaction Between Tetracycline and Oral Contraceptives. Various drugs, including antibiotics, may cause contraceptive failure and breakthrough bleeding in patients taking oral contraceptives. Janet F. Bacon and Gillian M. Shenfield[15-8] report the occurrence of pregnancy in a woman taking oral contraceptives and tetracycline.

Woman, 20, had been taking oral contraceptives for 4 years. Her only complaint was an increase in left-sided headaches. For the past 2 years she had been taking Microgynon 30 (ethinyl estradiol, 30 μg, plus D-norgestrel, 150 μg) with no breakthrough bleeding. She had normal withdrawal bleeding and 5 days later started both the next course of Microgynon and a 5-day course of tetracycline for sinusitis. She had no diarrhea or vomiting; however, only a very light 2-day menstrual flow occurred 25 days after beginning the course of oral contraceptives. She continued taking oral contraceptives for another 2 months until seen at a family planning center. The size of her uterus was then compatible with at least a 12-week gestation. This indicated that she must have ovulated either during the tetracycline therapy or in the following week.

The timing of events in this patient suggests that the tetracycline contributed to the failure of contraception. Breakthrough bleeding associated with tetracycline use has also been seen by one of the authors.

It is important that physicians be aware of the potential problem. Women using low-dose contraceptives should take extra precautions against conceiving in any cycle during which antibiotics are given.

► [Ampicillin and other antibiotics are at times responsible for decreased urinary estriol excretion in pregnancy. This effect is presumably due to interference with the enterohepatic circulation of estriol conjugates secondary to alterations in the intestinal bacterial flora. The current report does not prove anything, but raises the question of a relationship between the pill-failure pregnancy and tetracycline administration in this patient. A study of "pill-failures" looking specifically at other drugs taken by these women might be revealing, especially in this era of low-dose formulations.] ◄

Impaired Elimination of Caffeine by Oral Contraceptive Steroids. Caffeine is used extensively in treatment and is widely consumed in beverages. It affects many organ systems and has widespread effects on various metabolic processes through inhibition of phosphodiesterase and stimulation of cyclic adenosine monophosphate-mediated systems. Prolongation of caffeine elimination has been observed during pregnancy. Rashmi V. Patwardhan, Paul V. Desmond, Raymond F. Johnson, and Steven Schenker[15-9] (Vanderbilt Univ.) examined the effects of female sex and oral contraceptive steroids (OCS) on the disposition and elimination of caffeine in normal subjects of both sexes. Some of the females had been on OCS for over 6 months. Women not on OCS were studied at various stages of the menstrual cycle. An oral dose of 250 mg caffeine was given after an overnight fast.

(15–8) Br. Med. J. 1:293, Feb. 2, 1980.
(15–9) J. Lab. Clin. Med. 95:603–608, April 1980.

Caffeine absorption was rapid in all groups; peak blood concentrations were present within 30 to 60 minutes. The elimination half-time was significantly longer in females on OCS than in those not using OCS, and total plasma clearance was significantly less in OCS users. Plasma binding of caffeine and volumes of distribution were similar in the two groups of females. Free clearance or clearance of unbound drug was less in females on OCS. Plasma clearance and plasma binding were similar in females not on OCS and in the male subjects. No significant effects of age or stage of menstrual cycle on the pharmacokinetic parameters were observed.

Females on oral contraceptives have impaired elimination of caffeine. This should result in accumulation of caffeine with its long-term use. It is reasonable to recommend that women on oral contraceptives and pregnant women moderate their caffeine intake. These observations may be relevant to the therapeutic use of theophylline and other xanthines in patients using oral contraceptives.

▶ [In this interesting study, the plasma clearance of caffeine was nearly halved in patients taking oral contraceptives, presumably reflecting hormone-related inhibition of hepatic enzymes. If these acute effects persist under conditions of chronic caffeine ingestion, one could readily imagine that even relatively modest consumption by pill-takers could result in high blood levels. Does this mean that members of the Pepsi generation should avoid oral contraceptives and that pill-takers should eschew caffeine?] ◀

Interaction Between Anticoagulants and Contraceptives: Unsuspected Finding. E. de Teresa, A. Vera, J. Ortigosa, I. Alonso Pulpon, A. Puente Arus, and M. de Artaza[15-10] (Madrid) examined the effects of oral contraceptives on anticoagulant therapy by measuring prothrombin times in 12 patients while they took both agents simultaneously and while they took only anticoagulants. The drugs were acenocoumarion (nicoumalone) and an estroprogestogenic oral contraceptive. Eleven patients used oral preparations and 1 used a parenteral depot preparation. Mean age was 34.5 years. No subject had nephropathy, hepatopathy, or hypertension. Nine patients were given anticoagulants because they had Björk-Shiley valvular prostheses. Three had embolic mitral valve disease. Mean follow-up was 31.2 months. Patients took both agents during 250 months of follow-up and only anticoagulants for 144 months.

The mean prothrombin time ratio was significantly higher when both anticoagulants and oral contraceptives were used than when only anticoagulants were used. Anticoagulant requirements were less when oral contraceptives were used concurrently. Nearly 90% of all prothrombin time measurements were within the therapeutic range.

Therapeutic anticoagulation can be maintained during hormonal contraception. Oral contraceptives appear to potentiate the action of anticoagulants given orally, although the effect is not clinically significant. Slight adjustments in anticoagulant dosage are sufficient to maintain prothrombin activity within the therapeutic range. The synthetic estrogens in oral contraceptives may produce enzymatic in-

(15–10) Br. Med. J. 2:1260–1261, Nov. 17, 1979.

hibition in the hepatic microsomes, potentiating the action of anticoagulants through retarded metabolic degradation.

▶ [In our view, oral contraceptives and anticoagulants should only rarely be used in
the same patient, because patients at risk for thromboembolism usually should not
take hormonal contraceptives. The results of this study suggest that anticoagulant activity is potentiated, rather than diminished in pill-takers, so perhaps our opinion needs
reconsideration.] ◀

▶ ↓An effect of oral contraceptives on platelet activity is described in the following
abstract. Read on. ◀

**Effect of Oral Contraceptives on Platelet Noradrenaline and
5-Hydroxytryptamine Receptors and Aggregation.** Both 5-hy-
droxytryptamine (5-HT) and norepinephrine (NE) receptors have
been demonstrated on human platelets, and animal studies have
shown that estrogens alter the characteristics of 5-HT and NE platelet receptors. John R. Peters, J. Martin Elliott, and David G. Gra-
hame-Smith[15-11] (Oxford, England) examined the effects of the cyclic
use of the combined contraceptive pill on platelet NE and 5-HT receptors. Fifteen healthy women aged 22 to 30 years used combined preparations containing 30 μg of ethinyl estradiol and 150 or 250 μg of
levonorgestrel. Treatment was given over 2 to 24 cycles. Eight age-
matched controls had never used oral contraception. The α-adrenergic
receptor and serotonin receptor binding assays were performed, and
5-HT uptake was measured.

Subjects taking contraceptives showed a significantly higher α-adrenergic receptor binding capacity and a lower affinity on day 21 than
on day 28 of the cycle; controls showed no such differences. The capacity of both 5-HT receptor sites was higher on day 21 than on day
28 in the contraceptive group but not in controls. Uptake of tritiated
5-HT into intact cells was significantly higher on day 21 than on day
28 in the subjects taking contraceptives but not in controls. Both NE-
and 5-HT-induced platelet aggregation values were significantly
higher on day 21 in subjects using oral contraception. No differences
in platelet counts were found.

The use of a combined oral contraceptive increases receptors for 5-
HT and NE on human platelets, the aggregation induced by both bio-
genic amines, and the active uptake of 5-HT. The steroids presumably
modulate receptor binding characteristics through stimulating mes-
senger RNA production. The findings may provide a basis for enhanced platelet aggregability and a hypercoagulable state in women
taking oral contraceptives, but they cannot be directly extrapolated
to the clinical situation. Effects on analogous receptor sites in the
brain might explain such presumably hormonal effects as postpartum
and pill-associated depression.

▶ [Platelet adrenergic amine receptors increased during treatment with oral contraceptives, as did platelet aggregation induced by norepinephrine and serotonin.
Whether these findings explain the increase in thrombotic events in women taking the
pill is unknown.] ◀

**Comparison of Effects of Different Combined Oral Contra-
ceptive Formulations on Carbohydrate and Lipid Metabolism.**
Conflicting results have been reported in studies of the effects of es-

(15–11) Lancet 2:933–936, Nov. 3, 1979.

trogen-progestagen oral contraceptives on carbohydrate and lipid metabolism, in part because of varying dosages and components. V. Wynn, P. W. Adams, I. Godsland, J. Melrose, R. Niththyananthan, N. W. Oakley, and M. Seed[15-12] (St. Mary's Hosp. Med. School, London) performed oral glucose tolerance tests and measured serum cholesterol and triglyceride concentrations in 1,628 white women taking combined oral contraceptives and 577 controls. Contraception was used for at least 3 months. Estrogen doses were 30, 50, and 75 to 150 μg, and doses of *dl*-norgestrel were 150 and 500 μg. All women were aged 45 or under. None was over 150% of ideal body weight or had evidence of endocrine or metabolic disease.

Glucose tolerance deteriorated in all oral contraceptive groups using estrane progestagens or norgestrel, but it was unaltered by preparations containing a pregnane progestagen. Deterioration was most marked in subjects using a contraceptive containing 75 μg of estrogen or more. The early insulin response to glucose was impaired in these subjects. Insulin secretion was unaffected by use of a pregnane progestagen. Insulin secretion was increased in the other contraceptive groups, particularly when a gonane progestagen was used. Serum cholesterol concentration was elevated only with preparations containing 75 μg of estrogen or more and an estrane progestagen. It tended to be lower with gonane progestagen use. Hypertriglyceridemia was estrogen dose related, and this effect was potentiated by the pregnane progestagen. The gonane progestagen antagonized estrogen-induced hypertriglyceridemia.

The observations indicate the importance of the dose of estrogen and type of progestagen in oral contraception. The combination of an estrogen with a 17α-alkyl-substituted estrane or gonane progestagen confers diabetogenicity on an oral contraceptive. The estrogen-potentiating effect of pregnane progestagen may be related to the finding of a high incidence of thromboembolic disease in women taking pregnane-containing oral contraceptives. Further modification of oral contraceptive formulations is needed.

▶ [This large-scale study of various oral contraceptives shows that both the amount of estrogen and type of progestin influence their metabolic effects. Glucose tolerance was most affected by high-dose estrogen preparations that impaired insulin secretion. Lower-dose preparations were associated with *increased* insulin secretion and varying degrees of insulin resistance. Preparations containing norgestrel lowered cholesterol levels and had the least effect on increasing triglyceride levels. Although selecting a low-dose estrogen preparation makes sense on several counts, these metabolic data cannot tell us which progestin is "best." The issue is too complex.

In a much smaller series of previous gestational diabetes utilizing two low-dose progestagens (0.3 mg norethindrone in 15 and 0.5 mg lynestrol in 17), minimal changes in carbohydrate and lipid indices were noted. Norethindrone subjects exhibited a very slight deterioration in glucose tolerance compared with lynestrol in patients using an intrauterine device; none had any change in cholesterol or triglyceride levels (Pyorala et al.: Ann. Chir. Gynaecol. 68:69, 1979).] ◀

Risk of Vascular Disease in Women: Smoking, Oral Contraceptives, Noncontraceptive Estrogens, and Other Factors. Vascular disease underlies most of the major morbidity and mortality associated with the use of oral contraceptives, and a reduction in risk

---

(15–12) Lancet 1:1045–1049, May 19, 1979.

requires the identification of individuals already at high risk. Diana B. Petitti, John Wingerd, Frederick Pellegrin and Savitri Ramcharan[15-13] analyzed data from a cohort of 16,759 women aged 18–54 years, seen for routine health check-ups in 1969–71, to determine the relation between various factors and the risks of myocardial infarction, subarachnoid hemorrhage, other strokes, and venous thromboembolism. The population was predominantly white, suburban, and middle class. Average follow-up was $6^{1}/_{2}$ years.

Smoking significantly increased the risk for all four conditions evaluated. Oral contraceptive use was associated with an increased risk only for subarachnoid hemorrhage and venous thromboembolism. The use of noncontraceptive estrogens was not related to any increase in risk. The risk of myocardial infarction was increased in relation to hypertension, hypercholesterolemia, obesity, gallbladder disease and nondrinking of alcohol. Hypertension and hypercholesterolemia were associated with an increased risk for other strokes. The effects of smoking and oral contraceptive use in younger women appeared to be multiplicative. Only smoking was a clear risk factor in older women, but few of them were oral contraceptive users.

Cigarette smoking was by far the most important risk factor for vascular diseases in women in this survey. Smoking should be considered a contraindication to oral contraceptive use or, at the very least, women wishing to use oral contraceptives should be strongly urged not to smoke. Smoking and oral contraceptive use appear to act synergistically to increase the risks for subarachnoid hemorrhage, hemorrhagic stroke and myocardial infarction.

▶ [This type of study is hard to interpret. The authors conclude that oral contraceptive use increases the risk of venous thromboembolism and subarachnoid hemorrhage, but not of "other strokes" or myocardial infarction. Noncontraceptive estrogen use (presumably for menopausal replacement) was not associated with increased risk for the vascular diseases studied. Gallbladder disease increased the risk of myocardial infarction (both entities presumably reflecting abnormal lipid metabolism). The key risk factor for all four vascular diseases studied was cigarette smoking. We obstetrician-gynecologists, in our primary health care roles, must encourage our patients to kick the habit.] ◀

Progestogens and Cardiovascular Reactions Associated With Oral Contraceptives and Comparison of the Safety of 50- and 30-μg Estrogen Preparations. The increased risk of cardiovascular disease in women using combined oral contraceptives is usually attributed to the estrogenic component, but recent findings indicate a possible effect of norethisterone acetate. T. W. Meade, Gillian Greenberg, and S. G. Thompson[15-14] (Harrow, England) compared the effects of contraceptives containing 1, 2.5, 3, and 4 mg of norethisterone acetate combined with 50 μg of ethinyl estradiol and of agents containing 150 and 250 μg of levonorgestrel combined with 30 μg of ethinyl estradiol. Of 2,044 suspected cardiovascular and related reactions to oral contraceptives reported between 1964 and 1977, 6% were excluded from analysis.

(15–13) J.A.M.A. 242:1150–1154, Sept. 14, 1979.
(15–14) Br. Med. J. 1:1157–1161, May 10, 1980.

A significant positive association was found between dose of norethisterone acetate and deaths from stroke and ischemic heart disease (IHD), besides nonfatal cases of the two conditions. No association with hypertension or venous thrombosis was evident. The higher dose of levonorgestrel was associated with a possible excess of deaths, nonvenous plus venous, and with an excess of strokes. The dose of levonorgestrel was unrelated to hypertension or venous thrombosis. The lower dose of estrogen was associated with significantly fewer reports of death and IHD than the higher dose.

The findings indicate an association of norethisterone dose with nonvenous deaths. Although there are no grounds for major changes in oral contraceptive practice, the trend toward preparations with lower estrogen doses should be encouraged, and there is a case for minimizing the dose of progestogen to reduce the risk of thromboembolism.

▶ [Studies such as this which depend on sales figures to estimate drug use and on the reporting of adverse effects by a wide variety of sources may be interesting, but cannot be considered definitive. The suggestion here is that higher progestin dosage levels were associated with an increased risk of stroke and of ischemic heart disease, but not of hypertension or of venous thrombosis or embolism. We would guess that the type of oral contraceptive prescribed is not uniform throughout the population, at least it is not within our own practices. A woman in her late 20s who has taken a particular pill of "moderate" strength for several years without problems will probably have it prescribed again; a teenager placed on oral contraceptives for the first time will probably receive a "weaker" preparation. The patients undoubtedly differ in their cardiovascular risk status on the basis of age differences, independent of the particular pill they are taking. Any subsequent analysis of the effects of a particular pill would have to consider this nonrandom assignment of a particular pill to a particular patient.] ◀

Oral Contraceptives and Fatal Subarachnoid Hemorrhage. Previous studies have suggested an association between oral contraceptive use and fatal cerebrovascular disease. William H. W. Inman[15-15] (London) carried out a case-control study of deaths from subarachnoid hemorrhage (SAH) in women aged 15–44 years in England and Wales in 1976. The dead women were matched with healthy living controls in the same practice for age, and matching was also close in other respects. A small, nonsignificant excess of oral contraceptive use was found in women who died of SAH, compared with controls. Hypertension was present in 34 of 134 women who died of SAH and in 6 of their controls. Renal disease and preeclamptic toxemia were more commonly associated with hypertension in the dead women than in controls.

No change in annual mortality from SAH has been observed in the past 20 years, such as might be expected were the risks high. Current or past use of oral contraceptives may have increased the blood pressure and risk of SAH in a few women, but hypertension is the chief factor determining this risk. Subarachnoid hemorrhage probably should not be considered a serious cause for concern in healthy normotensive women using oral contraceptives. It would be prudent to monitor blood pressure in women using oral contraceptives and to

(15–15) Br. Med. J. 2:1468–1470, Dec. 8, 1979.

change the method of contraception where hypertension cannot be controlled.

▶ [The subject of the cerebrovascular risks associated with oral contraceptives is confusing and the literature is divided on this issue. The present article indicates that hypertension is a risk factor for subarachnoid hemorrhage, but that the pill probably is not.] ◀

Epidemiology of Hepatocellular Adenoma: Role of Oral Contraceptive Use. The hypothesis of an association between oral contraceptive use and the development of hepatocellular adenoma has been supported by findings in several case series. Judith Bourne Rooks, Howard W. Ory, Kamal G. Ishak, Lilo T. Strauss, Joel R. Greenspan, Annlia Paganini Hill and Carl W. Tyler, Jr.[15-16] report the results of a case-control study of hepatocellular adenoma conducted by the Center for Disease Control and the Armed Forces Institute of Pathology. Interviews were completed with 79 women aged 16–61 years, diagnosed in 1957–76 as having hepatocellular adenoma, and 220 age- and neighborhood-matched controls. Limited information was obtained on 9 other patients who had died.

The mean age at diagnosis of hepatocellular adenoma was 30.4 years. Patients with hemorrhage had greater risks of morbidity and death than those with other symptoms. About 34% of patients had intraperitoneal bleeding, 15% hemorrhaging into their tumors before diagnosis. The overall death-to-case ratio was 8.1%, excluding 2 patients in whom tumor was found incidentally at autopsy. Six women were pregnant or within 6 weeks post partum at the time hepatocellular adenoma was diagnosed. An increasing duration of oral contraceptive use increased the risk of hepatocellular adenoma. No significant difference was found between oral contraceptives containing ethinyl estradiol or mestranol with regard to frequency of tumor development. Among oral contraceptive users, bleeding was 6 times more frequent in women reporting over 3 years of oral contraceptive use. Of 32 women who continued to use oral contraceptives for at least a year after tumor resection, 4 had a recurrence of the tumor or experienced the development of another hepatocellular adenoma. Women who had never used oral contraceptives were older than those who had; in addition, they were more often nulliparous, and many had difficulty becoming pregnant.

The estimated annual incidence of hepatocellular adenoma in long-term oral contraceptive users is 3–4/100,000. The risk may be less if an oral contraceptive having low potency is used. Women over age 30 probably should avoid long periods of oral contraceptive use, and those who have had an hepatocellular adenoma should discontinue oral contraceptive use permanently. The differential diagnosis of vague abdominal symptoms, or symptoms suggesting gallbladder disease, in an oral contraceptive user should include hepatocellular adenoma.

▶ [This retrospective case-control study provides significant new observations regarding the association between oral contraceptives and liver adenomas. It confirms suggestions from earlier reports of correlations with both high-dose preparations and pro-

(15–16) JAMA 242:644–648, Aug. 17, 1979.

longed usage. It does not, however, confirm a relationship with mestranol as opposed to ethinyl estradiol when the times of introduction of these two estrogens are taken into account. As pointed out in an editorial comment in the 1977 YEAR BOOK (p. 383), the suggestion of Edmondson et al. (N. Engl. J. Med. 294:470, 1976) that mestranol is the culprit could well reflect the earlier and more widespread use of this agent than was the case with ethinyl estradiol. How nice it is to have one's suspicions confirmed!

Perhaps the greatest value of this article is the estimate of risk of 3 or 4 cases per 100,000 users.] ◀

Mode of Action of *dl*-Norgestrel and Ethinyl Estradiol Combination in Postcoital Contraception. A high rate of severe side effects results from postcoital estrogen treatment, and the failure rate with norgestrel, another postcoital contraceptive agent, has been relatively high. William Y. Ling, Alfred Robichaud, Isamil Zayid, William Wrixon and S. Clair MacLeod[15-17] (Dalhousie Univ., Halifax) evaluated combined oral contraception with ethinyl estradiol and *dl*-norgestrel in 12 healthy women, 6 of whom measured basal body temperature daily for 2 consecutive menstrual cycles and had luteal phases of consistent length. Four were of proved fertility. Six other women did not undergo prelimininary basal body temperature screening. An oral dose of 0.1 mg ethinyl estradiol and 1.0 mg *dl*-norgestrel was given to all 12 women at the predicted time of ovulation and again 12 hours later. Hormone levels were measured by specific radioimmunoassays from the 8th day of the cycle to onset of menses.

The medication elicited varied individual pituitary and ovarian responses. Three women had significantly reduced luteinizing hormone peaks. The mean luteal phase was shortened to 2 days in treatment cycles, compared with an average of 11 days after the peak level of luteinizing hormone occurred in control cycles. One woman had a much prolonged treatment cycle in which ovulation appeared to be delayed for about 13 days. Two others had a much shortened luteal phase. Endometrial biopsies showed significant changes in endometrial development, with dissociation of maturation of the glandular and stromal components. No significant changes in serum prolactin levels were observed. Ten women experienced side effects ranging from severe vomiting to leg cramps.

The combined postcoital contraceptive of ethinyl estradiol and *dl*-norgestrel acts either by suppressing ovulation, or by disrupting luteal function through a direct action on the corpus luteum or by interfering with appropriate endometrial responses to ovarian steroids.

▶ [An abstract in a previous edition of the YEAR BOOK indicated that Ovral, two tablets taken twice 12 hours apart, was an effective postcoital contraceptive. This report looks at possible mechanisms of action. There apparently are several. If given prior to the LH surge, ovulation can at times be delayed or eliminated. The endometrium showed glandular-stromal dissociation in all cases, whether the "interceptive" was given before or after the LH surge. Luteolytic and other effects are possible as well. It is this diversity of sites of action that probably explains the clinical effectiveness of this sort of therapy.] ◀

Intranasal Gonadotropin-Releasing Hormone Agonist as a Contraceptive Agent. The luteinizing hormone-releasing hormone (LRH) analogue D-Ser(TBU)^6-EA^{10}-LRH is a potent LRH agonist,

---

(15–17)   Fertil. Steril. 32:297–302, September 1979.

SUMMARY OF RESULTS

Intranasal dose (μg)	Subjects (no.)	Treatment (mo)	Anovulatory treatment (mo)	Amenorrhœa during treatment (No.)
400	13	43	42	5
600	14	46	45	1
Total	27	89	87	6

which can paradoxically inhibit ovulation in regularly menstruating women. Christer Bergquist, Sven Johan Nillius, and Leif Wide[15-18] (Univ. of Uppsala) administered the LRH agonist every day intranasally to 27 women for 3 to 6 months. The subjects were regularly menstruating women aged 21 to 37 years. All but 4 had been pregnant. One women used an intrauterine device also. Thirteen women received a daily dose of 400 μg, whereas 14 received 600 μg daily, beginning on the first day of menstrual bleeding.

All but 2 of 89 treatment cycles were anovulatory (table). The 2 women with evidence of ovulation had technical problems with their nasal spray bottles and probably received an insufficient amount of analogue in the first treatment cycle. Nine women had slightly elevated serum progesterone concentrations during treatment, indicating luteinization of follicles. No woman conceived during the study. Twenty-one women had one or more small bleeds resembling menstruation at intervals of 19 to 61 days, but no dysfunctional uterine bleeding occurred. Biopsies of 3 of these women showed weak endometrial proliferative activity. There were no hyperplastic changes. The 6 women who were amenorrheic had lower serum estradiol concentrations than those who had bleeding. All women ovulated and had menstrual bleeding after treatment was discontinued. Most women found the nasal spray was convenient and practical. Some had cold symptoms during treatment. Three women reported having short-lived headaches in the first week of treatment.

Luteinizing hormone-releasing hormone agonists have a specific action on pituitary gonadotropes. They will probably have fewer adverse effects than oral contraceptives, but side effects may occur after several years of treatment as a result of anovulation. Long-term intranasal therapy was well accepted by all subjects in this study, and most wished to continue this form of contraception.

▶ [Luteinizing hormone-releasing hormone (LRH) is being used experimentally to induce ovulation in anovulatory infertile women who fail to respond to clomiphene. In this study, an LRH analogue was tested as a contraceptive. It apparently inhibits gonadotropin release from the pituitary, thereby preventing ovulation. One fifth of the study subjects were amenorrheic during treatment. Dysfunctional bleeding or symptoms of estrogen deficiency were not problems in this small series, but would seem to be likely adverse effects of this treatment. Some concern exists, too, about possible antibody formation against the polypeptide. This is an interesting approach to contraception, but much more study is needed.] ◀

(15–18) Lancet 2:215–217, Aug. 4, 1979.

Intrauterine Device Termination Rates and Menstrual Cycle Day of Insertion. Most clinicians apparently prefer to insert the intrauterine device (IUD) during the bleeding phase of the menstrual cycle. Michael K. White, Howard W. Ory, Judith B. Rooks, and Roger W. Rochat[15-19] examined the benefits and risks of inserting the copper T-200 IUD at various times during the cycle, with emphasis on events occurring within the first 2 months after insertion.

For 9,094 women the rates of pregnancy, IUD expulsion, and IUD removal, specific for age, parity, months after insertion, and menstrual cycle day of insertion, were calculated. Reasons for removal included pain or bleeding, pelvic inflammatory disease, as well as other medical or personal reasons. The largest category of women, 39.5%, were between 20 and 29 years of age and nulliparous.

Of the 9,094 insertions, 52.1% were done between cycle days 1–5, and 84.1% prior to day 11. Expulsion rates decreased significantly from 50.3 to 22.0 per 1,000 as insertions were done later in the cycle.

Pregnancy rates and removal for pain and bleeding increased as IUDs were inserted later in the cycle. The increase was significant for pain and bleeding removals, but not for pregnancy rates. The increases in these categories were associated primarily with insertions done on or after day 18. There were no significant differences in removals for pelvic inflammatory disease or other medical or personal reasons with respect to day of insertion.

The trends for expulsion, accidental pregnancies, and removals for pain and bleeding which were found in the first two months after insertion were not seen in the third and fourth months.

IUD expulsion rates showed a significant downward trend both as insertions were done later in the cycle and as the woman's age increased.

It is estimated that there will be 9 or more IUD terminations per 1,000 insertions done before day 11 due to expulsion, pain or bleeding, or pregnancy, compared to insertions done after day 11. If all reasons for termination are included, the difference increases to 29 excess terminations in women having early insertions. However, late cycle insertions may subject 4 women per 1,000 to the risk of an unplanned pregnancy with an IUD in situ.

If a woman is not likely to be pregnant, the copper T-200 can be inserted with relative safety regardless of day in her menstrual cycle.

▶ [From this study, it looks as though you "pays your money and you takes your choice" with respect to when the IUD (at least the copper T-200) should be inserted. The later in the menstrual cycle insertion takes place, the less likely expulsion becomes but the more likely removal for pain or bleeding and pregnancy become. Before making too much of these data, however, it should be noted that the patients were not randomly assigned to time of insertion and it is possible, therefore, that some other variable (eg, variation in technical skills among early and late inserters) might be operative.] ◀

Quantitative Menstrual and Intermenstrual Blood Loss in Women Using Lippes Loop and Copper T Intrauterine Devices. Uterine bleeding is the most common side effect that leads to removal

(15–19)   Obstet. Gynecol. 55:220–224, February, 1980.

of plastic and copper intrauterine devices (IUDs) and thus contributes substantially to failure of this family planning method. S. T. Shaw, Jr., A. T. L. Andrade, J. Paixão de Souza, L. K. Macaulay, and P. J. Rowe[15-20] compared intermenstrual with menstrual blood loss in women before and after insertion of the "inert" Lippes Loop C and the copper-bearing Tatum T IUDs. A total of 127 parous women were included in the study; most were multiparas. Over half had used combined oral contraceptives within the past year.

Menstrual blood loss was nearly doubled by insertion of the Lippes Loop C and was increased by about 40% after insertion of the Copper T. Quantifiable intermenstrual bleeding occurred in the first postinsertion cycle in 90% of women with loops and 84% of those with Copper Ts. Only 7 women had intermenstrual bleeding in the second cycle, and such bleeding was negligible in subsequent cycles. Hemoglobin concentrations were essentially unchanged 1 year after insertion of the IUDs.

Intermenstrual bleeding and spotting, though contributing significantly to discontinuance of IUD use, are not significant causes of overall blood loss or iron loss after IUD insertion. A study using serum ferritin assays is in progress to evaluate iron balance in women with IUDs.

▶ [This report confirms a general clinical impression that copper-containing IUDs are associated with less bleeding, both during and between menses, than inert IUDs, Menstrual blood loss on the average doubled with the Lippes loop but increased by less than 50% with the copper T. The incidence and volume of intermenstrual bleeding was more nearly similar with the two devices.] ◀

Naproxen Sodium in Uterine Pain Following Intrauterine Contraceptive Device Insertion. Massey et al. (1974) reported a reduction in discomfort after intrauterine device (IUD) insertion in patients given the prostaglandin synthetase inhibitor naproxen. Veasy Buttram, Allen Izu, and Milan R. Henzl[15-21] evaluated naproxen sodium in IUD users in whom uterine cramping or increased discomfort developed after they were fitted with the devices. Naproxen and placebo were compared during episodes of uterine pain in a double-blind study of 35 patients. Either 550 mg naproxen sodium or placebo was taken at the first sign of menstrual distress, followed by 275 mg every 6 hours as needed during the period of uterine pain.

Naproxen was evaluated in 17 patients and placebo in 16. The groups were comparable in age, obstetric history, and history of dysmenorrhea. All patients but one had used analgesics for uterine pain, but only three had obtained a notable effect. Naproxen-treated patients had greater pain before intake of the study drug than did placebo patients. Naproxen afforded significantly greater relief from pain than placebo. Patients with the earliest symptoms of dysmenorrhea benefited most from active treatment. More placebo patients required additional analgesia, but the difference was not significant.

Naproxen sodium is clearly superior to placebo in alleviating uterine cramping pain that is caused or aggravated by IUD insertion.

(15-20) Contraception 21:343-352, April 1980.
(15-21) Am. J. Obstet. Gynecol. 134:575-578, July 1, 1979.

Elevated endometrial prostaglandin E has been observed after IUD insertion; if this contributes to dysmenorrhea in women practicing intrauterine contraception, the use of a prostaglandin synthetase inhibitor seems logical as a means of counteracting the pain.

▶ [A number of recent reports have noted prostaglandin synthetase inhibitors to be efficacious in treating primary dysmenorrhea. To our knowledge, this is the first indication of value in uterine pain associated with the IUD.] ◀

Comparative Study of the Effect of Progestasert and Gravigard IUDs on Dysmenorrhea. Pain probably is the second most common reason for removing intrauterine devices (IUDs). Ernesto Pizarro, Carlos Gomez-Rogers (Univ. of Chile), and Patrick J. Rowe[15-22] (WHO, Geneva) obtained information on dysmenorrhea in 146 women using the progesterone T 65 μg daily IUD (Progestasert) and 149 using the copper 7 IUD (Gravigard). Follow-up extended to 12 months in both groups. Information on pain was obtained to the end of the study in 112 patients using the progesterone T and 102 using the copper 7 IUD. Four medical removals of the Progestasert were carried out in a total observation time of 1,569 patient-months, only one for pain. No copper 7 IUDs were removed because of pain during 1,558 patient-months of observation.

Menstrual cramps were reduced significantly during one year of IUD use in both groups. The reduction was slightly greater in the progesterone T group. No significant differences were noted when comparing premenstrual and intermenstrual cramps. Eight progesterone T patients reported severe menstrual pain at the outset and 1 after 12 months. Five copper 7 users reported severe pain at insertion and 2 at the end of the study.

It remains unclear whether the Progestasert device actually reduces premenstrual cramps or menstrual pain, or whether the Gravigard IUD reduces dysmenorrhea. More exact and detailed questionnaires are need to ascertain the presence and characteristics of pain.

▶ [This carefully designed study suggests that the progesterone T and copper 7 are similar with respect to menstrual cramps. The former device has been advocated as being superior in this regard. Both devices were associated with decreasing symptoms over 12 months of use. Admittedly, pain is a hard complaint to judge, but it seems to us that, generally speaking, carefully controlled, randomized, blinded studies of IUDs have tended to show that the performances of those devices currently available are more similar than they are different.] ◀

Real-Time Ultrasound in Locating Intrauterine Contraceptive Devices. Spontaneous expulsion of and uterine perforation by the intrauterine device (IUD) have led to a search for a reliable means of locating the IUD when the strings are not visible at the cervical os. Lewis H. Nelson and Joel B. Miller[15-23] assessed the location of IUDs in nongravid patients by use of real-time ultrasonography. Sixty-eight subjects at a family planning clinic were scanned. Criteria for the presence of an IUD were harsh intrauterine echoes from the midportion of the uterine cavity. A "stair-step" pattern was identified as a Lippes Loop and a single harsh midline echo as a Copper-7, al-

(15–22) Contraception 20:455–466, November 1979.
(15–23) Obstet. Gynecol. 54:711–714, December 1979.

though a similar pattern was expected for the Saf-T-Coil. A real-time scanner with a 3.5- or 5.0-MHz transducer array was used.

Thirty-seven evaluable patients with IUDs and 24 controls were compared. Ten patients with IUDs were erroneously thought not to have them. All 20 patients with a Copper-7 were correctly identified, although the type was not correctly identified in 11. No patient with a Saf-T-Coil was correctly identified as having an IUD. In 2 patients without an IUD, a device was thought to be present.

The type of IUD must be known for reliable blind detection of the presence or absence of an IUD by use of real-time ultrasound. Accuracy may be increased through improvement in transducer arrays by mechanical and electric focusing.

▶ [Real-time ultrasound was not particularly effective in locating IUDs in this study. False negative results were more common than false positive ones, and the results varied according to the type of device present. In our view, the simplest way to handle a patient with "missing strings," if pregnancy is not suspected, is to pass a sound into the endometrial cavity and to palpate the characteristic grating of the sound against the intrauterine device. Though invasive, this procedure has the advantages of speed, efficiency, and low cost. For those in whom it is unsuccessful, hysteroscopy has been found by some to be of great value.] ◀

Trophoblastic Markers in Women Using Intrauterine Contraception. It has been suggested that the contraceptive action of the intrauterine device (IUD) is largely mediated through local interference with the early implanted blastocyst. O. Ylikorkala, Marita Siljander, I. Huhtaniemi, A. Kauppila, and M. Seppälä[15-24] investigated the occurrence of human chorionic gonadotropin (hCG) and pregnancy-specific β-glycoprotein in the serum of 214 women using copper T-200 IUDs. The frequency of cycles with positive markers was compared to both the known frequency of pregnancies in a similar population using no contraception and to the reported rate of pregnancies among copper IUD users.

A blood sample was drawn from each woman between 25 and 35 days of the cycle. No contraceptive measures were employed other than the copper IUD. The IUDs had been in place for 1 to 36 months.

In 3 (1.4%) of the 214 cycles, human chorionic gonadotropin was found; pregnancy-specific β-glycoprotein was found in 7 (3.3%). Both markers were found in the same sample from 2 women (0.9%). In all 8 samples with positive trophoblastic markers, the progesterone value exceeded the normal ovulatory level. An apparently normal menstrual flow occurred in all but 1 woman; she reported a 5-day delay in onset.

Because hCG appears in the maternal blood only after implantation, a positive reading for this substance suggests that implantation with subsequent subclinical abortion occurred in those 3 cycles, because a normal menstrual-like bleeding followed.

The authors estimate that 93% of the volunteers would have had at least one implantation in a year if no contraception were used. The incidence of established pregnancies for copper IUDs is 1.6/100 woman-years in a population similar to that of this study. Further,

(15–24) Obstet. Gynecol. 55:329–332, March 1980.

based on the present data, they estimate an annual rate of occult pregnancies of 16.8%, which is only 18% of the expected implantation rate in the absence of contraception. This finding suggests that the copper IUD prevented pregnancy before implantation in 82% of potential pregnancies. However, the estimated occult pregnancy rate of 16.8% is ten times the incidence of established pregnancies among women using copper IUDs.

If only the 2 women with both markers in the serum are considered to have had implantation, the annual subclinical abortion rate would be calculated as 10.8%, or seven times the established rate of pregnancy among IUD users.

These calculations show that the IUD prevents pregnancy in most women before significant quantities of trophoblastic markers are secreted into the maternal bloodstream.

▶ [The subclinical abortion rate in IUD users reported here varied according to the criterion selected as indicating implantation (elevated hCG, pregnancy-specific β-glycoprotein, or both). The occult pregnancy rate was much higher than that found in certain earlier studies. It would be of interest to test other contraceptive methods in the same experimental design and also to test patients using no contraception in cycles where conception *apparently* did not occur.

In a related study, Custo and associates (Contraception 21:311, 1980) measured hormone levels in 12 subjects through four consecutive cycles of Progestasert IUD usage. None exhibited detectable hCG, implying that the action of progestin IUDs is different from nonmedicated devices or at least acts at an early enough stage to prevent hCG formation.] ◀

16. Abortion

Prospective Study of Spontaneous Fetal Losses After Induced Abortions. Susan Harlap, Patricia H. Shiono, Savitri Ramcharan, Heinz Berendes and Frederick Pellegrin[16-1] prospectively observed the incidence of spontaneous abortions among 31,917 women who were members of the Kaiser Foundation Health Plan who were followed from their first prenatal visit from 1974 to 1976. These women experienced 661 first-trimester and 753 second-trimester miscarriages. A total of 3,942 women (10.9%) reported having had one or more induced abortions, including 2,019 (14.4%) of 14,061 nulliparous women and 1,493 (8.3%) of 17,852 women who had previously borne children.

Life-table analysis showed that losses in the first trimester were not significantly affected by previous induced abortions, and no change in risk of second-trimester losses was detected among parous women who had had induced abortions after childbirth. However, the incidence of second-trimester losses among nulliparous women with previous induced abortions was increased (Fig 16–1). The age-adjusted rate of loss, per 100,000 women at risk per day, was 59.9 among nulliparous women with previous induced abortions and 24.2 among nulliparous women who had not had previous abortions (P < .001).

In nulliparous women, relative risk of miscarriage increased with

Fig 16–1.—Spontaneous abortions according to week of pregnancy, parity, and previous induced abortions. Loss rate is average number of daily spontaneous abortions per 100,000 women at risk, adjusted on the basis of age and woman-days of observation. (Courtesy of Harlap, S., et al.: N. Engl. J. Med. 301:677–681, Sept. 27, 1979.)

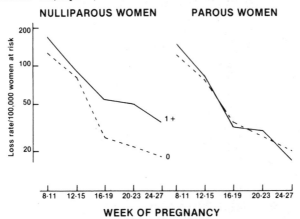

(16–1) N. Engl. J. Med. 301:677–681, Sept. 27, 1979.

number of previous induced abortions and was not explained by the distribution of demographic and social variables. The risk decreased from 3.27 after abortions induced before 1973, when dilation and curettage was the predominant method used, to 1.42 after abortions done since 1973, when the more gentle technique of insertion of laminaria several hours before the abortion was introduced. Thus, there is apparently little or no risk of spontaneous fetal loss after abortions induced by current techniques.

▶ [This large study of the risk of spontaneous abortion following induced abortion is generally reassuring. Only nulliparous women who had had an induced abortion were at increased risk, and these only for a second-trimester spontaneous loss. This presumably reflects damage to the nulliparous cervix during dilatation. For patients with induced abortions since 1973 (from which time laminaria tents were commonly used), the relative risk of subsequent spontaneous abortion was markedly reduced. A caveat in all of this is that 90% of the induced abortions took place in the first trimester. These reassuring findings do not, therefore, necessarily apply to induced abortions in the second trimester of pregnancy. For more information—or perhaps to become further confused—read on.] ◀

Association of Induced Abortion With Subsequent Pregnancy Loss. It has been suggested that spontaneous abortion is more frequent in women with a history of induced abortion. Ann Aschengrau Levin, Stephen C. Schoenbaum, Richard R. Monson, Phillip G. Stubblefield, and Kenneth J. Ryan[16-2] (Boston) compared the reproductive histories of women having a fetal loss up to 28 weeks' gestation with those of women having term deliveries in a case-control study. Women seen between 1976 and 1978 with a spontaneous abortion before 20 weeks' gestation or premature delivery at 20 to 27 weeks were included in the study. A total of 240 cases were compared with 1,072 controls.

Women who had had two or more previous induced abortions had about a twofold to threefold increase in risk of first-trimester spontaneous abortion. The increased risk was present for women in whom legal abortions were induced after 1973. It could not be related to smoking status, history of prior spontaneous fetal loss, method of abortion, or degree of cervical dilatation. No increase in risk of pregnancy loss was found for women with only a single prior induced abortion. Vacuum aspiration or suction had been used in over two thirds of all groups. The risks of having a first-trimester loss, an incomplete abortion or missed abortion at 14 to 19 weeks, or a premature delivery at 20 to 27 weeks' gestation all increased progressively with an increasing frequency of prior spontaneous losses.

The findings suggest a direct relation between number of previous induced abortions and subsequent risk of a pregnancy loss. Although women who have had multiple induced abortions could have difficulty carrying a pregnancy to viability, the findings do not indicate that such women are ultimately unable to achieve a successful pregnancy or to achieve their desired total family size. Prevention of unwanted pregnancies appears to be increasingly important for women who have had one or more prior induced abortions.

▶ [The results of this study indicate that patients with two or more (but not one) pre-

(16–2) JAMA 243:2495–2499, June 27, 1980.

vious induced abortions are at increased risk for spontaneous abortion or premature delivery before 28 weeks' gestation compared with a "control group." Different conclusions have been reached by others (1979 YEAR BOOK, p. 438). The chief problem in a study of this sort concerns the nature of the control group. In our experience, patients with multiple induced abortions have certain differences in personality traits and lifestyles from other patients of apparently similar socioeconomic backgrounds. In other words, is it the previous procedures or is it the patient herself that makes the difference? Cervical trauma is apparently not the whole answer, as both first-trimester abortions and second-trimester missed abortions were more common in patients with a history of two or more induced abortions. Cervical incompetence cannot explain this sort of increased risk.] ◄

Disappearance of Human Chorionic Gonadotropin and Resumption of Ovulation Following Abortion. It has been reported that resumption of ovulation after term pregnancy occurs later than after first-trimester induced abortion. Richard P. Marrs, Oscar A. Kletzky, Wilbur F. Howard, and Daniel R. Mishell, Jr.[16-3] (Univ. of Southern California) investigated the disappearance of human chorionic gonadotropin (hCG) and resumption of cyclic pituitary ovarian function in 13 patients following different methods of pregnancy termination.

Four patients (group A) had first-trimester termination of pregnancy by dilation and curettage under light general anesthesia. Five patients (group B) had second-trimester termination by use of prostaglandin $F_{2\alpha}$ followed by sharp curettage. Hysterectomy was the method used in 4 second trimester patients (group C); 1 of these patients had early ligation of the uterine blood vessels and minimal manipulation of the uterus during surgery. Patients in the first two groups used nonhormonal methods of birth control after the abortion.

Serum levels of luteinizing hormone, follicle-stimulating hormone, the β subunit of hCG, and progesterone were measured by radioimmunoassay.

In group A, a mean time of 37.5 ± 6.4 days was required for hCG levels to plateau at 2 mIU/ml, regardless of initial baseline values. Levels of follicle-stimulating hormone were low or undetectable for 3 to 7 days following abortion, then increased to an ovulatory peak between 20 and 25 days. The maximum rise of serum luteinizing hormone was concomitant with the rise in follicle-stimulating hormone level. Serum hCG levels were still measurable in all 4 patients at the time of probable ovulation.

In group B, the mean time to reach a plateau of 2 mIU/ml of hCG was 27.4 ± 4.8 days, a significantly shorter time than in group A. These patients also had measurable levels of hCG at time of ovulation.

In the patients who underwent routine hysterectomy, the mean time for the hCG value to drop to the plateau level was 39.7 ± 5.3 days, similar to findings in group A, but longer than in group B. The patient who had early ligation of the uterine blood vessels and minimal manipulation of the uterus required only 12 days to reach the plateau level of hCG, significantly less than any other patient in the study.

(16–3) Am. J. Obstet. Gynecol. 135:731–736, Nov. 15, 1979.

The time of disappearance of hCG in relation to the total baseline level was also evaluated. Only those patients with an hCG baseline of less than 10,000 mIU/ml had a significantly shorter disappearance curve than the other groups.

These data indicate that the disappearance of hCG after first and second trimester abortions occurs at a predictable rate; the time of complete disappearance depends upon the procedure used for termination and to some degree on stage of gestation. Ovulation occurred within 3 weeks, thus adequate contraceptive measures should be taken within two weeks of termination. The most sensitive pregnancy tests, radioreceptor assays, may remain positive for 10 to 15 days following pregnancy termination, whereas agglutination-inhibition tests can remain positive for approximately 1 week after abortion.

▶ [It is of interest that hCG disappeared more rapidly following second-trimester abortions (induced with prostaglandin $F_{2\alpha}$ and incorporating sharp curettage) than it did following first-trimester suction procedures. Ovulation and presumed fertility returned rapidly in these patients—as early as 21 days following the abortion.] ◀

Local versus General Anesthesia: Which Is Safer for Performing Suction Curettage Abortions? Despite the wide prevalence of suction curettage abortion, little is known of the relative safety of local paracervical vs general anesthesia for these procedures. David A. Grimes, Kenneth F. Schulz, Willard Cates, Jr., and Carl W. Tyler, Jr.[16-4] (Center for Disease Control) compared the safety of these anesthetic techniques in 36,430 women who received local anesthesia and 17,725 given general anesthesia for suction curettage abortion in the United States during 1971–1975. Local anesthesia consisted of paracervical anesthesia with or without administration of a sedative or analgesic. Operations were done at or before 12 weeks' gestation. About 55% of abortions took place in hospitals. The women given local anesthesia tended to be younger, were less likely to be married, and were of lower gravidity. They also were more likely to report preexisting medical conditions. The gestational age distribution was similar for the two groups.

Major complication rates did not differ significantly for the two anesthetic groups. The relative risk of complications from general anesthesia was 1.2 times greater than with local anesthesia, but the difference was abolished by adjusting for type of facility. Uterine hemorrhage was 1.7 times more likely with general anesthesia, and the risk of uterine perforation was 2.2 times higher. The relative risk of intra-abdominal hemorrhage was 8.2. Cervical injury also was more frequent with general anesthesia, the relative risk being 2.9. The risk of fever was greater with local anesthesia, even after adjustment for antibiotic prophylaxis, and convulsions were more frequent. Endometritis and retained products of conception were comparably frequent after both forms of anesthesia. Rates of readmission to a hospital did not differ significantly.

Both local and general anesthesia for suction curettage abortion appear to be safe. General anesthetics that depress uterine contractil-

(16–4) Am. J. Obstet. Gynecol. 135:1030–1035, Dec. 15, 1979.

ity, such as halothane and enflurane, should be avoided to minimize the occurrence of uterine hemorrhage.

▶ [The results of this study are predictable. With the awake patient under local anesthesia, the operator may tend to be more gentle, to use less force in dilating the cervix, and perhaps to be less thorough in emptying the uterus. This would result in fewer cervical tears, less chance of perforation, and less bleeding, but an increased likelihood of retained tissue and subsequent infection.] ◀

Gestational Trophoblastic Disease Within an Elective Abortion Population. Barry A. Cohen, Ronald T. Burkman, Neil B. Rosenshein, Milagros F. Atienza, Theodore M. King, and Tim H. Parmley[16-5] (Johns Hopkins Med. Inst.) examined the occurrence of gestational trophoblastic disease in 4,829 patients undergoing suction curettage for elective first-trimester abortion from 1973 to 1976. About 75% of subjects had gestations of 12 weeks or less. Criteria for gestational trophoblastic disease included the presence of placental villi with edema, loss of vasculature, and trophoblastic proliferation.

Eight cases of hydatidiform mole were diagnosed during the 3-year study, for a frequency of about 1 in 600 cases. Six patients were aged 16 and under. Five were nulliparous. Socioeconomic characteristics were similar to those of the general abortion population. Two patients reported mild vaginal spotting, and 1 presented with galactorrhea. Tissues raising suspicion of molar pregnancy were identified grossly in 6 cases. All patients had normal titers of the β-subunit of human chorionic gonadotropin in serum within 6 weeks, and none required chemotherapy. One patient later underwent hysterectomy for myomas, and pathologic study showed no evidence of trophoblastic disease. Another patient has presented three times since for pregnancy termination without problems. In the patient with galactorrhea, symptoms resolved several weeks after evacuation of the molar pregnancy.

The clinical course of patients with hydatidiform mole appears to be benign, but gross examination of tissue obtained at suction curettage and liberal use of histologic evaluation in questionable cases are necessary for the diagnosis. If fetal parts are absent or any tissue appears to be abnormal, histologic evaluation is mandatory.

▶ [The incidence of hydatidiform mole found in this series of nearly 5,000 first-trimester pregnancy terminations, 1 in 600, is somewhat higher than that normally quoted. Whatever the true incidence is, the importance of recognizing trophoblastic disease is unquestioned. Ideally, all abortion tissue should be examined microscopically, for only in this way can trophoblastic disease be identified and other serious conditions such as ectopic pregnancy suspected. Cost factors, however, are a deterrent to routine microscopic study. As a minimum, tissue obtained by suction curettage should be carefully inspected; if fetal parts cannot be identified grossly or if there is any suspicion of abnormal tissue, the specimen should be submitted for full histologic examination.] ◀

(16–5) Am. J. Obstet. Gynecol. 135:452–454, Oct. 15, 1979.

17. Breast Diseases

Danazol Treatment of Chronic Cystic Mastopathy. Clinical and Hormonal Evaluation. Chronic cystic mastitis is a common condition that may be incapacitating and may require medical treatment. Greenblatt et al. obtained success with danazol in the therapy of mastitis, endometriosis, and gynecomastia. M. Dhont, L. Delbeke, J. van Eyck, and L. Voorhoof[17-1] (State Univ., Ghent) evaluated the clinical and hormonal effects of danazol in the short-term management of chronic cystic mastitis in 16 premenopausal women in an open trial. The mean age was 32 years. All patients had mild to severe mastodynia for at least 3 months. Danazol therapy was begun on the first day of the menstrual cycle in a dose of 400 mg daily and continued for 2 months. Assessments were made after 2, 4, and 8 weeks of therapy, and 4 weeks after discontinuance of the drug. A double-blind trial of danazol and placebo was also carried out in 25 women with moderate to severe mastalgia.

Nine patients were completely relieved by danazol, with the others reporting considerable improvement after 2 months of therapy. Decreased nodularity was apparent in all patients. Three women had recurrent mastodynia a month after therapy was stopped. Four women became amenorrheic during treatment, and the rest had irregular bleeding. All patients gained weight during treatment. Blood pressures remained unchanged. Regular menses resumed within a month after treatment, and all side effects resolved. Gonadotropin levels increased during danazol therapy. The serum prolactin level decreased significantly, as did the total urinary estrogen concentration. The results of the double-blind trial are given in the table.

Danazol was significantly more effective than placebo in relieving mastalgia. Three patients became amenorrheic during treatment. In both trials, danazol completely relieved mastalgia in 52% of patients and led to improvement in another 41%.

RESULTS OF DOUBLE-BLIND RANDOMIZED CLINICAL TRIAL OF DANAZOL (400 mg DAILY FOR 2 MONTHS) VERSUS PLACEBO IN CHRONIC CYSTIC MASTOPATHY

	n	Dropped out	Partial or complete relief of symptoms	Decreased nodularity
Placebo	12	3	3/9	0/9
Danazol	13	2	9/11*	6/11*

*$P < .005$ (chi-square).

(17–1) Postgrad. Med. J. 55(Suppl. 5):66–70, 1979.

These findings confirm the beneficial effect of danazol in the treatment of chronic cystic mastopathy. The effect may be related to inhibition of ovulation, with low, nonfluctuating estrogen production, or to a direct effect on breast tissue through competition for estrogen receptor sites. The decreased prolactin level may enhance the effect of the drug on benign breast tissue.

▶ [The results of this study suggest the possibility of another use for danazol. Similar effects have been noted by Mansel et al. (Postgrad. Med. J. 55 (Suppl. 5):61, 1979), Baker and Snedecor (Am. Surg. 45:727, 1979), and Nezhat and associates (Am. J. Obstet. Gynecol. 137:604, 1980). Side effects (menstrual disruption and weight gain) and cost are potential problems.

The endocrine effects of danazol noted in the table are virtually opposite those found in an article in the "Endocrinology" chapter of this YEAR BOOK.] ◀

Low-Dose Mammography. Application to Medical Practice. Stephen A. Feig[17-2] (Thomas Jefferson Univ. Hosp.) discusses recent advances in mammographic technology, accuracy of the technique, its risks, and current recommendations for its use.

Two new imaging systems, reduced-dose xeromammography and screen-film combinations specifically designed for mammography, have resulted in reduction of the radiation doses required and enhancement of image quality. For a typical two-view examination, the midbreast tissue dose is 0.08–0.74 rad, less than the previous estimate of 2 rad for the low-dose technique. Because the hypothetical risks from low-dose medical radiation is immeasurably small, these figures indicate that mammography can be undertaken with little risk.

The improved accuracy of the technique is demonstrated by comparing the results of two large screening programs begun at different times. The earlier screening project was conducted from 1963–1967; the later one, started in 1973, was completed recently. Both studies included physical examinations and mammography. Although the two populations are not strictly comparable, there is a difference in cancer detection rates. In the earlier study 55% of all cancers were detected by mammography with or without associated physical findings; in the later study 93% of all cancers were discovered by mammography.

The most important factor in breast cancer survival is axillary lymph node status at time of surgery. In the later study, mammography was more reliable than physical examintion for both normal and abnormal nodes. Of cancers in patients with normal lymph nodes, 50% detected by mammography were undetected by physical examination.

It is not known whether the extremely low doses of radiation associated with current mammographic techniques could cause breast cancer; however, the risk, if it exists, is small and has never been measured in human populations exposed to low doses of gamma radiation.

In all human populations studied, the breasts of older women were considerably less sensitive to radiation. The natural breast cancer in-

(17–2) JAMA 242:2107–2109, Nov. 9, 1979.

cidence is double at the age of 70 as compared to that observed at the age of 40. Considering that half of these cancers might be detectable by mammography at an early stage, the benefits seem to outweigh the risks of the procedure.

Physical examination and mammography represent complementary methods of detection. Younger women have more glandular breasts which can be more difficult to interpret by mammography, but improved technology has made this less of a problem.

The American College of Radiology recommends that mammography be an integral part of patient evaluation if symptoms or physical findings are suggestive of cancer. For screening asymptomatic women, a baseline examination should be performed between 35 and 40 years of age. Subsequent examinations should be at 1- to 3-year intervals, unless more frequent examinations are medically warranted. After age 50, mammographic examinations should be carried out annually or at other regular intervals.

▶ [Feig presents a strong case for increased use of mammography in breast cancer detection. The American College of Radiology, the American College of Obstetricians and Gynecologists, and the American Cancer Society have all made recommendations in this area. Women over age 50 years should have breast examinations including mammography annually or at "other regular intervals." Women between ages 35 and 50 should have a baseline mammogram and subsequent x-ray studies at intervals to be determined by the physician (the radiology group suggests 1- to 3-year intervals). We find that we are making increased use of mammography in our own patients. Given the evidence available to this point, we think this practice is appropriate although we do not know that cost-benefit proof has been established.] ◀

▶ ↓ The following two abstracts attest to the value of mammography in early detection of breast cancer. ◀

Sensitivity of Mammography and Physical Examination of Breast for Detecting Breast Cancer. The average woman has about a 7% chance of having breast cancer, the foremost cause of cancer deaths in women. The prognosis is, in general, better with earlier detection and treatment. Mary Jane Hicks, John R. Davis, Jack M. Layton, and Arthur J. Present[17-3] (Univ. of Arizona) evaluated mammography and physical examination of the breast as screening measures for detecting breast cancer using local biopsy data obtained from women enrolled in a national breast cancer screening program. Over 10,000 women were enrolled from 1975–1979. In women under age 40, mammography was done only on a physician's order or if there was a history of previous breast cancer. Women aged 40–49 were examined if there was a family history of breast cancer. Women aged 50 and over were routinely screened by mammography. Thermography was also done on many screenees.

The sensitivities of mammography and physical examination in detecting the 113 breast cancers were 62% and 24%, respectively (Table). The sensitivity of the two methods combined was 75%. Thirty-seven lesions were in situ or only minimally invasive, and 81% of these small cancers were detected by screening. Node metastases were present in 8 of 28 cancers detected by self-examination and interval biopsy, and in 18 of 85 lesions detected by screening. Forty-

(17–3) JAMA 242:2080–2083, Nov. 9, 1979.

COMPARISON OF SENSITIVITY OF
MAMMOGRAPHY AND PHYSICAL
EXAMINATION IN BREAST CARCINOMA
CASES

Carcinoma	Sensitivity
Physical Examination	
Small*	10%
>1 cm	27%
Overall	22%
Mammogram	
Small*	72%
>1 cm	57%
Overall	63%

*In situ or invasive carcinoma ≤1 cm in size.

eight cancers were detected by mammography alone. Eight patients had suspicious physical findings but benign mammographic findings. Two patients died of disseminated breast cancer; 1 had refused treatment, and the other had recurrent disease when entered into the study.

Mammography is more sensitive than physical examination as a screening instrument for breast cancer. Together these methods remain important complementary screening measures for breast cancer detection. A beneficial effect on survival may be anticipated through the high rate of discovery of early, small cancers.

Prognostic Factors of Breast Neoplasms Detected on Screening by Mammography and Physical Examination. Stephen A. Feig, Gordon F. Schwartz, Rudolph Nerlinger, and Jack Edeiken[17-4] (Thomas Jefferson Univ.) analyzed neoplasms in 183 women, aged 45 to 64 years, with breast cancer detected on screening by xeromammography and/or physical examination.

Most neoplasms (113) were of the invasive ductal type; 51 were in situ ductal, microinvasive ductal, and tubular carcinoma. These latter have been associated with high five-year survival rates (96% to 100%), and most were detected by mammography in this study (85% to 93%). Neoplasms representing infiltrating lobular carcinoma were among the largest of all lesions detected and were the only group in which detection by physical examination exceeded detection by mammography.

Two reasons were used for placing a breast cancer in a favorable prognostic category: (1) an early cancer as determined by size, high proportion of in situ growth, or no axillary nodes; (2) a lesion with less inherent metastatic potential because of tubule formation or low histologic grade. Mammography consistently detected lesions based on each of these factors at a higher rate than physical examination. For each prognostic factor, lesions included in the most favorable category were much more likely to have been detected by mammography, but not by physical examination, than those in less advanta-

(17-4) Radiology 133:577-582, December 1979.

geous categories, mean lesion size in each category being the important factor.

Most early cancers appear to be relatively aggressive, since factors suggesting less metastatic potential were seldom present. For example, only 20% of all tubular and ductal cancers of 2.0 cm or less were of histologic grade I (Fig 17-1). Also, only 15% of all tubular and invasive ductal lesions of 2.0 cm or less had 90% to 100% tubule formation. Nearly all of these preponderantly tubular lesions were included in histologic grade I.

Virtually all breast cancers began to manifest their aggressive behavior at an early stage. The proportion of in situ lesions decreased dramatically with even slight increase in lesion size.

After changing from in situ to invasive growth, lymphatic vessel invasion and axillary node metastasis can occur (Fig 17-2). At first,

Fig 17-1 (top).—Proportion of cancers in each size group according to histologic grade. Each of the 164 ductal and tubular cancers was given a single grade based on its dominant histologic picture. Most grade I cancers were seen in the lower size ranges, but even there, they represented a relatively small percentage of cases.

Fig 17-2 (bottom).—Frequency of axillary lymph node metastasis according to lesion size in 171 breast neoplasms. Note the sharp increase in metastasis occurring with a lesion larger than 2.0 cm.

(Courtesy of Feig, S. A., et al.: Radiology 133:577–582, December 1979.)

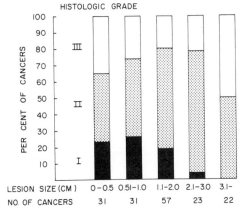

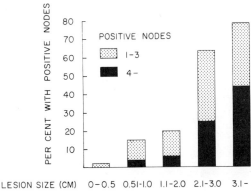

the incidence of these is low, but axillary metastases were seen in 71% of lesions of more than 2.0 cm and in only 13% of lesions of 2.0 cm or less. For all tumors of 2.0 cm or less, 82% were found by mammography but only 40% by physical examination.

Women below age 50 years showed little difference in percentage of tumors that could not be palpated compared to the number of lesions detected; this was not significantly different from the findings for women above 50. Mammographic screening should lead to improved survival rates in women aged 45 to 49 years as well as those older.

▶ [This article and the preceding one indicate, not surprisingly, that mammography is superior to physical examination in breast cancer detection, particularly with small (< 1 cm) lesions. Many small lesions show lack of differentiation, which suggests an aggressive tendency, yet the prevalence of positive nodes clearly relates to the size of the lesion. Therefore, early identification of these small cancers holds considerable promise as a means of decreasing breast cancer mortality. Nonetheless, the two techniques, physical examination and mammography, are complementary; the report of Hicks and associates included 8 cases identified by abnormal physical findings in the face of negative x-ray findings.] ◀

Use of Ultrasonography in Management of Masses of the Breast was reviewed by Hind S. Teixidor[17-5] (Cornell Univ.). Patients with a mass at least 1 cm in diameter that did not have a typical mammographic appearance were referred for ultrasonography. Contact B mode scanning of the area in question was performed with a gray-scale unit and a 5-MHz transducer. Longitudinal and transverse sections were obtained at low- and high-gain settings. A total of 260 patients were examined by both mammography and ultrasonography, and 145 lesions were confirmed pathologically after mastectomy, excision biopsy or needle aspiration. The findings in 1 patient are shown in Figure 17-3.

All 63 fluid-filled cysts were correctly diagnosed by ultrasound, and

Fig 17–3.—Palpable mass in tail of breast in woman, aged 42 years. **A,** mammogram showing mass with nondiagnostic features *(arrows).* Its ill-defined borders make it suspicious for malignant growth. **B,** gray-scale B mode sonogram of same mass at high-gain setting showing typical cyst. Note absence of internal echoes, sharp far wall, and enhancement of sound deep to mass *(arrows).* Cyst proved by aspiration. (Courtesy of Teixidor, H. S.: Surg. Gynecol. Obstet. 150:486–490, April 1980.)

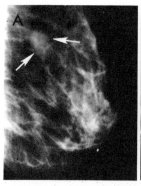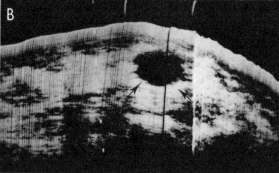

all but 2 of 39 carcinomas were correctly identified as solid masses. The 2 exceptions were 1 and 1.5 cm in diameter. All but 2 of 20 fibroadenomas were identified as solid masses. Eleven of 17 cases of mammary dysplasia were correctly diagnosed by ultrasound as not being discrete masses. The false positive rate in this group was 35.3%. Much overlap exists between the ultrasonic features of circumscribed carcinomas and those of benign solid masses. Abscesses were easily diagnosed by ultrasonography, especially when they were well localized.

Contact B mode ultrasonography of breast masses is a simple, safe means of accurately distinguishing cystic from solid masses measuring 1 cm or more in diameter. A sonographically solid mass should be biopsied unless it has an unequivocally benign appearance on mammography. An asymptomatic, purely cystic mass need not be biopsied for diagnostic purposes. Ultrasonography is preferable to needle aspiration for diagnosis of breast cysts. When it is properly used and when the results are carefully related to the clinical and mammographic findings, ultrasonography can eliminate over one third of all breast operations.

▶ [According to these results, gray-scale ultrasonography seems very accurate in differentiating cystic and solid tumors of the breast as long as the tumor is larger than 1 cm in diameter. Since cysts are nearly always benign, this capability could prove useful in many cases. Ultrasonography avoids the ionizing radiation of mammography, and in some instances (such as that illustrated in Fig 17-3) is more definitive. Within the group of solid masses, however, ultrasound is substantially less accurate than mammography.] ◀

Case-Control Study of Menopausal Estrogen Therapy and Breast Cancer. A hormonal role in the cause of breast cancer is highly probable, and it is likely that several hormones, particularly estrogens, are important. Ronald K. Ross, Annlia Paganini-Hill, Vibeke R. Gerkins, Thomas M. Mack, Robert Pfeiffer, Mary Arthur, and Brian E. Henderson[17-6] undertook a case-control study of the association between estrogen replacement therapy and breast cancer in two Los Angeles area retirement communities. A total of 138 study cases of breast cancer in residents aged 50 to 74 years were compared with age- and race-matched community controls. Two controls were selected for each index case.

The risk ratio for a total cumulative estrogen dose of over 1,500 mg was estimated as 2.5 in women with intact ovaries (table). The excess was present when various independent sources of drug use information were used, but it was inconsistent at low dosages and undetectable in oophorectomized women. No important sources of confounding were identified. No risk modifiers were apparent other than a history of surgically confirmed benign breast disease. The risk ratio for women with such disease, intact ovaries, and a high cumulative dose was 5.7, compared with nonusers who had normal breasts. The results were not significantly influenced by interval from first estrogen use to diagnosis, interval from menopause to first use, or age at first use.

(17-6) JAMA 243:1635–1639, Apr. 25, 1980.

TOTAL MILLIGRAM ACCUMULATED DOSE (TMD) OF CONJUGATED ESTROGEN
USE BY OVARIAN STATUS

| | TMD | | | | | One-sided P |
	0	1-1,499	1,500+	Unknown	Ever	(χ^2 for Trend)
Ovaries intact						
Cases	50	21	28	2	51	
Control subjects	103	56	23	5	84	
Matched risk ratio	1.0	0.9	·2.5	. . .	1.4	.02
95% confidence interval	. . .	0.4-1.7	1.2-5.6	. . .	0.7-2.4	
Ovaries removed						
Cases	13	6	7	0	13	
Control subjects	29	15	21	1	37	
Unmatched risk ratio*	1.0	0.9	0.7	. . .	0.8	NS
95% confidence interval	. . .	0.2-3.2	0.2-2.4	. . .	0.5-3.5	
All†						
Cases	64	28	37	2	67	
Control subjects	134	73	48	7	128	
Matched risk ratio	1.0	0.8	1.9	. . .	1.1	.03
95% confidence interval	. . .	0.5-1.5	1.0-3.3	. . .	0.8-1.9	

*Matched analysis omitted because only three sets were informative when matched on prior oophorectomy.
†Includes persons with ovarian status unknown.

It is estimated that a woman undergoing natural menopause at age 50 who receives 1.25 mg of replacement estrogen therapy daily for about 3 years has an increase in lifetime risk of developing breast cancer by age 75 from 6% to 12% if no latency is required, to nearly 10% if a 5-year latency is required, and to 9% if allowance is made for a 10-year latency period. These figures imply sizable mortality effects, and the benefits from estrogen therapy would have to be great to warrant such risk. The cost-benefit ratio of lower dosages is clearly more favorable.

▶ [Although case-control studies concerning the relationship between exogenous estrogens and endometrial cancer have generally shown a significant association, the situation regarding breast cancer is not at all clear. The present report does not solve things. In patients with ovaries there was a suggestion of increased breast cancer risk with high levels of estrogen exposure. In patients whose ovaries had been removed, however, there was no increased risk with estrogen therapy (the risk was actually less than in controls, although not significantly so in a statistical sense). Moderate levels of estrogen exposure in patients with ovaries were not associated with an increased risk of developing breast cancer. There is no clear-cut message here for the practitioner, other than that the issue is unresolved.

In a related study, Bland and associates (Cancer 45:3027, 1980) reviewed the effect of exogenous estrogen on mammographic findings in 405 postmenopausal women. There was no evidence that estrogen altered the mammographic parenchymal pattern or increased the risk of breast cancer.] ◀

Relationship of Estrogen-Receptor Status to Survival in Breast Cancer. Estrogen-receptor (ER) status has been shown to be a useful predictor of the response of breast cancer to endocrine therapy, but survival after mastectomy has not been clearly shown to be influenced by the ER status of the primary tumor. H. M. Bishop, R. W. Blamey, C. W. Elston, J. L. Haybittle (Nottingham, England), R.

I. Nicholson, and K. Griffiths[17-7] (Cardiff, Wales) determined the ER content of primary breast cancers in 133 postmenopausal women who underwent simple mastectomy and triple node biopsy during 1973–1977. All had follow-up for at least 2 years. No adjuvant therapy was used. Patients with symptomatic distant metastases received tamoxifen and local radiotherapy. Those who failed to respond received combination chemotherapy, as did patients who relapsed after responding.

Of the 133 study patients, 59% were ER positive. Thirty-nine patients have died. Those with ER-positive tumors lived longer than those with negative tumors, and the difference was significant. The effect of ER status was apparent only in patients with node invasion at mastectomy.

The presence of ER in a tumor seems to be an index of tumor cell differentiation, well-differentiated tumors containing ER. This may largely account for the better prognosis of patients with ER-positive breast tumors. No relationship is apparent between ER status and either tumor size or tumor stage. The disease-free interval is longer in ER-positive cases, and these tumors respond better to endocrine treatment.

▶ [Estrogen-receptor positivity in breast cancers in postmenopausal women was associated with improved survival in this study. The effect of the estrogen-receptor status was limited to those patients with positive lymph nodes at the time of mastectomy. According to the authors, well-differentiated tumors are more likely to be estrogen-receptor positive than are poorly differentiated ones. For an apparently contrary view, read on.] ◀

Relative Importance of Estrogen Receptor Analysis as Prognostic Factor for Recurrence or Response to Chemotherapy in Women With Breast Cancer. Several reports have suggested that earlier recurrence of breast cancer and shorter survival are associated with lesions that contain no estrogen receptor (ER) on assay. Russell Hilf, Michael L. Feldstein, Scott L. Gibson, and Edwin D. Savlov[17-8] (Univ. of Rochester) have performed ER assays in cases of primary breast cancer since 1970, using sucrose gradient centrifugation techniques. Data were analyzed for 111 patients not treated after mastectomy, 52 patients given adjuvant therapy with melphalan or with cyclophosphamide, methotrexate, and 5-fluorouracil and 70 patients with advanced disease who received combination chemotherapy.

Among patients untreated after mastectomy, recurrences were seen earlier in those with node-positive cases but could not be related to ER status. The group without recurrence included a somewhat higher proportion of patients with smaller tumors. All 27 patients in whom adjuvant therapy failed had node involvement, and 18 had ER. No significant relation was found between recurrence rates and ER status of the primary lesion. No relation of ER status to prognosis was apparent in the group with advanced disease, in terms of response to combination chemotherapy.

The findings indicate no striking prognostic value of ER status with

(17–7) Lancet 2:283–284, Aug. 11, 1979.
(17–8) Cancer 45:1993–2000, Apr. 15, 1980.

respect to recurrence of breast cancer, either in patients untreated after mastectomy or in those given adjuvant chemotherapy after operation.

▶ [This report and the preceding one seem contradictory with respect to the prognostic import of estrogen receptor status in breast cancer patients. In the study by Bishop et al., patients who were ER positive had a better prognosis than those who were ER negative, although the difference was limited to those with positive nodes. This report of Hilf and associates, by contrast, found no clear difference with respect to ER status in (1) time to recurrence in patients receiving no therapy postoperatively, (2) course in patients given adjuvant chemotherapy, and (3) response of advanced disease to cytotoxic chemotherapy. It should be noted, however, that endocrine therapy was not used in the latter series, and perhaps the response to hormonal manipulation (oophorectomy, adrenalectomy, antiestrogens, androgens, etc.) might correlate with estrogen-receptor status.] ◀

Psychologic Response to Breast Cancer: Effect on Outcome. Some clinicians believe that the coping responses adopted by cancer patients may influence the prognosis. S. Greer, T. Morris, and K. W. Pettingale[17-9] (King's College Hosp. Med. School, London) conducted a prospective multidisciplinary 5-year study of 69 consecutive patients with early breast cancer. All were under age 70 years and had no past history of malignant disease. Simple mastectomy was performed in each case; 25 patients also received prophylactic postoperative radiotherapy to the ipsilateral axillary nodes. Psychologic responses to the diagnosis were assessed 3 months postoperatively by a structured interview and then related to the outcome 5 years after surgery.

Of sixty-seven patients who were assessed 3 months postoperatively, 33 were alive and well 5 years after surgery, 16 were alive with metastases, and 18 had died of breast cancer. The outcome was similar in patients given radiotherapy and in those who had only mastectomy. The outcome at 5 years was not significantly related to patient age, social class, reaction on discovering the breast lump, delay in seeking medical advice, or the habitual reaction to stressful events. Depression and hostility scores, psychologic stress, sexual adjustment, interpersonal relationships, work record, and extraversion and neuroticism scores also failed to relate to the outcome. Patients who were unmarried or who reported poor marital relations at the time of diagnosis tended to have a less favorable outcome. Psychologic responses to the diagnosis of cancer (as assessed 3 months after surgery) were significantly related to the 5-year outcome, with a favorable outcome being related to denial or a fighting spirit, compared with either stoic acceptance or a helpless, hopeless response. The latter reactions were seen in 14 of 16 patients who died and in only 13 of 28 women who were well at follow-up.

This study showed a significant relationship between psychologic response to the diagnosis of breast cancer and the outcome at 5 years. It is possible that particular responses were themselves the result of occult metastatic disease, but it is more likely that the psychologic responses of these patients affected their outcome. Such an effect could be mediated via neuroendocrine or immune pathways.

(17–9) Lancet 2:785–787, Oct. 13, 1979.

▶ [These observations are fascinating. Among patients with early breast cancer, outcome was better in patients who responded with either denial or a "fighting spirit" than in those who stoically accepted their disease or felt helpless. Is this mind over matter, or do patients with occult metastases subconsciously "recognize" their situation?] ◀

Subject Index

Index to Authors

The number after each entry is the reference number of the author's article in the text. The reference number indicates the chapter in which the article appears and its numerical order within the chapter.